The Nuts and Bolts of Cardiac Resynchronization Therapy

T0206028

Tom Kenny

Vice President Clinical Education & Training
St Jude Medical, Austin, Texas

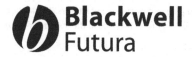
Blackwell
Futura

© 2007 St Jude Medical

Published by Blackwell Publishing
Blackwell Futura is an imprint of Blackwell Publishing

Blackwell Publishing, Inc., 350 Main Street, Malden, Massachusetts 02148-5020, USA
Blackwell Publishing Ltd, 9600 Garsington Road, Oxford OX4 2DQ, UK
Blackwell Science Asia Pty Ltd, 550 Swanston Street, Carlton, Victoria 3053, Australia

First published 2007

1   2007

ISBN: 978-1-4051-5372-0

Library of Congress Cataloging-in-Publication Data

Kenny, Tom, 1954-
  The nuts and bolts of cardiac resynchronization therapy / Tom Kenny.
    p. ; cm.
  Includes bibliographical references and index.
  ISBN 978-1-4051-5372-0 (alk. paper)
  1. Heart failure--Treatment. 2. Cardiac pacing. I. Title.
  [DNLM: 1. Heart Failure, Congestive--therapy. 2. Cardiac Pacing,
Artificial. 3. Defibrillators, Implantable. 4. Pacemaker, Artificial.
WG 370 K36n 2007]

  RC685.C53K46 2007
  616.1'23025--dc22
                        2006035499

A catalogue record for this title is available from the British Library

Commissioning Editor: Gina Almond
Development Editor: Fiona Pattison
Editorial Assistant: Victoria Pitman

Set in 9.5/12 pt Minion by Sparks, Oxford – www.sparks.co.uk

For further information on Blackwell Publishing, visit our website:
www.blackwellcardiology.com

The publisher's policy is to use permanent paper from mills that operate a sustainable forestry policy, and which has been manufactured from pulp processed using acid-free and elementary chlorine-free practices. Furthermore, the publisher ensures that the text paper and cover board used have met acceptable environmental accreditation standards.

Contents

Preface

A lot has happened since the day I was involved in caring for my first patient with an implanted cardiac rhythm management device. Back then, about the only devices available were fairly simple VVI pacemakers – at least, they look simple today. Back then, we thought adjustable programmable rates and output inhibition were very sophisticated concepts. I can remember how incredible the first dual-chamber pacemakers seemed, and can still recall learning about AV delays and other dual-chamber timing cycles.

When implantable defibrillators were introduced, they were just that: implantable defibrillators. Some of those first patients who needed both pacing and defibrillation ended up with two devices! Today, you cannot find an implanted defibrillator on the market without very advanced pacing functionality.

The cardiac resynchronization therapy (CRT) system is a device I would never have foreseen back in my rookie year as a clinician. Comparing those simple single-chamber pacemakers I worked with then with today's CRT devices is like comparing a wagon with a space ship.

This is by far the longest and most complex book I have ever written. Spurred by the success of *The Nuts & Bolts of Cardiac Pacing* and *The Nuts & Bolts of ICD Therapy*, I wanted to tackle the latest type of device that is turning up in clinics around the world. The CRT device is the most promising, most powerful and most complicated implantable cardiac device available today.

For that reason, I want to go on the record by saying that this book was written at the advent of CRT devices. Unlike my books on pacing and ICDs, which were written after decades of successful clinical application of these devices, writing about CRT is a little like writing about the future.

There are aspects to these devices that we still do not understand. Algorithms and features are still evolving. In fact, even a few years from now, this book may seem out of date. Manufacturers have evidenced a strong commitment to put the most advanced and useful tools into the hands of clinicians. That means a steady stream of new products and features!

My main concern is that clinicians from all types of practices understand the basics – the nuts and bolts – of these CRT devices. It is hard to imagine any sort of clinical practice that will not encounter CRT systems sooner or later. But while these systems may be new and even a bit complicated, they work on some fundamental concepts that clinicians can readily understand. It is my goal to try to make these concepts and the device functions that address them as simple and understandable as possible.

This book could not have been written without the outstanding contributions of many of my colleagues. I want to particularly recognize the work of Dr Angelo Carboni of the University of Parma, Italy, for his pioneering educational efforts in CRT training. I would also like to thank Dr. Mark Kroll for his insights into the nature of defibrillation. In my own office, I must thank David Andreasen for assisting me in a review of the manuscript. I am also grateful to the 'behind-the-scenes' team of Jo Ann LeQuang, who helped prepare the manuscript, Belinda Kinkade who handled the art work, and my gracious editor, Fiona Pattison.

Of course, the biggest debt of gratitude I owe is to my family, all of whom have more or less come to terms with having an author in the family. They have generously given me time to devote to my new passion of writing and have been my best critics and strongest allies.

It is my sincere hope that you find this book of immediate practical use. I welcome your comments and opinions, and I appreciate the tremendous support and confidence that readers have shown me.

Tom Kenny
October, 2006
Austin, Texas

Chapter 1

Understanding Heart Failure

Although heart failure (HF) was observed in ancient times (ancient physicians called it 'dropsy'), medical science has been slow to respond to its challenge. Unlike other things that concern cardiologists, HF is a syndrome rather than a disease, i.e. it is a constellation of symptoms. There remains no straightforward way to diagnose the disease; classification systems are more subjective than objective and we are only recently beginning really to understand what goes on when the human heart begins to fail.

The name of the syndrome itself is something of a misnomer. The heart does not 'fail' in a sudden spasm. The failure is a gradual, stepwise degeneration. Not too many years ago, all we clinicians could do in the face of progressive HF was keep the patient comfortable in the face of the inevitable decline. Even today, the prognosis for HF patients is not good. However, new treatment options are changing how we think about HF and that includes not just trying to stop the progressive deterioration but actually to fight to reverse it. As clinicians, we are not always successful in the fight against HF, but every year we become better and better equipped. In fact, Dr John G. F. Cleland stated recently in an interview that at this point in medical history, 'I think it's realistic to talk in terms of remission of heart failure'.[1]

Most clinicians have heard the term congestive heart failure (CHF). Although you still hear it, it is starting to sound old-fashioned. Congestion is a troublesome and extremely obvious symptom of advanced HF. Today we know that patients can have HF without congestion. In fact, by the time fluids start to accumulate, the heart has withstood considerable assault. Early treatment of HF involves diagnosing and managing the syndrome long before fluid overload becomes a problem. In fact, Dr. Jonathan Sackner-Bernstein wrote that not treating a heart failure patient until fluid accumulation oc-

curred was similar to waiting for metastasis rather than screening for a primary tumor.[2]

The American College of Cardiology and American Heart Association define heart failure as 'a complex clinical syndrome that can result from any structural or functional cardiac disorder that impairs the ability of the ventricle to fill with or eject blood'.[3] There is no objective definition of HF because there are no currently agreed-upon cut-off values in terms of cardiac dysfunction, such as change in flow, pressure, dimension or volume. The main symptoms are shortness of breath and fatigue, which often manifests as exercise intolerance. Fluid retention may be observed and, even if present, may not dominate the clinical presentation. A straightforward diagnosis is not possible and, when diagnosed, HF should not be the sole finding.

HF impairs the heart's ability to pump blood and that, in turn, causes an inadequate blood supply to the body's main organs. This lack of oxygen-rich blood flow to the brain, liver and kidneys is responsible for some of the symptoms of HF. As the heart's pump becomes less effective, blood can pool in the heart and stagnate. It can back up into the veins or clots may form, increasing the patient's risk of stroke. The symptoms relate to an inadequate oxygenated blood supply to the body, including:

• Dyspnea (shortness of breath)
• Fatigue, feeling overtired
• Edema or fluid accumulation.

Types of heart failure

Since the definition of HF is vast, it is not unusual for clinicians to describe HF further to help describe the type and stage of the condition. Some of the adjectives used with HF include: chronic, acute, congestive, decompensated, systolic, diastolic, right-sided and left-sided.

Acute heart failure (AHF) is used to describe two different things. Sometimes the term is heard for new-onset cases of HF. However, the term is often applied when a patient with heart failure experiences a sudden and dangerous worsening of symptoms, typically characterized by pulmonary or peripheral congestion (or both). Patients with chronic heart failure may have bouts of AHF, sometimes requiring emergency hospitalization.

Decompensation is a term that means 'failure to compensate'. It describes quite well what happens as heart failure progresses. In the early stages of HF, the heart develops some radical methods to compensate for its failings and still provide the body with an adequate supply of oxygenated blood. As the heart continues to fail, the heart loses its ability to compensate and starts to pump inadequately. Decompensated HF is an advanced form of HF.

Chronic HF (which confusingly sometimes uses the same acronym as congestive heart failure or CHF) describes most of what we clinicians know as HF. Not long ago, it was common to talk about patients being 'in heart failure' or 'out of heart failure' as if HF was something that might clear up. While symptoms can be alleviated, today we recognize that HF is a chronic condition.

Systolic and diastolic HF will be discussed in more detail in a later chapter, but they refer to the portion of the cardiac cycle where the heart can no longer pump effectively. Systolic HF may be thought of as the inability to eject blood effectively during the cardiac cycle (aligning with systole), while diastolic HF generally refers to the heart's inability to fill effectively with blood prior to pumping (matching diastole). While these terms and conditions are important to know, systolic and diastolic HF are not mutually exclusive. Many patients have both together and, over the long term, it is difficult to imagine a patient with systolic HF who does not have impaired diastolic function and vice versa. Thus, when the adjectives 'systolic' or 'diastolic' appear together with HF, they tend to describe what is more dominant and observable in the patient at that particular point in time.

Left-sided and right-sided HF are sometimes used, but these terms do not indicate which ventricle is the more damaged. Left-sided HF does indeed refer to the left ventricle's ineffective pumping action of blood and manifests as congestion in the pulmonary veins. Right-sided HF involves impaired right-ventricular pumping action, causing congestion in systemic circulation. Left-sided HF is by far the more common type, although cases of 'true right-sided HF' have been documented. Over the long term, patients may develop both forms of HF, in that left-ventricular dysfunction eventually causes right-sided failure.

Classification of HF

When classifying heart failure, the most commonly used method is not necessarily the most elegant. The New York Heart Association (NYHA) came up with a four-level classification scale which is still in broad use around the world today.[4] Although subjective and based on symptoms, the NYHA scale has proven to be exceedingly useful in helping to quantify a syndrome that seems to defy hard definitions. The NYHA scale maps the degree of exertion required to elicit symptoms (see Table 1.1).

The American College of Cardiology (ACC) and American Heart Association (AHA) proposed an alternative classification system for HF which is not in widespread use despite its obvious clinical value. This system allows for the classification of the asymptomatic and mildly symptomatic patient as well as those with more advanced cases of HF without relying on exertion to provoke symptoms. One reason for this new classification system is that we truly do not understand why exercise should provoke symptoms. For instance, it has been observed that some patients with markedly impaired left-ventricular function may be asymptomatic during exercise. Other patients may have symptoms with exercise because of mitral valve regurgitation, pulmonary disease or general poor condition. Thus, the presence of dyspnea with exercise is not necessarily a reliable yardstick.

The ACC and AHA have proposed another classification system[3] (see Table 1.2) which offers the

Table 1.1 New York Heart Association classification system

NYHA class	Effort required to elicit symptoms
I	Exertion that would limit normal individuals
II	Ordinary exertion
III	Less than ordinary exertion
IV	Rest

Table 1.2 American College of Cardiology (ACC)/American Heart Association (AHA) classification

ACC/AHA class	Definition
A	Patients at high risk of developing left-ventricular (LV) dysfunction
B	Patients with LV dysfunction who have not developed symptoms
C	Patients with LV dysfunction with current or prior symptoms
D	Patients with refractory end-stage HF

advantage of including asymptomatic (actually, it would be more accurate to say pre-symptomatic) patients without neglecting the progressive nature of the condition.

While the presence of left-ventricular (LV) dysfunction is common in HF patients and is the basis of the ACC/AHA classification scale, the presence of LV dysfunction does not define HF, nor does its absence preclude it.

Incidence, prevalence, populations

Incidence is a public health term used to define the number of new cases of a disease each year in a particular population. The incidence of HF has been growing steadily from 250 000 annually in 1970 to 400 000 annually in 1990.[5] The AHA says the number in the year 2000 is 550 000 new cases a year.[6] HF is one of the few forms of heart disease actually increasing in incidence. In the population of Americans < 75 years old, men are more likely to develop HF than women. At age ≥ 75 years, the incidence becomes more balanced between the genders. Hospital discharges (patients alive or dead at time of discharge) show that heart failure is increasing over time, more than doubling from 1980 to 2003 (see Fig. 1.1).

Prevalence is another public health term used to describe the number of people who have a condition at any given time. HF is increasing in prevalence mainly because the population, overall, is aging and HF is a chronic condition. Of people above the age of 65, about 6–10% have some form of HF[7] (see Fig. 1.2). As better medical treatment allows people to live longer and as we know how to manage HF better, the prevalence of the syndrome will continue to increase. While the incidence of HF is higher among men (at least up until age 75), the prevalence statistics show that in the USA, more females have HF than males. That is partly due to the fact that women live longer and that many women have a less severe form of HF known as diastolic dysfunction.

HF contributes to more than 287 000 deaths annually. The real extent of the devastation caused by

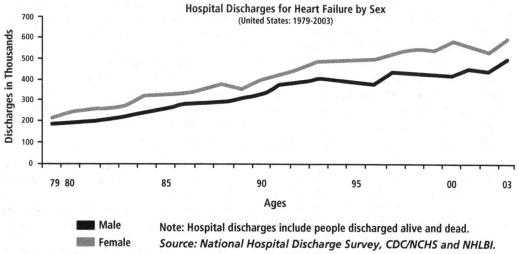

Figure 1.1 Hospital discharge rates for heart failure. The number of discharges of people from US hospitals with the diagnosis of heart failure has increased steadily since 1979. The gap between male and female patients has widened over time.

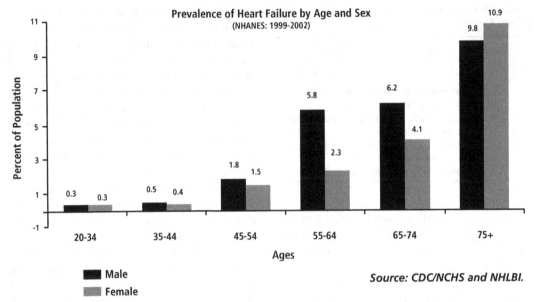

Figure 1.2 Heart failure prevalence by age and sex. The prevalence of heart failure increases sharply with advancing age. Up to age 74, more men than women have heart failure. This reverses at ages above 75, when slightly more females have heart failure than males. Women tend to develop heart failure later in life and to live longer than men.

HF is probably better captured in what it costs society. HF costs the world about $60 billion a year and accounts for 12–15 million office visits and 6.5 million hospital days.[8] In the USA, HF is the single most common Medicare diagnosis-related group (DRG) and Medicare spends more on HF than on any other disease.[9]

HF is a progressive disorder that can affect more than just the heart: it often affects the lungs, liver and kidneys. As a patient's functional status deteriorates, his or her chance of survival decreases. In the earlier stages of the disease, HF is associated with a higher incidence of sudden cardiac death, while in later stages, worsening HF is more likely to be the cause of death. The main objective in treating HF patients has been to improve symptoms, reduce the risk of death and disease progression and enhance the patient's quality of life.

One of the latest innovations for HF treatment is cardiac resynchronization therapy, which is a device-based treatment. However, HF requires a multidisciplinary approach and rarely is any HF patient well served by one drug or even one therapeutic approach. It is a complex syndrome which requires careful management.

References

1   Stiles S. CARE-HF: CRT improves survival, symptoms and remodeling—and sometimes achieves HF "remission". Available at http://theheart.org/printArticle. do?primaryKey=399895. Accessed March 22, 2005.

2   Sackner-Bernstein J. Heart failure treatment options. In: Resynchronization and Defibrillation for Heart Failure: A Practical Approach. Hayes DL, Wang PJ, Sackner-Bernstein J, Asirvatham SJ, eds. Oxford, UK: Blackwell Futura (Blackwell Publishing) 2004:2.

3   Hunt SJ, Baker DW, Chin MH et al. ACC/AHA Guidelines for the evaluation and management of chronic heart failure in the adult: executive summary. Circulation 2001; 104:2996–3007.

4   The Criteria Committee of the New York Heart Association. Diseases of the Heart and Blood Vessels: Nomenclature and Criteria for Diagnosis, 6th edn. Boston, MA: Little Brown 1964.

5   Jaski BE. Basics of Heart Failure: A Problem-Solving Approach. Norwell, MA: Kluwer Academic Publishers 2000.

6   American Heart Association. 2002 Heart and Stroke Statistical Update. Dallas, TX: American Heart Association 2001.

7   ACC/AHA Guidelines for the Evaluation and Management of Heart Failure, October 24, 2002.

8   Zevitz ME. Heart Failure. Available at http://www.
    emedicine.com/med/topic3552.htm. Accessed April 23,
    2003.

9   Weintraub NL, Chaitman BR. Newer concepts in the
    medical management of patients with congestive heart
    failure. *Clin Cardiol* 1993; **16**:380–390.

The nuts and bolts of understanding heart failure

- Heart failure (HF) is not a disease with a specific diagnostic test. It is a complex syndrome of symptoms and conditions.
- HF is increasing in incidence and prevalence. In the USA, Medicare spends more on HF than on any other condition. Worldwide, HF costs about $60 billion annually.
- While there are many 'types' of HF, the main one of concern for device-based therapy is chronic HF. It may or may not be accompanied by significant congestion.
- HF affects the heart's ability to pump blood effectively. It can be systolic (impairs ability to pump blood out) or diastolic (impairs ability of heart to fill with blood). Having one form of HF does not preclude the other. Some patients have both systolic and diastolic HF.
- The most commonly used system to rank HF patients is the New York Heart Association (NYHA) classification, where Class I is the least symptomatic and Class IV is the most symptomatic. These classes are not static and are based on somewhat subjective criteria.
- The American College of Cardiology (ACC)/American Heart Association (AHA) have proposed an alternative classification system of four stages, A–D, where A indicates patients at high risk of developing HF and Class D end-stage refractory HF patients. The ACC/AHA scale is based on degree of left-ventricular dysfunction. Although this is an important classification system, it is not as widely used as the NYHA classes.
- In populations <75 years old, more men than women get HF every year (incidence). At ≥76 years old, the incidence is about equal for men and women. However, more women than men have HF at any given point in time (prevalence), partly because women live longer and partly because they are more likely to have less severe diastolic forms of HF.
- The hallmark symptoms of HF include shortness of breath, fatigue and fluid accumulation. Exercise intolerance is frequently the way patients are classified (the NYHA classification system is based on symptoms that occur based on levels of exertion). While left-ventricular (LV) dysfunction and congestion are common in HF patients, neither one defines HF. In fact, many people with HF may have neither LV dysfunction nor congestion.
- On the other hand, LV dysfunction cannot occur without some degree of HF being present, even if the patient is not (yet) symptomatic.
- The best way to think of HF is as a deterioration of the heart's ability to pump blood effectively.
- Many other organs can be affected by HF besides the heart, mainly the lungs, liver and kidneys.
- HF is associated with many other conditions (co-morbidities), including diabetes, hypertension and atrial fibrillation.

Chapter 2

Cardiovascular Anatomy of the Healthy Heart

When talking about pacemakers or defibrillators, it is useful to think of the heart as consisting of an atrium and a ventricle. The heart has four chambers: upper chambers called atria and larger, more muscular, lower chambers called ventricles. Traditional pacemakers and implantable cardioverter defibrillators work with the right side of the heart (right atrium and right ventricle). As we start to talk more about cardiac resynchronization therapy systems, we will involve the left ventricle also (see Fig. 2.1).

When thinking about heart failure (HF), it is more useful to think of the heart as being right-sided and left-sided. Both sides consist of an atrium and a ventricle and both sides are complete pumping units. The right side of the heart receives oxygen-depleted blood from the body's venous system. Its job is to pump that blood out over the lungs where it can be re-oxygenated. The left side of the heart receives that oxygen-rich blood from the lungs and pumps it out through the arterial system to the rest of the body. In the healthy individual, the right side and the left side work together efficiently (see Fig. 2.2).

Blood enters the right side of the heart from two vessels, the superior vena cava (SVC) and the inferior vena cava (IVC). The terms superior and inferior actually mean 'upper' and 'lower' rather than bigger or smaller. Blood enters the right side of the heart, is pumped out over the lungs, collects again in the left side of the heart and from there is pumped out to the rest of the body.

The body would be unable to move blood through this two-sided pump efficiently without the valves. The heart has four valves, which prevent backflow of blood. When oxygen-depleted blood is delivered to the heart, it enters the right atrium by way of the venous system. Blood passively fills the right ventricle by flowing over the tricuspid valve—so named from the fact that it is has three leaflets. The tricuspid valve separates the right atrium from the right ventricle. When the right ventricle contracts to send blood over the lungs, that blood travels through the pulmonary valve into the pulmonary artery and from there is passed over the lungs.

The blood drains from the lungs by way of pulmonary veins, which collect the blood and feed it back to the left atrium. Blood flows passively into the left ventricle by passing over the mitral valve (so called from the miter or a Catholic bishop's traditional tricornered hat). The mitral valve connects the left atrium and the left ventricle. When the left ventricle contracts, blood flows out over the aortic valve, which is placed between the left ventricle and the aorta, the body's main blood conduit. From the aorta, blood is delivered to all parts of the body, even the extremities (see Fig. 2.3).

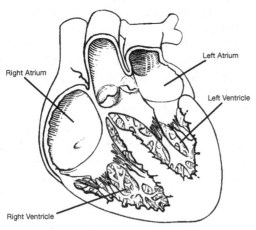

Fig. 2.1 Image of four-chambered heart (cross section). The heart is composed of four chambers: two upper chambers called atria (right atrium, left atrium) and two lower chambers called ventricles (right ventricle, left ventricle). Conventional pacemakers stimulated only the right side of the heart. Cardiac resynchronization therapy systems work to help both right and left ventricles contract.

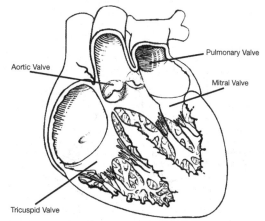

Fig. 2.3 Heart and valves. There are four main valves in the healthy heart: the tricuspid and mitral valves separate atrium from ventricle (tricuspid on the right, mitral on the left). Blood pumped out of the right side of the heart travels through the pulmonary valve to enter the lungs; blood pumped out of the left side of the heart travels through the aortic valve to enter the rest of the body. Valve malformations or dysfunction can seriously affect cardiac performance.

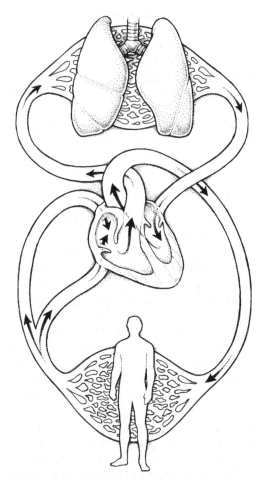

Fig.2.2 Heart and lungs. The path blood takes through the body can be best diagrammed starting with the image of the man at the bottom. Oxygen-depleted blood from the body flows to the right side of the heart. The right heart pumps this blood out over the lungs, where the blood receives oxygen. From the lungs, the oxygen-infused blood travels back to the heart, this time to the left side of the heart. It is from the heart's powerful left ventricle that this oxygen-rich blood is then pumped out to nourish the body. When the body has used up the oxygen in the blood, the blood returns to the right side of the heart to be re-oxygenated over the lungs.

The opening and closing of these four valves produces most of the heart sounds clinicians hear when they place a stethoscope over a patient's heart. When the heart is healthy, the valves close effectively and seal off the chambers. Valvular disease occurs when these valves cannot seal well. The two main types of valvular disease are stenosis (when the valve is stiff and blood has difficulty passing over the valve) and insufficiency (when the valve cannot close well and blood flows back or regurgitates). Mitral regurgitation (MR) in particular occurs when blood flows from the left ventricle backward up into the left atrium. This limits the outward flow of blood. MR is not uncommon in HF patients.

The heart is a muscle and, like any other muscle, it needs an adequate supply of oxygenated blood. The main vessels feeding the heart muscle are coronary arteries (named because they form a crown or corona around the heart). There are four main coronary arteries which wrap around the exterior of the healthy heart: the left main coronary artery, the left anterior descending, the left circumflex coronary artery and the right main coronary artery (see Fig. 2.4). Blood from the coronary arteries drains into the coronary veins and then empties into a structure called the coronary sinus. The coronary sinus is a small structure situated between the atria and ventricles. From the coronary sinus, blood then drains into the right atrium.

The venous system around the anterior (front side) of the heart includes the great cardiac vein,

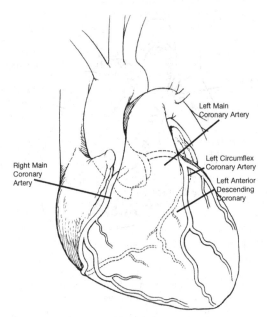

Fig. 2.4 Coronary arteries. The coronary arteries encircle the outside of the heart, and they guide the flow of blood away from the heart. The main coronary arteries are the right main, the left main, the left circumflex and the left anterior descending artery.

the left lateral vein and the anterior vein. On the posterior (back side), the middle cardiac vein and

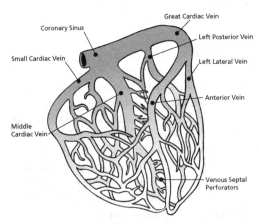

Fig. 2.5 Coronary veins. The coronary veins deliver oxygen-depleted blood back to the heart muscle. The main coronary veins are the great cardiac vein (GCV), the left lateral and anterior vein on the anterior side of the heart's exterior. On the posterior side, the main coronary veins are the middle cardiac, left posterior and main veins. There are also smaller, and often very tortuous, tributaries.

the left posterior vein are the main veins (see Fig. 2.5).

The heart also has nerves and the innervation of the heart is coming under increasing study as we learn more about cardiac rhythm disorders. The parasympathetic nervous system (PSNS) influences the heart through the vagus nerve, which has the ability to slow the heart rate and weaken the strength of the cardiac contraction. The sympathetic nervous system (SNS) also influences the heart, but mainly through the hormones epinephrine and norepinephrine. These hormones can increase heart rate, increase contractility (the vigor of a cardiac contraction) and constrict blood vessels, which in turn raises blood pressure.

By far the most intriguing aspect of the heart's unique structure is its elaborate electrical system. A healthy heart literally generates its own electricity and delivers it on an efficient pathway through the heart in such a way that it precisely and appropriately controls the cardiac cycle. The electrical energy originates from a small group of cells in the high right atrium called the sinoatrial (SA) node. In a healthy heart, the SA node is the 'natural pacemaker' because of its property of automaticity. It generates electricity at exactly the right time to cause the heart to beat in such a way that it keeps up with our metabolic demand. The property that enables a cell to generate electrical energy spontaneously is known as automaticity. The SA node possesses automaticity, but actually all cardiac cells have some degree of automaticity.

Cardiac cells are particularly adept at transferring electrical energy allowing a charge which originates in the upper portion of the heart to travel swiftly along the cardiac conduction pathways. The typical route is an outward and downward motion over the atria, causing them to depolarize and contract in a phase of the cardiac cycle called atrial systole.

The cardiac conduction system then funnels this electrical energy over a specialized bundle of cells called the atrioventricular (AV) node, located at the approximate center of the heart (it is below the atria, above the ventricles and in the middle). The electrical conduction properties of the AV node cells is somewhat different than the rest of the heart, which causes the electrical energy to slow down slightly be-

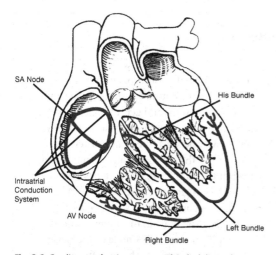

Fig. 2.6 Cardiac conduction system. The dark lines show the typical conduction pathways of electrical energy in a healthy heart. The electrical impulse is initiated at the upper portion of the right atrium (the sinoatrial or SA node) and travels through the intra-atrial conduction pathway and from there goes down the septum and then back upward through the right and left ventricles. The normal flow of conduction in the healthy heart is from the top (upper right atrium) downward and then slightly back upward. Cardiac pacing can distort the conduction pattern.

fore moving on to the ventricles. The result of this slowdown is that the atria can contract completely before the ventricles even begin to depolarize. This ability to change the speed of the electrical energy through the heart allows the AV node to function as a sort of 'gate keeper'.

Once the electrical energy travels through the AV node, it then descends the ventricles through the bundle of His and the Purkinje network, a group of fibers that divide into the right and left bundle branches. This Purkinje network helps the electrical energy travel rapidly outward, across and down so that the ventricles depolarize in a synchronous and efficient way, leading to uniform and coherent contraction (see Fig. 2.6).

On an ECG, the electrical conduction sequence can be observed clearly in the form of the P-wave (atrial contraction), the PR segment (the period of rest while the electrical energy is slowed through the AV node), the QRS complex (the ventricular contraction) and the T-wave (the ventricular repolarization) and the flat line between complexes when the heart is at rest (see Fig. 2.7).

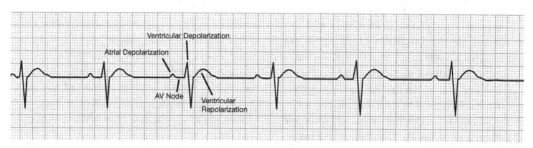

Fig. 2.7 The healthy heart on ECG. This is a classic unpaced ECG showing the P-wave (atrial depolarization), the QRS complex (the ventricular depolarization) and the T-wave (ventricular repolarization). The small segment of flat line between the P-wave and QRS complex reflects the heart's natural atrioventricular (AV) delay when the electrical impulse is delayed briefly at the AV node.

The nuts and bolts of cardiovascular anatomy

- The heart has two upper chambers (atria) and two lower chambers (ventricles), but for heart failure (HF) it may be better to think of the heart as right-sided and left-sided. The right side of the heart pumps de-oxygenated blood out over the lungs, while the left side of the heart receives oxygen-replenished blood from the lungs and pumps it via the aorta to the rest of the body.
- Blood is moved through the heart in a complex system of valves (tricuspid, pulmonary, mitral and aortic), chambers and a network of vessels. In that way, the heart can be thought of as having a plumbing system. But this network of chambers works because of the heart's elaborate conduction system. In that way, the heart can also be thought of as having an electrical system. Both have to work together for the heart to function effectively.
- The valves are what clinicians hear when they place a stethoscope over the heart. Common valve problems involve stenosis (the valve is stiff), insufficiency (the valve does not close well) and regurgitation (backward flow of blood). Mitral regurgitation or the flow of blood from the left ventricle backward into the left atrium is common in people with HF.
- The heart is a muscle that also needs oxygen-rich blood. It is fed by a network of exterior vessels known as coronary veins and coronary arteries, so-named because they wrap around the outside of the heart like a crown (the word coronary is related to coronation).
- Blood from the coronary arteries drains into the coronary veins and gets funneled into the coronary sinus. The coronary sinus is a tiny sinus cavity between the atria and ventricles. Blood from the coronary sinus is funneled into the right atrium, from where it gets pumped by the right ventricle over the lungs.
- The heart's conduction system begins at the sinoatrial (SA) node in the upper portion of the right atrium. The SA node or the 'natural pacemaker' spontaneously generates an electrical impulse, which travels outward and down, causing an atrial depolarization and contraction. The electrical energy regroups at the atrioventricular node, a special collection of cells located between atria and ventricles, which slows down the electricity long enough to allow the atrial contraction to complete. From there, the electrical energy travels outward and downward over the bundle of His and the Purkinje fibers, a network of increasingly fine fibers. The Purkinje network can be divided into right and left bundle branches.
- Automaticity is the special property of cardiac cells to generate spontaneously an electrical impulse. The best example of cardiac automaticity is found in the cells of the SA node, but all cardiac cells possess some degree of automaticity.

Chapter 3

Cardiac Physiology and Heart Failure

The heart is a pump with an electrical system

The cardiac cycle is the proper term for what everybody knows as a single heartbeat. Actually, heartbeat is something of a misnomer. The heart does not beat as a unified whole. Instead, the upper chambers contract first, followed by the lower chambers. One complete cycle starts with the atrial contraction and ends with the ventricular contraction. When patients feel their heart beating, they are typically sensitive to the larger ventricular contraction. But every heartbeat involves two separate rounds of contraction and relaxation: atrial and ventricular.

The healthy heart beats when the sinoatrial (SA) node generates an electrical impulse which travels outward and down the right and left atria. This electrical energy causes a cellular phenomenon known as depolarization. At the cellular level, the polarity or charge of the individual cells is reversed. Depolarization and its reverse, repolarization, involve the opening and closing of various ion channels in a complex, precisely timed, elaborate system. An electrical impulse of sufficient magnitude (and often it need not be more than 1 or 2 V) is enough to start cardiac depolarization. Depolarization occurs at the cellular level, but it is accompanied by a very real physiological response: contraction of the cells. When depolarization occurs in a coherent, uniform pattern, all of the muscle cells in the heart contract together. The result is the pumping effect of the heart. The electrical charge is sufficient to depolarize the cells for only a brief moment; the cells quickly repolarize or try to go back to what is known as resting membrane potential. As they repolarize, the muscle cells relax and the heart muscle regains its old shape.

In the healthy heart, the SA node fires an electrical impulse, which causes an atrial depolarization and subsequent repolarization. Meanwhile, the electricity collects and pauses at the atrioventricular node before traveling down to the ventricles, where it causes a ventricular depolarization and contraction.

These phases of the cardiac cycle—contraction and relaxation—are typically called systole (contracting or pumping) and diastole (relaxing or resting). Every cardiac cycle involves an atrial systole and diastole and a ventricular systole and diastole (see Fig. 3.1). With all of these precisely timed mechanisms required for the heart to pump properly, it is no wonder that cardiac disorders can occur!

The main job of the heart is to pump blood and the volume of blood pumped with each cardiac contraction is an important factor in efficient pumping. The volume of blood the heart can pump in 1 min in milliliters is called cardiac output (CO). A typical CO value might be 5000 ml/min (or 5 l/min).

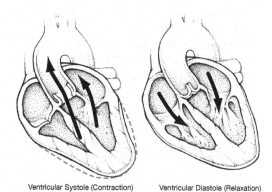

Ventricular Systole (Contraction)   Ventricular Diastole (Relaxation)

Fig. 3.1 Ventricular systole and diastole. Ventricular systole refers to the contraction of the ventricles, which forces blood out of the heart and over the pulmonary valve to the lungs (right side) or over the aortic valve and out to the rest of the body (left side). Ventricular diastole refers to the time the heart relaxes and blood flows back into the heart.

The heart is designed to pump at peak capacity, i.e. maximum volume, all of the time. The volume of blood pumped through the heart is in part determined by how well the upper and lower chambers work together. In the resting or diastolic phase of the cardiac cycle, blood rushes into the heart in what is called 'passive filling of the ventricles'. The blood pours in and the lower chambers as well as the upper chambers are filled. Then the valves between atria and ventricles close. The atria receive more blood and are filled to maximum capacity. In the healthy heart, the atria now depolarize and contract just as the valves to the lower chambers open. The result is that the atria squeeze all of their blood into the lower chambers. This 'atrial contribution to ventricular filling' has been well nicknamed 'atrial kick'. Since the muscular walls of the ventricle stretch, the lower chambers literally bulge out to accommodate this additional bolus of blood. The muscle fibers stretch. They possess a property called contractility, which means that the more they stretch, the more vigorously they snap back into shape. (A rubber band is also contractile; the harder you stretch it out, the harder it snaps back.) There is a brief pause in the cardiac cycle (measured in thousandths of a second), then the ventricles contract.

The added volume of blood from 'atrial kick' combined with cardiac contractility means that the maximum amount of blood gets pumped out into the circulatory system.

During periods of exertion or stress, the body needs more oxygenated blood as fuel. Since the heart is designed to pump at maximum capacity all of the time, the only way to increase the volume of blood in circulation is to increase the heart rate. As a person exercises, his heart rate speeds up and the volume of blood delivered to the body increases as well. The cardiac output increases due to more vigorous contractility as well as the faster heart rate. At rest or during sleep, the heart rate slows down because the body needs less oxygen-rich blood for fuel. Heart rate (HR) is defined as the number of cardiac cycles that occur in 1 min. Healthy individuals can have heart rates that vary widely, from relatively slow rates during sleep to very rapid rates during running or strenuous exercise. Other factors, such as certain medications, fever or emotional stress, can also cause significant changes in heart rate. It

is not just physical exertion that can cause the heart rate to accelerate. All of us have been startled and felt our heart start to pound, even though we were not exerting ourselves physically.

The amount of blood pumped in a cardiac cycle is called the stroke volume (SV). A healthy individual might have a SV of about 70 cm^3 of blood per cycle. SV can increase with more vigorous contractility, typically during physical exercise.

Clinicians use a formula to describe the heart's pumping function:

***Cardiac output* = HR × SV**

Using that formula, a healthy individual with a heart rate of 72 beats/min and SV of 70 cm^3 per cycle pumps 5040 cm^3 (or about 5 l) of blood per minute. In managing HF patients, it is important to bear in mind the enormous quantity of blood that must stay in constant circulation to keep a healthy human being functional.

Of course, cardiac output will vary depending on the size of the patient. For example, 5 l of blood a minute may be perfectly adequate to supply oxygen-rich blood to a small person, but barely sufficient for a much larger one. The degree to which oxygenated blood saturates the body's tissues and organs is known as perfusion. Clinicians have developed a cardiac indexing system, which attempts to adjust cardiac output values required for adequate perfusion based on the size of the patient. The cardiac index divides cardiac output (ml/min) into the body surface area (see Fig. 3.2). A normal-range cardiac index is from 2.5–4.0 l/min. As a general rule of thumb, a cardiac index < 2.5 l/min suggests inadequate perfusion.

While the heart always passively fills with as much blood as flows in, SV can be affected by three variables: preload, afterload, and contractility.

The cells of the heart muscle itself are called myocytes and they have some degree of natural stretchiness. Preload defines the amount of stretch in the myocytes at the end of ventricular filling (ventricular diastole). During that period in the cardiac cycle, blood passively flows into the ventricles and fills them. The actual volume of inflowing blood defines the preload. The actual volume of inflowing blood, in turn, is influenced by the total amount of blood in the body and by something called 'venous compliance', which means how help-

Afterload defines the amount of resistance the left ventricle must overcome in order to pump blood out into the body. In this way, afterload determines how much oxygen-rich blood the body actually gets. When the afterload is large, the heart has to work very hard to get blood to the body. One of the factors influencing afterload is blood pressure and the vascular condition of the arteries, i.e. whether they are constricted or dilated. If a patient has hypertension and constricted blood vessels, there is considerable afterload and the heart has to work much harder to send oxygen-rich blood to the body.

Although most clinicians are well aware of hypertension, the fact is that the body's system of regulating blood pressure is a sophisticated way of moving blood from areas of higher pressure to those of lower pressure. As such, it is a sensitive and interconnected system which responds to subtle variations. When managing HF patients, there are actually several types of blood pressure of crucial importance.

When a clinician 'takes blood pressure' using the cuff manometer, he is actually measuring systolic and diastolic blood pressure values (the famous '120 over 80' numbers we put in charts). Systolic blood pressure measures blood pressure during systole or contraction. It represents the highest pressure against the walls of the arteries. Diastolic blood pressure measures the lowest pressure on the arteries. These two values provide a maximum and minimum value for what is going on within the arteries, which direct blood flow away from the heart.

Pulse pressure is a term that describes the difference between the diastolic and systolic blood pressure values. It is normal that pulse pressure increases as we age. However, in HF patients, it is common for pulse pressure to decrease. For example, a younger healthy person might have a pulse pressure of 40 mmHg (120/80 mmHg), whereas an older person without HF might have a pulse pressure of 70 mmHg (blood pressure of 160/90 mmHg). But a person with HF might present with a pulse pressure of just 30 mmHg (blood pressure of 90/60 mmHg). Pulse pressure can be a useful way of evaluating the degree of severity of the HF.

For HF patients, it is also crucial to know the pressure in the left atrium. During hemodynamic monitoring, an invasive electrophysiology procedure involving a balloon catheter, the electrophysiologist

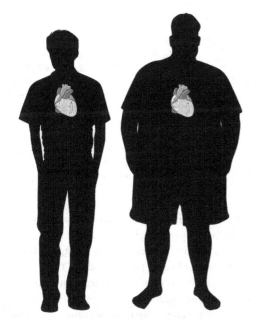

Fig. 3.2 The cardiac index. While two people may have the same size heart, they do not necessarily have the same cardiac index. The cardiac index is obtained by dividing the cardiac output (ml/min) into the body surface area. Normal cardiac index values range from about 2.5 to 4.0 l/min.

ful the veins are in routing the blood back into the ventricles. Clinicians define preload by measuring the end diastolic index (EDI), which defines how much blood is contained per mm² of ventricle. The average healthy adult at rest might have an EDI of around 60–110 ml/mm².

For a healthy individual, the greater the EDI (i.e. the bigger the preload), the more contractility the heart muscle will have and the more vigorously it will contract. Of course, there is a limit to how far myocytes can be made to stretch. They are not capable of infinite contractility! If a patient has a low preload, perhaps owing to low blood volume or dehydration, then his cardiac output will suffer. By the same token, excessive preload can also negatively impact the cardiac output because overly stretched myocytes may be unable to regain their original shape and eventually lose the ability to contract forcefully. Ironically, a very high preload is actually the problem for many HF patients. They retain fluids, which increases blood volume and causes the preload to stretch the heart muscle out of shape so that it cannot contract properly.

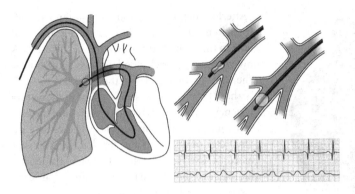

Fig. 3.3 Pulmonary capillary wedge pressure (PCWP). To obtain the PCWP value, a balloon catheter is passed into the pulmonary artery during an invasive electrophysiological procedure. The balloon is wedged into the pulmonary capillary and then pressure in the left atrium is measured. Heart failure patients typically have higher-than-normal PCWP values.

wedges a small balloon catheter in the branch of the pulmonary artery and measures the pressure in the left atrium (see Fig. 3.3). It is thought that this pressure represents the pressure in the pulmonary capillaries. If the patient has a healthy mitral valve, pulmonary capillary wedge pressure (PCWP) will equal left-ventricular end diastolic pressure. However, many people with HF have damaged mitral valves and may have high PCWP values.

Resistance to the flow of blood through the body involves the state of the body's enormous network of blood vessels. From veins and arteries to tiny capillaries, the vessels are the 'pipes' through which the heart delivers its oxygen-rich blood to the organs and tissue or returns oxygen-depleted blood to the lungs. The nervous system has considerable control over the diameters of these blood vessels, which can dilate (increase in diameter) or constrict (decrease in diameter) with changing conditions. Vasoconstriction or the narrowing of the diameters of the body's blood vessels may dramatically increase the resistance against which blood pumps. Yet some degree of vasoconstriction may be necessary to help move blood efficiently through the body. Dilated (sometimes called dilatated) vessels offer less resistance but are not always effective at channeling blood properly. Vasoconstriction is closely interrelated with blood pressure. In fact, one way the body works to regulate blood pressure is by changing the degree of constriction of the blood vessels.

Another factor that influences afterload is the viscosity (thickness) of the blood itself. Thick blood is harder to move through the body's vessels than thin blood. Blood viscosity is defined by the number of red blood cells or hematocrit and plasma proteins in the fluid. A 'blood count' test measures hematocrit.

For patients with congestive heart failure, blood viscosity becomes of crucial importance since the use of diuretics involves a delicate balancing act. Diuretics are prescribed to rid the body of excess fluids, but removing too much fluid from the blood can increase the hematocrit level, making the blood too thick to circulate easily. For that reason, it is important to monitor the blood of HF patients on diuretics.

Besides viscosity, the total volume of blood is another important piece of the puzzle. The body will attempt to compensate for large increases or decreases in blood volume in order to keep itself in proper balance. If blood volume increases, the heart muscle will stretch and the vessels will dilate. If blood volume decreases, the vessels will contract to maintain sufficient blood pressure (this is a compensatory mechanism). Either extreme—too much or too little blood volume—increases the workload for the heart.

Contractility is probably the best known of the factors influencing SV. It describes how much and how well myocytes can shorten (contract) and lengthen (relax). While preload can impact contractility, contractility can be impaired even in a patient with normal range preload values.

The ventricles are unable to pump out their entire contents during a single contraction. In fact, they actually pump out just a percentage of the blood they hold; this percentage is called the ejection fraction (the fraction or percentage of the blood ejected in one contraction). Usually, the value of the left-ventricular ejection fraction (LVEF) is the one of key interest. The ejection fraction is calculated by dividing the SV by the left-ventricular end diastolic volume (LVED), better known as the preload.

An LVEF score of 55–70% is considered normal, while scores of ≤ 40% generally indicate some degree of left-ventricular dysfunction. Many clinical trials have made a low LVEF score an entrance criterion (MADIT II used 30% or below[1], SCD-HeFT 35% or below[2]). A low LVEF score indicates some degree of left-ventricular or systolic dysfunction.

Not only is the heart a complex electrical pumping system, the body further relies on a network of vessels to move blood properly through the body so that it can deliver the oxygen the body needs to survive. The proper movement of blood through the body is called hemodynamics, and it is governed by blood pressure, the qualities of the blood itself (how thick it is) and the state of the vessels or 'pipes' through which the blood has to navigate.

References

1   Moss AJ, Wojciech Z, Hall WJ *et al.* Prophylactic implantation of a defibrillator in patients with myocardial infarction and reduced ejection fraction. *N Engl J Med* 2002; **346:**877–83.

2   Bardy GH, Lee KL, Mark DB *et al.* Sudden Cardiac Death in Heart Failure trial (SCD-HeFT) Investigators. Amiodarone or an implantable cardioverter-defibrillator for congestive heart failure. *N Engl J Med* 2005; **352:**225–37.

The nuts and bolts of cardiac physiology in heart failure

- The cardiac cycle consists of four distinct parts: an atrial systole (contraction) and diastole (relaxation) followed by a ventricular systole and diastole. To make that happen, the heart has a precise electrical system which causes the depolarizations (which lead to contractions) and repolarizations (which lead to relaxation).
- A healthy heart relies on the atrial contribution to ventricular filling (atrial kick) to help maximize the inflow of blood into the ventricles, enhancing contractility and leading to more vigorous and effective pumping action of the ventricles.
- Cardiac output is the amount of blood the heart puts in circulation in a minute. It can be defined as the heart rate times the stroke volume. (The stroke volume is how much blood the heart ejects in a single cardiac cycle.)
- Cardiac output is stated as l/min, but it needs to be indexed or related to the person's physical size to be meaningful. For example, a cardiac output of 5 l/min may be adequate for a person of average size, but inadequate for a very large-framed individual. The cardiac index divides cardiac output into body surface area.
- Stroke volume is influenced by preload, afterload and contractility. Preload refers to how much blood flows into the ventricle; afterload describes how much resistance the heart has to pump against; contractility is a property of cardiac (and many other muscles) cells to stretch and then recover their original shape.
- If preload is too low or too high, the heart muscle cells (myocytes) may have difficulty contracting. A small preload may fail to stretch the myocytes enough to allow a vigorous contraction as a response. A large preload can stretch the myocytes too much, so that they are unable to contract vigorously. Many people with heart failure (HF) have a large volume of blood (because of fluid accumulation), which increases preload.
- The preload is calculated as the left-ventricular end diastolic volume (LVED).
- Afterload is affected by blood pressure and the state of the vessels (constricted or dilated). Hypertension and constricted blood vessels increase afterload.
- Contractility refers to the ability of many muscle cells in the body (including cardiac cells) to stretch and then contract vigorously. In fact, they contract more vigorously the further they are stretched up to a point. Think of the myocytes in the heart like rubber bands. Stretch them a little, and they snap back slightly. Stretch them a lot, and they snap back vigorously. Stretch them too much and they can break or not go back into shape at all.
- An ejection fraction (EF) defines the percentage of blood ejected or pumped out in one cardiac

Continued p. 16.

Continued.

cycle. The most typical score is the left-ventricular ejection fraction (LVEF). It can be calculated by dividing the stroke volume by the LVED.
- An LVEF of 55–70% is considered normal and scores <40% indicate some degree of left-ventricular dysfunction. HF and a low LVEF score have a strong association, but are not absolutely linked. That is, it is possible for a patient to have HF and a normal LVEF score and vice versa.
- Blood pressure is an important factor in hemodynamics. Routine blood pressure measurements capture the systolic and diastolic values, which can also be thought of as maximum and minimum blood pressures during a cardiac cycle. The difference between them (systolic minus diastolic scores) is called the pulse pressure. It is typical for HF patients to have low pulse pressures, while older people without HF often have higher pulse pressures.
- The measurement of blood pressure in the left atrium is taken in an invasive EP procedure known as pulmonary capillary wedge pressure (PCWP). An EP guides a balloon catheter into the pulmonary artery and wedges it in place to rate the pressure in the pulmonary capillaries. In a person with a normal mitral valve, PCWP is taken as the same as left-ventricular end diastolic pressure. It is then used to calculate preload or LVEF scores.
- Blood viscosity (thickness) is measured in a blood count of hematocrit (red blood cells) and plasma proteins. Viscous blood is more work for the heart to pump.
- The vessels of the body dilate (increase in diameter) or constrict (decrease in diameter) under control of the nervous system. Vasoconstriction is one of the ways the body tries to self-regulate blood pressure.
- Blood volume can also affect how much work the heart has to do in order to pump effectively. Too much or too little blood volume can make it harder for the heart to work efficiently.

Chapter 4

Causes of Heart Failure

Heart failure (HF) is a syndrome with a predictable course. Knowing the course of HF can help us make treatment decisions and it may allow for pre-emptive treatments that reduce symptoms and improve quality of life. To understand how HF develops over time, it is important to understand where and why it begins.

Since HF is a syndrome, not a disease, there is no single cause. The syndrome is not defined by any objective criterion, nor can it be limited to symptoms. Rather, heart failure describes a constellation of conditions which impair the heart's ability to pump blood effectively. If the heart cannot pump blood sufficient for the patient's metabolic needs, HF is present. It is quite frequently associated with left-ventricular dysfunction, low ejection fractions, fluid accumulation and shortness of breath, but none of those defines the syndrome. It is possible (although uncommon) to have HF without those signs and symptoms.

HF begins with an injury to the heart. The human body is extremely resourceful in developing compensatory mechanisms to help us overcome physical limitations. The heart is an outstanding example of using compensatory techniques to manage the body's complex circulatory system, even when the heart cannot perform optimally. Changes in heart rate, contractility, blood pressure, even the body's chemical balance can all help a wounded heart to maintain adequate or at least nearly adequate cardiac output. While these compensatory mechanisms work well in the short term, none of them is good over the long term. In fact, many of these compensatory fixes introduce gradual deterioration which plays out in the symptoms we relate to HF.

It may be impossible to pinpoint the precise cause of HF in any given patient. However, the following lists the main conditions that clinicians see in patients who are at high risk of developing HF or who

may already have some degree of HF (even if they do not yet have symptoms). These conditions include cardiomyopathy, coronary artery disease, myocardial infarction, systolic dysfunction, diastolic dysfunction and co-morbid conditions such as atrial fibrillation and diabetes.

In all cases, what happens is that some condition or state occurs which causes an injury to the heart, which reduces the number of functional myocardial cells. This loss causes the heart to compensate. These compensatory mechanisms may work well in the short term, but eventually they can lead to profound changes in the heart muscle or function. Eventually, the heart loses its ability to pump effectively. That is why HF is a progressive syndrome; it begins with a simple injury to the heart and progresses gradually toward pump failure.

Cardiomyopathy

The word itself says it all: it means disease (pathy) of the heart (cardio) muscle (myo). When the muscle portion of the heart becomes impaired, a cardiomyopathy occurs and that sets the stage for HF. There are actually several types of cardiomyopathy, depending on how the heart muscle is affected.

Dilated cardiomyopathy occurs when the heart becomes large, distended and flabby. The shape of the heart changes from the football-like shape of a healthy heart to the more rounded shape of a basketball. This floppy heart muscle is no longer sufficient to serve as an efficient pumping unit. Dilated cardiomyopathy occurs in a large number of patients and is common in HF sufferers. For reasons we do not entirely understand, it is more common in men than in women.

The causes of dilated cardiomyopathy are not well understood. Most patients have idiopathic dilated cardiomyopathy, an impressive sounding medical term which means we do not actually know why they developed a stretched-out heart muscle. Certain viral infections or a disease called myocarditis may also lead to dilated cardiomyopathy, but such etiologies are rarer.

Hypertrophic obstructive cardiomyopathy (HOCM) is another form of cardiomyopathy with an entirely different shape. Patients with HOCM have hearts that become overly stiff. The muscular walls of the left ventricle thicken, sometimes to the extent that it limits the storage capacity within the chamber. These rigid, thick walls have trouble pumping blood effectively.

HOCM is associated with abnormal muscle fibers which cause the myocardium to become thicker than normal. The greatest thickening typically occurs in the left ventricle or in the ventricular septum, the wall between the right and left ventricles. HOCM can be idiopathic (i.e. of unknown origin), but it is also known to be a genetic disorder. Although HOCM can affect patients of any age, it is commonly associated with young athletes with heart problems.

There are also two broad types of HF: systolic HF and diastolic HF. Systolic HF involves the heart's impaired ability to pump blood out of the heart. Diastolic HF involves the heart's impaired ability to receive blood into the heart. As a general rule of thumb, dilated cardiomyopathy results in systolic HF (impaired pumping out), while HOCM is associated with diastolic HF (impaired blood flow into the heart). However, HF is almost never simple. It is possible for patients to exhibit both types of HF and both types of cardiomyopathy!

Systolic and diastolic dysfunction

When the heart cannot pump blood effectively, some degree of left-ventricular systolic dysfunction (sometimes shortened to LV dysfunction or systolic dysfunction) is present. The typical marker for systolic dysfunction is a low left-ventricular ejection fraction (LVEF) score (generally $\leq 40\%$), but systolic dysfunction in its early stages may not produce an alarmingly reduced LVEF score. Since systolic dysfunction and HF are closely interrelated (most HF patients have some degree of LV impairment), it is common to hear about LVEF scores in conjunction with HF patients (see Table 4.1)

However, it is important to remember that a patient may have HF without any systolic abnormality. Diastolic dysfunction occurs when the heart's pumping ability is impaired because it cannot accept enough blood into the chamber to pump out effectively. A patient with diastolic dysfunction may also have a low LVEF score, but that score is because of the heart's limited intake of blood rather than reduced pumping function. In fact, patients with

Table 4.1 Systolic versus diastolic heart failure (HF)

Characteristic	Systolic HF	Diastolic HF
Size of left ventricle (LV)	Dilated	Normal
Condition of LV	Flabby, floppy	Rigid, stiff
Wall thickness of LV	Normal	Thick
Wall motion of LV	Reduced	Normal
Ability of LV to fill with blood	Efficient	Impaired
Ability of LV to pump out blood	Impaired	Efficient
Principal evidence patient has this type of HF	Low ejection fraction, typically < 40%	Low index of ventricular filling
Gender	More common in men	More common in women
Coronary artery disease	More likely	Less likely
Non-ischemic cardiomyopathy	Less likely	More likely
Percentage of total HF patients who have this disorder	60–80%	20–40%
Amount of randomized clinical trials on this specific population	Many	Few

diastolic dysfunction may have normal or even enhanced contractility of the heart.

Even in people without HF, diastolic function declines with age. Diastolic dysfunction also increases with hypertension, which also is more common in older people. As a result, diastolic HF is not as rare as many clinicians may think. In addition, it is possible for a HF patient to have both systolic and diastolic HF simultaneously. In fact, in advanced cases of HF, systolic and diastolic components are almost assuredly present.

Coronary artery disease

The most common cause of HF is the presence of ischemic coronary artery disease (CAD), a build-up of fatty deposits and plaque in the arteries that supply the heart muscle with oxygen-rich blood. When plaque (a mixture of cholesterol, fatty deposits and other waste materials) builds up in the veins, the condition is called atherosclerosis. Our grandparents knew this condition as 'hardening of the arteries'. As plaque builds up, it narrows or occludes the inner diameter of the blood vessel. Occlusion is typically reported as a percentage of blockage. In most cases, symptoms do not show up with CAD until vessels are 70% occluded or more!

Ischemia refers to the restriction of oxygen to an organ or tissue that may cause damage, dysfunction or even death to that area. Ischemic CAD involves the disruption of the supply of oxygen-rich blood to a body organ or area, which causes damage. Unfortunately, ischemic tissue does not repair itself.

When CAD occludes blood vessels, the patient may experience chest pains (angina pectoris). If a clump of plaque breaks free (ruptures), it can form a blood clot (thrombus) which can block the flow of blood through the vessel downstream. If the thrombus is able to totally block the flow of blood to an area of the heart, a myocardial infarction (MI) occurs. Depending on the location, severity and speed of receiving treatment, an MI can be mild to fatal.

If the thrombus breaks free and manages to navigate its way out of the heart region to another part of the body, it is called an embolus or embolism. The term thromboembolism refers to plaque that breaks free from an occluded vessel and circulates out into the body; if it travels to the heart, it is a thrombus, but if it goes elsewhere, it is an embolism. One of the most deadly (and, sadly, common) destinations for an embolism is the brain. If an embolism blocks the flow of blood to the brain, a stroke occurs. Strokes can be thought of as a form of 'cerebral vascular accident'. Strokes can be relatively minor (some tiny strokes may occur without symptoms) to lethal; most cause some degree of debilitation, often permanent.

Myocardial infarction

MI or the common 'heart attack' can be grouped together with CAD, since an MI traces back to coronary arteries blocked by CAD. When this blockage restricts the myocardium from receiving the oxygen-rich blood it needs, a portion of the myocardial tissue dies. The MI is mild or severe (or lethal) depending on how much of the myocardium is 'starved to death' during the attack.

A heart attack survivor has CAD, which immediately puts him or her at risk of HF. The fact that an MI has occurred introduces another risk factor into the mix. A heart attack causes an ischemic area of tissue to form, which actually presents as a lesion or scar-like area. If part of the heart's normal conduction system ran through this area, the lesion now interferes with it. In fact, the conduction system may have to 're-route' around the lesion. The areas immediately adjacent to the lesion can become alternative conduction routes, such that they form 'substrates' or aberrant conduction pathways. These substrates can introduce conduction pathways, which facilitate re-entry or other mechanisms that can support a tachycardia. In fact, the MADIT II study in particular has demonstrated that heart attack survivors are a population at special risk of dangerous ventricular tachyarrhythmias.[1]

For heart attack survivors, the MI weakens the heart muscle, the CAD contributes to cardiac dysfunction and the myocardial lesions may increase the likelihood of life-threatening ventricular tachyarrhythmias.

Ischemic and non-ischemic heart disease

The distinction between ischemic and non-ischemic heart disease is sometimes important to make in HF patients. Ischemic coronary artery disease (with or without an MI) is by far the most common cause of HF. In fact, it is so commonly associated with HF that clinical studies have often looked at ischemic HF to the exclusion of the non-ischemic variety. Today, we recognize that non-ischemic HF can occur as well, such as in patients with cardiomyopathy but no restricted blood flow. Again, for reasons we do not yet understand, ischemic heart disease is more common in males than in females.

Ischemia refers to any condition that involves tissue damaged by lack of oxygen. In the case of the heart, CAD or MI can kill certain areas of the myocardium. These dead patches of the myocardial muscle are ischemic.

Non-ischemic heart disease involves heart disease in which there is no reduction in blood flow to the tissue, so that there is no ischemic or damaged tissue. The most common form of non-ischemic HF is dilated cardiomyopathy.

Blood pressure

High blood pressure or hypertension is another common condition associated with HF. Hypertension is sometimes called the silent killer because it can occur and worsen to even severe states without any symptoms at all. Hypertension is more common with age and is generally associated with an increasing stiffness in the proximal region of the aorta. The aorta is the main conduit for the blood's distribution network through the body. It runs down the center of the body and is by far the largest of all of our many blood vessels. The presence of coronary artery disease and age will cause this 'pipe' to thicken and grow rigid. Blood pressure increases, causing the heart to work harder to pump the same amount of blood. As the heart increases its work against the stiff aorta, the heart muscle may stiffen or hypertrophy. The result is that the ventricular muscle is so rigid that it cannot really relax well. The result can be diastolic HF (the inability of the heart to fill well with blood for pumping).

Metabolic diseases

Metabolic conditions can also set the stage for HF. The body's complex system of hormones and other chemicals directly affects how the heart works. When disorders disrupt the endocrine system, there can be ramifications on the heart. Diabetes and hypothyroidism are both associated with HF, although they do not directly cause it.

Hypothyroidism (reduced thyroid function) can lead to decreased myocardial function. Hyperthyroidism (overactive thyroid) in the presence of some underlying heart disease can lead to systolic compromise. Patients with hyperthyroidism often suffer from cardiac arrhythmias, which can include atrial fibrillation (AF). Again, in the presence of some structural heart disease, hyperthyroidism and AF can set the stage for HF.

Rhythm disorders

Likewise, cardiac rhythm disorders are associated with HF, although they do not necessarily 'cause' HF. The arrhythmia most commonly associated with HF is AF. AF is progressive arrhythmia and eventually becomes permanent and refractory to all treatment. At its worst, AF involves a seemingly chaotic atrial rhythm which no longer permits the atrial contribution to ventricular filling and may cause the ventricles to beat erratically and overly rapidly in a futile effort to keep pace. While the rapid ventricular response to AF is responsible for most of the typical AF symptoms, the quivering action of the atria causes blood to pool and stagnate in the upper chambers, rather than pump through the system. Clots can develop and, if they do manage to pump out of the atrium, can lead to stroke. In fact, patients with AF are at a dramatically increased risk of stroke for that very reason.

If a patient has only AF, the AF can eventually cause the heart to pump ineffectively and thus gradually bring about HF. For people with some degree of HF already, AF makes the heart an even more inefficient pump by weakening its electrical system and depriving the heart of atrial kick. Many HF patients have some degree of AF; in fact, it is the most common comorbidity for HF.

Valvular disorders

The four main valves of the heart are one-way valves to keep the blood moving forward through the heart (from right atrium to right ventricle and out over the lungs, then back from the lungs from left atrium to left ventricle and into the aorta for distribution to the body). Valvular disorders occur when a valve does not close properly or becomes very stiff. This compromises the heart's ability to pump, because an incomplete seal means that some of the blood within the heart's chamber will move backward through the system.

Another valve problem commonly associated with HF is aortic stenosis, a narrowing of the aortic valve. The aortic valve separates the left ventricle from the aorta, the body's main conduit for blood flow. With aortic stenosis, pressure builds up on the left ventricle, giving it increasingly more force to 'work against' as it pumps oxygenated blood out over the body.

The most common valvular disorder associated with HF is mitral regurgitation (MR; sometimes called mitral valve regurgitation). The mitral valve is strategically positioned between the left atrium and left ventricle. When it cannot close properly, due either to a birth defect or to disease (such as calcification of the leaflets), blood can flow backward from the left ventricle into the left atrium. This backward 'sloshing' of blood impairs cardiac output, so that the heart works just as hard as it should to pump blood, but with less result. Over time, MR can cause the heart rate and cardiac contractility to increase in an effort to compensate for the backflow of blood. While these compensatory mechanisms work well in the short term, over the long term, the heart muscle can become distorted.

Other causes

Heart failure can also be caused by toxins (such as acute alcohol poisoning) or a viral infection. These are relatively rare.

Reference

1 Moss AJ, Zareba W, Hall WH *et al.* Prophylactic implantation of a defibrillator in patients with myocardial infarction and reduced ejection fraction. *N Engl J Med* 2002; **346**:877–83.

The nuts and bolts of causes of heart failure

- Heart failure (HF) is a syndrome with no one single cause for all patients; however, as a disease, it has a predictable course.
- HF is a constellation of conditions that impair the heart's ability to pump blood effectively. It is most frequently associated with left-ventricular dysfunction, low ejection fractions, fluid accumulation and shortness of breath.
- HF begins with an injury to the heart, for which the body tries to compensate, which over the long term leads to impaired pumping capability.
- Some factors which may 'cause' HF include cardiomyopathy, coronary artery disease, myocardial infarction, systolic or diastolic dysfunction. Co-morbid conditions include metabolic disorders (hyperthyroidism and diabetes) and atrial fibrillation.
- Cardiomyopathy refers to a disease of the heart muscle itself. It may be dilated (a flabby heart) or hypertrophic obstructive (a rigid, thick-walled heart). Dilated cardiomyopathy is quite common in HF patients, is more common in men than women and is frequently of

unknown etiology. Hypertrophic obstructive cardiomyopathy (HOCM) is not as common, can be genetic and is frequently the underlying heart disease in young athletic cardiac patients.
- Systolic dysfunction refers to the heart's inability to pump blood out effectively; diastolic dysfunction refers to the heart's inability to fill with blood adequately, which, in turn, impairs its ability to pump an adequate amount of blood out. It is possible for a patient to have both systolic and diastolic dysfunction. It is also possible for a patient to have systolic HF or diastolic HF, although pure diastolic HF (with no systolic component) is rare.
- Coronary artery disease (CAD) is a build-up of fatty deposits and plaque in the arteries that supply the heart muscle with oxygen-rich blood. CAD blocks or occludes these vessels. When a clump of plaque in a vessel breaks free, it can form a thrombus (clot) which can block blood flow to the heart (myocardial infarction) or an embolus (clot) which lodges in the brain (stroke).
- A myocardial infarction (MI) creates scar tissue

Continued p. 22.

Continued.

on the myocardium, which can cause substrates to form, which encourage and sustain certain re-entry-type tachycardias.

- Ischemic heart disease refers to any heart disease in which tissue in the heart is damaged because it is deprived of oxygen for a short time. Typical ischemic heart disease is CAD or MI. Non-ischemic heart disease also occurs, which involves diseases that do not trace back to reduced blood flow to cardiac tissue. An example of non-ischemic heart disease is dilated cardiomyopathy. Note that HF patients may have both ischemic and non-ischemic heart conditions simultaneously.
- HF can be ischemic (involving CAD or a prior MI) or non-ischemic (involving dilated cardiomyopathy). Many of the clinical studies done to date have focused on the ischemic HF patient and excluded or minimized non-ischemic HF patients.
- Hypertension, which increases with age, is associated with HF, in that it can lead to a thickening of the aorta and diastolic HF.
- Two metabolic conditions are associated with (but do not directly cause) HF. They are hyperthyroidism and diabetes.
- The most common co-morbid condition with HF is atrial fibrillation (AF). AF can lead to HF and can exacerbate existing HF. Likewise, HF can exacerbate existing AF.
- Mitral regurgitation (MR) is associated with HF, in that it impairs the heart's ability to pump effectively.
- Although HF can be caused by toxicity (such as acute alcohol poisoning) or a virus, these cases are relatively rare.

Chapter 5

The Neurohormonal Model of Heart Failure

Not long ago, doctors thought of heart failure (HF) as pump failure and delayed any sort of diagnosis or treatment until fluid accumulation had set in. Today we know that HF is a complicated and progressive syndrome which can be effectively treated and even held at bay by recognizing how it proceeds. One of the great breakthroughs in our understanding of HF is recognizing the neurohormonal contribution to the syndrome.

HF begins with injury to the heart that impairs the heart's ability to pump. The heart launches compensatory mechanisms to help take up the slack for this compromised pumping function. While there are a number of compensatory mechanisms at work, one of the most fundamental is the body's neurohormonal response. It is our recent understanding of the neurohormonal system which has led to new treatment strategies (mostly drug therapy) for HF.

To understand the neurohormonal model of HF, we need to go back to the basics of the body's nervous system. The nervous system is not just a system of nerves crisscrossing the entire body; it is a communications network which involves transmitting messages cell-to-cell to cause various reactions. These communications are transmitted mainly by special chemical substances manufactured by the body and sent out to relay specific messages. These chemicals include neurohormones and other substances. Thus, the body's nervous system is run by a finely tuned balance of interacting chemical substances. This is the primary reason why pharmacological therapy has been and remains the backbone of HF treatment: a lot of what is going on with HF is chemical and can be addressed at the chemical level.

The nervous system can be grouped into two main divisions: the sympathetic nervous system (SNS) and the parasympathetic nervous system (PSNS). Healthy individuals have both an SNS and a PSNS, which interact.

The SNS regulates many of the body's functions not under conscious control, such as respiration, digestion, body temperature and even cardiac activities such as heart rate and contractility. These 'non-conscious' functions are also known as autonomic functions, and they allow us to function without having to think constantly about breathing or digesting food or causing our heart to beat. In a healthy individual, the SNS is always working efficiently in the background. When danger strikes, it is the SNS which launches the body's 'fight or flight response' by flooding the body's chemical system with a wave of hormones that trigger heightened emergency responses.

The PSNS could be thought of as the more peaceful twin. In a healthy individual, the PSNS acts as the checks-and-balances to the SNS and keeps the system in proper balance. In a healthy person, the PSNS is the dominant branch of the nervous system, while the SNS hums along in the background and only rarely initiates one of its fight-or-flight responses.

When a person develops HF, the compensatory mechanisms involved cause the PSNS to slip into a diminished role, while the SNS becomes deranged and ends up on chronic red alert. How does this happen? It is a logical cascade effect of HF. HF decreases cardiac output, which causes less blood volume to enter the arterial tree or network of blood vessels that feed the body. The result is a reduced quantity of blood flowing through the system, lowering blood pressure. The body actually monitors blood volume in a very clever way by using baroreceptors, which measure the stretch of certain blood vessels at the aortic arch, the carotid sinus and the cardiac chambers. The lowered blood pressure, combined with less stretch measured by the baroreceptors, is enough to stimulate the brain (technically, the medulla, which regulates the vasomotor system) and launch the SNS into response mode.

SNS releases two neurotransmitters, chemical substances designed to relay a special message through the nerves. These substances are called norepinephrine and epinephrine; the former is familiar even to lay people as adrenalin. Norepinephrine and epinephrine cause the heart rate and contractility to increase and the blood vessels to constrict. The vasoconstriction increases blood pressure (afterload) and forces more blood to return to the heart (preload), which in turn increases stroke volume and raises cardiac output.

While this increase in preload and afterload do achieve the desired effect of elevating blood pressure in the short term, they also significantly increase cardiac workload. This puts greater strain on the heart and, in the long term, can actually reduce cardiac output.

This SNS activity involves the body's adrenergic system, which is further subdivided into the α-adrenergic system and the β-adrenergic system. In a healthy individual, adrenergic activity was intended to allow fight-or-flight responses to danger. However, people with HF are exposed to prolonged periods of high adrenergic activity.

One result of this adrenergic activity is that the heart is stimulated to beat more quickly in an effort to help maintain sufficient cardiac output. This increased heart rate and boosted cardiac output meanwhile increase the heart muscle's need for oxygen. The failing heart may not be able to get all of the oxygen it needs, because the increased heart rate shortens the diastolic period, reducing the amount of available oxygen, and lowers stroke volume, reducing the amount of blood available for the next systole. Thus, patients with HF are confronted with an increased demand for oxygen at the same time they are experiencing a decreased availability of oxygen. This lack of sufficient oxygen or fuel for the heart muscle can be described as decreased myocardial perfusion. Decreased myocardial perfusion can lead to ischemia and may provoke dangerous arrhythmias.

This elevated heart rate persists in HF patients even at rest, which means they may not be able to increase heart rate adequately to exert themselves. This results in the exercise intolerance or shortness of breath common in HF patients. In a healthy person, there is a high degree of heart rate variability, meaning that the heart beats at different rates at different times and in appropriate response to metabolic demand: for example, a healthy person's heart may beat 50 beats/min at rest, 70 beats/min during office work, 90 beats/min moving around the office and 120 beats/min playing tennis. HF patients have a decreased heart rate variability, in that their hearts are always trying to beat as fast as they can to maintain proper cardiac output (and respond to the fight-or-flight adrenergic activity going on).

However, that is not all that is going on with the SNS. The SNS also regulates the renin–angiotensin–aldosterone (RAA) system. The RAA system is activated when blood perfusion to the kidneys drops as a result of the diminished cardiac output associated with HF. Baroreceptors, which measure stretch in cells, notice that the kidneys are not receiving adequate blood, which activates the body to release an enzyme known as renin.

Renin, in turn, converts a plasma protein known as angiotensinogen into a substance called angiotensin-I (A-I). Another enzyme, known as the angiotensin-converting enzyme (ACE) can change A-I into angiotensin-II (A-II). A-II is a powerful vasoconstrictor, which has the immediate effect of boosting blood pressure. A-II further stimulates the release of another chemical into the mix, a substance known as aldosterone. Aldosterone's main effect is to encourage the kidneys to retain sodium and water. In the short run, fluid and salt retention increases blood volume and raises arterial pressure. The increased blood volume stretches the muscle fibers of the myocardium and increases cardiac output.

While this may sound good as an immediate solution, prolonged stimulation of the RAA system overloads a weakened heart. A-II increases preload and afterload, both of which add to the workload on the heart. A-II has been associated with low serum sodium levels (hyponatremia). Aldosterone causes fluid retention, leading to congestion with all of its unpleasant symptoms. In patients with advanced HF, the excess fluid escapes from the circulatory system and starts to accumulate in the tissues, causing swelling and edema.

In a healthy individual, the SNS helps regulate blood pressure and cardiac activity and is very adept at managing crises of short duration. Prolonged activation of these SNS emergency systems and high levels of these specific chemicals expose HF patients to considerable stress and wear-and-tear on their heart.

As the heart tries to cope with increased workload and elevated volume and rate, the ventricular muscle stretches to distribute wall stress more evenly and maintain cardiac output. The left ventricle (the body's main blood pump) looses its ability to pump, which increases diastolic pressure. In turn, that increased diastolic pressure causes the left ventricle to dilate. This change in myocardium is known as ventricular remodeling. It can occur in two main forms: eccentric hypertrophy and concentric hypertrophy.

Eccentric hypertrophy occurs with progressive dilation of the left ventricle, reducing its contractility and lowering the left-ventricular ejection fraction. This results in left-ventricular or systolic dysfunction. The heart shape is 'eccentric,' which in this case means 'off-center' or asymmetrical.

However, sometimes the increased workload on the heart causes the ventricle to hypertrophy or become thicker. Increased afterload decreases stroke volume. The body strives to maintain stroke volume (and to respond to an increase in left systolic pressure) with a thickening of the muscle in the ventricular wall. The left ventricle, in particular, thickens inward. Unfortunately, this thicker, stiffer ventricular wall reduces the size of the ventricular filling chamber and causes the wall to become too stiff to pump effectively. The ventricles become unable to relax appropriately during diastole (causing diastolic dysfunction). This form of ventricular remodeling causes the heart to change shape in a more rounded fashion and is known as concentric hypertrophy (concentric, in this case, means, centered).

The neurohormonal model of HF answers many previously unsolved riddles about heart disease. For example, it explains why the disease is progressive and why people with HF often do well for protracted periods of time before succumbing to debilitating conditions and even death. It also helps us appreciate how complicated the syndrome can be and that a simplistic approach (a monotherapy) simply does not work. It also shows us that HF begins long before the familiar symptoms of congestion set in. This understanding of the genesis of HF can help us find ways to treat it more effectively by treating it early.

The nuts and bolts of the neurohormonal model of heart failure

- Today we recognize the neurohormonal contribution to heart failure (HF). In fact, much of the drug therapy for HF is based on the neurohormonal model.
- The body has a parasympathetic nervous system (PSNS) and a sympathetic nervous system (SNS). In a healthy individual, the PSNS is dominant and the SNS (which manages functions not under conscious control, such as respiration, digestion, heart rate and so on) kicks in primarily in times of stress. This SNS 'emergency response' is often called the 'fight or flight' response. HF patients have a deranged nervous system, such that the SNS is dominant and largely in control. This means that HF patients live with an abnormally high level of neurohormonal 'fight or flight' chemicals in their system.
- One reason that the SNS becomes activated is that HF decreases cardiac output, which decreases blood volume. Baroreceptors (which measure stretch of blood vessels) detect the lower-than-normal blood volume and signal production of epinephrine and norepinephrine (commonly known as adrenalin). These are neurotransmitters, which signal the body to increase heart rate, constrict blood vessels and increase the contractility of the myocardium.
- Another portion of the SNS system involves the α- and β-adrenergic systems. The adrenergic response to lowered cardiac output (typical in HF patients) is to increase the heart rate. This in turn, causes the heart to increase its need for oxygen, although oxygen-rich blood is in short supply. This can lead to reduced myocardial perfusion, which may even provoke arrhythmias.
- The SNS raises the heart rate, so that HF patients often have decreased heart rate variability. This means their hearts beat at maximum rate most of the time and cannot ramp up to accommodate stress or exertion.

Continued p. 26.

Continued.

- When blood flow to the kidneys is reduced, it activates another part of the SNS, namely the body's renin–angiotensin–aldosterone (RAA) system. The RAA system works in a cascade: renin is released, which converts a plasma protein (angiotensinogen) into a substance called angiotensin-I (A-I). An enzyme is released which transforms A-I into angiotensin-II (A-II). A-II is a powerful vasoconstrictor, which immediately elevates blood pressure and stimulates the RAA system to release aldosterone, which encourages the renal system to store water and sodium. This causes fluid accumulation.
- While the actions of the SNS system work well in the short term to help the body compensate for reduced cardiac output and diminished blood volume, over the long run they produce significant changes in the heart. The most notable of these include changes to the shape and functionality of the myocardium.
- The ventricle changes shape as HF progresses in a condition known as 'ventricular remodeling'. There are two main types: eccentric hypertrophy and concentric hypertrophy.
- A person with eccentric (or 'off-center,' i.e. asymmetrical) hypertrophy experiences progressive dilation of the left ventricle, reducing its contractility and lowering the ejection fraction. The heart becomes flabby and enlarged.
- A person with concentric (or 'on-center') hypertrophy experiences a thickening of the interior of the ventricular walls, which reduces the capacity of the heart's pumping chambers. The heart becomes rounded with very stiff walls, and loses its ability to relax completely during diastole.
- The neurohormonal model of HF does not present the entire picture of the syndrome, but it does indicate why the disease progresses the way it does and it also helps clinicians determine appropriate pharmacological approaches. Since much of HF happens at the chemical level, there is value in treating the syndrome chemically as well as with other approaches.

Chapter 6

An Overview of Heart Failure Drugs

An understanding of cardiac resynchronization therapy (CRT) has to involve the basics of heart failure (HF) drug therapy, simply because HF patients need to take certain drugs as the foundation of their care. For HF patients, treatment is not limited to either drugs or devices. Treatment first involves drugs, with device therapy a possible addition for certain patients. Adjunctive device-based treatment does not eliminate the need to maintain a sound pharmacological regimen.

Even the most responsive CRT patient cannot stop taking medication!

Our understanding of the pharmacological management of HF patients is based on the neurohormonal model of the syndrome. In other words, we counteract what is occurring at a chemical level by introducing other chemicals into the system. In one way, some of the discussion of drugs for HF patients will sound logical and straightforward.

In reality, managing the drug therapy of a typical HF patient can be very tricky. Most HF patients need to submit to polypharmacy, i.e. taking multiple drugs. Drugs can interact with other drugs. As the syndrome worsens or improves, drug dosages may have to be adjusted. Not all of the main HF drugs are well tolerated; some patients will experience side effects, occasionally severe enough to require discontinuing one drug in favor of an alternative. There is even new evidence of racial and gender differences in drug response. In short, keeping the right drugs in the right amounts is a juggling act.

These main types of drugs should be considered for HF patients:[1]

- Loop diuretic
- Angiotensin-converting enzyme (ACE) inhibitor or, if not tolerated, an angiotensin-receptor blocker (ARB)
- β-Blocker
- Spironolactone

- Digoxin
- In some cases, amiodarone.

While there are other drugs HF patients may take and new drugs are being investigated, this chapter will focus on these 'first-line' drugs.

Diuretics are one of the most commonly prescribed drugs for HF patients and no other drug can relieve symptoms faster than diuretics. A diuretic drug can often reduce congestion in a matter of hours. Diuretics improve dyspnea and exercise tolerance in a very short time. Loop diuretics are probably the best-known type of diuretic for HF patients. However, for patients with milder symptoms, less powerful diuretics such as thiazide or metolazone should be used.[1]

While we often think of HF as a cardiac condition, it also affects the renal and respiratory systems. The heart, lungs and kidneys all work together to keep the body fed with oxygen-rich blood and to remove carbon dioxide waste products from the body. In a healthy person, a quarter of the total blood supply is at the kidneys at any given time. Besides filtering the blood, the kidneys are also in charge of regulating blood volume and blood composition. As the heart fails, the kidneys no longer receive the volume of blood they need; they can no longer maintain the proper blood volume and composition. Baroreceptors in the renal system activate the body's renin–angiotensin–aldosterone (RAA) system to produce chemicals that will cause the body to try to hold onto sodium and water. In the short run, this is a compensatory mechanism which works to boost blood volume, but over time, it can lead to fluid accumulation, compromised renal function and even kidney failure.

Loop diuretics are so-named because they work on a portion of the kidney cell known as the loop of Henle. The kidneys are composed of about one million highly specialized filtration cells called nephrons. Each nephron contains a tiny blood vessel and a miniature tube called a tubule. The tubule connects to a network of other tubes that eventually lead to the bladder. As blood is filtered through the nephrons, waste material is collected through the tubule and ultimately excreted. The loop of Henle is a part of the tubule of an individual nephron which acts like a miniature sodium pump. The loop of Henle works to be sure that the body retains sodium instead of excreting all of it in the urine. A loop diuretic works on the sodium pump at the loop of Henle to encourage sodium excretion. As the body releases sodium, diuresis or an increased production of urine occurs, which, in turn, relieves fluid overload, decreases pulmonary congestion, decreases jugular venous pressures and may even lower body weight by getting rid of excess water in the system. Diuretics work quickly and the rapid relief of edema and congestion provide significant symptomatic relief.

While most patients tolerate diuretics well, there are some risks and potential side effects. While loop diuretics, in particular, are effective at getting rid of excess fluid, they can also deplete serum potassium levels, which can lead to a condition called hypokalemia. Reduced potassium in the body can have serious and even fatal clinical consequences. Over the long term, diuretics can deplete the body's electrolyte household. Symptoms of an electrolyte imbalance include hypotension, kidney failure, rashes and even hearing problems.

Loop diuretics are the most powerful diuretics available. There are three main types: bumetanide, furosemide and torsemide. Patients on milder diuretics would probably take thiazide or metolazone, but whatever diuretics a HF patient may take, there are some important safeguards. All patients on diuretics should be monitored regularly. It is not uncommon to have to adjust the dosage from time to time to help keep up with fluid accumulation. Serum potassium levels and electrolyte levels should be checked often and kidney function evaluated, since these are things that diuretics can affect adversely. The most recent guidelines for HF patients advise that diuretics should be given only to HF patients already taking ACE inhibitors (or another similar drug, if ACE inhibitors are not tolerated) and β-blockers.[1]

While there have been many major randomized drug trials, there have been no large-scale studies of diuretics, so we have no hard evidence of their morbidity or mortality benefits in HF patients. The reason that there is a lack of evidence for such familiar drugs may seem simplistic. Diuretics are so basic to the care and well-being of HF patients that it is considered inhumane to withhold them, even for the purposes of a randomized clinical trial. We therefore lack hard evidence that there is any mortality benefit attached to diuretics. However, smaller studies show a trend for the notion that diuretics improve survival in HF patients[2] and most clinicians who care for HF patients observe the clear benefits of diuretic therapy on their patients.

Diuretics are some of the oldest drugs in HF treatment, whereas spironolactone is one of the newest. Spironolactone has a mild diuretic effect, but technically it is an aldosterone blocker. Its main function, when prescribed, is to block the effects of aldosterone, part of the sympathetic nervous system (SNS). In so doing, it also increases urinary output and decreases fluid accumulation. But spironolactone is what has come to be called a 'potassium-sparing diuretic'. Regular diuretics cause the body to excrete potassium, to the point that sometimes patients are advised to take potassium supplements to avoid hypokalemia. Spironolactone has a diuretic effect but does not lower the body's potassium levels. Thus, a patient on spironolactone should probably not be taking potassium supplements. In fact, any patient taking spironolactone should be carefully monitored for serum potassium levels. However, the degree to which spironolactone spares potassium in the system depends on dosage; lower doses may not have much potassium-sparing effect at all.

Hyperkalemia or potassium overload can develop in patients taking spironolactone, particularly if they are taking potassium supplements or are not under regular care by a physician. Hyperkalemia, like hypokalemia, can become a very dangerous condition.

Potassium is one of many minerals in the body, but unlike other minerals, most (98%) of the body's potassium store is contained within cells and only a tiny amount (2%) is extracellular. It is this ratio of intracellular to extracellular potassium which can drastically affect the body: it impacts cell membrane polarization, nerve conduction speeds and muscle contractility (including cardiac contractility). Even a tiny shift in the body's potassium ratios can cause serious clinical consequences.

While spironolactone is not one of the 'corner-stones' of pharmacological management of HF patients, it is increasingly seen in clinical practice. The combination of diuretic effect and aldoster-one blocker has made it very attractive. Note that in the USA, only one potassium-sparing diuretic (spironolactone) is currently available commercial-ly, while in other parts of the world there are several drugs in this particular category.

While spironolactone is new to HF, it is not a new drug. A large randomized clinical trial of spironol-actone (RALES) found that it reduced the risk of sudden cardiac death or HF death by 35% in certain Class III and Class IV HF patients.[3]

One of the mainstays of drug treatment for HF is the ACE inhibitor. An ACE inhibitor is a drug which inhibits a naturally produced enzyme in the body (the angiotensin-converting enzyme) which is supposed to convert the inactive substance an-giotensin-I (A-I) into the powerful vasoconstric-tor angiotensin-II (A-II). In terms of how the drug works, it does not block A-II at all; it merely inhibits the body's ability to produce A-II.

A-II is a formidable substance. Not only is it a vasoconstrictor, it is also associated with sodium retention (leading to edema). It has a toxic effect on cardiac cells and is known to contribute to ven-tricular remodeling. A healthy individual has a low level of A-II in his system, which does not have any particular adverse effect. HF patients have very high levels of A-II. Taking an ACE inhibitor helps bring these high levels of A-II under control.

There are many different types of ACE inhibitors on the market, most of which have a generic com-pound which ends in '-pril'. Examples of ACE in-hibitors include enalapril (the best known), capto-pril, lisinopril and ramipril. There are others. There have been many large, randomized clinical trials with ACE inhibitors, primarily enalapril. There is evidence that ACE inhibitors have what is known as a class effect, meaning that drugs in this particular class have the same effect. In other words, study re-sults from enalapril are likely to apply to other ACE inhibitors.[4] From the CONSENSUS study, we have evidence that ACE inhibitors reduce mortality[5] in certain Class IV HF patients.

According to the most recent HF guidelines, HF patients with systolic dysfunction should be taking an ACE inhibitor even if they have no symptoms.[1]

They are literally a first-line of defense drugs for all HF patients with some degree of LV impairment (typically expressed as a left-ventricular ejection fraction of < 40%). They are to be given unless the patient does not tolerate them. While there are alter-natives to ACE inhibitors, the ACE inhibitor should be attempted first and an alternative selected only if the ACE inhibitor produces unmanageable side effects.

Most HF patients tolerate ACE inhibitors well, but the most common side effect is a non-produc-tive cough. If patients can tolerate it, many HF spe-cialists will try to keep them on the ACE inhibitor despite the cough. Other, but much less frequently occurring side effects include an allergic reaction involving a swelling of the throat, lips or eyes, as well as hypotension and dizziness. ACE inhibitors can cause potassium retention and thus may worsen renal failure, so they should be given with care to such patients. In all cases, renal function should be monitored for patients taking ACE inhibitors.

If an ACE inhibitor must be discontinued, the most common alternative is an ARB. In theory, an ARB does the same thing as an ACE inhibitor, but in a different way. Both ACE inhibitors and ARBs attempt to reduce the effects of high levels of A-II in the body. An ACE inhibitor stops the body from making A-II out of A-I. An ARB allows the body to make A-II (and thus does not diminish the level of A-II in the body), but it blocks the ability of the A-II to do its job. In order for A-II to transmit its message to the body (typically to constrict blood vessels), it must 'plug into' receptor cells. Every neurotransmis-sion in the body involves a substance that relays the messages (in this case, A-II) and a way for that mes-sage to be received (the receptor). When a chemical substance meets its appropriate receptor, it fits like a key in a lock. This allows the substance to transmit its message. ARBs work by blocking the receptors that allow A-II to complete its mission. Patients tak-ing ARBs still have high levels of A-II in the body, but the A-II is rendered ineffective.

ARBs are much newer drugs than ACE inhibitors and lack the same body of clinical evidence favor-ing their morbidity and mortality benefits in HF patients. Generic ARBs are drugs that end in '-sar-tan,' including candesartan, irbesartan, losartan and valsartan, among others. Most HF specialists do not regard ARBs as equivalent to ACE inhibitors (which are the gold standard); instead, ARBs are a valuable alternative if and when ACE inhibitors cannot be used in a particular patient.

Another cornerstone of HF drug therapy is the β-blocker, a drug that block the body's β-adrenergic system, part of the body's 'fight-or-flight' response. The β-adrenergic system is best known for producing two powerful neurohormones: epinephrine and norepinephrine. In a healthy person, these two neurohormones have three main effects on the heart:

- A positive chronotropic effect (increasing heart rate)
- A positive dromotropic effect (increasing electrical conduction velocity within the heart)
- A positive inotropic effect (causing the heart muscle to contract more vigorously).

In a healthy patient, these three effects are beneficial. In a HF patient, these three effects increase the heart's demand for oxygen and other nutrients in the blood. This sets up an oxygen-deficit, which can lead to ischemia. If the HF patient has developed abnormal cardiac cells (as a result of ventricular remodeling), increasing their automaticity can lead to irregular and potentially dangerous heart rhythms. Norepinephrine has also been associated with apoptosis or programmed cell death. For reasons we do not fully understand, the nucleus of a cardiac cell contains instructions to destroy itself at a certain point in the future. Norepinephrine is thought to trigger premature apoptosis in cardiac cells.

β-Blockers have been used for decades in HF patients and their morbidity and mortality benefits have been well established in numerous large, randomized clinical trials. While studies and clinical experience show that β-blockers can and do reduce HF symptoms, they do not provide symptomatic relief in all patients. Initially, patients starting β-blockade may experience worsening symptoms, in particular fatigue and increased fluid retention. Physicians prescribing β-blockers to a new patient are advised to 'start low and go slow'. In time and with careful management, most HF patients who experience problems with β-blockers at the outset can be successfully up-titrated to proper doses with diminished side effects. However, even if the patient derives no symptomatic relief, β-blockers are still vital.

β-Blockers have been shown in a large, randomized clinical trial to reduce mortality.[6–9] However, unlike ACE inhibitors with a class effect, there is evidence that different β-blockers have different clinical effects.[10] For that reason, the most commonly used β-blockers are those for which we have excellent clinical evidence: bisoprolol, carvedilol and metoprolol.

HF patients on β-blockers should also be receiving diuretics, in particular because it is likely that β-blockade will increase fluid retention.

Another drug in the HF medicine chest is digoxin, which is not routinely administered to all patients. Part of the family of cardiac glycosides, digoxin has been familiar to cardiologists for over a century and remains widely prescribed because of its positive inotropic properties, which cause the heart muscle to contract more vigorously. Digoxin is also a negative chronotrope, meaning that it slows the heart rate. Taken together—slower rate, more vigorous contraction—these effects make the heart a more efficient pump. Digoxin does not work directly on the neurohormonal system, but it does contribute to the overall well-being of many HF patients.

However, digoxin is not appropriate for patients with AV block (unless they already have a pacemaker) or for patients with acutely decompensated HF. The main effect of digoxin is symptomatic relief, so digoxin is not typically prescribed to asymptomatic patients. While there is evidence of the morbidity benefits of digoxin and of the fact that it can reduce HF hospitalizations,[11] it has not been proven to reduce mortality.

Dosing digoxin requires careful monitoring. There is a very narrow therapeutic range, and digoxin can be toxic (even fatal) at high levels. Given at proper dosage, digoxin is safe, effective and has long-established morbidity benefits.

Antiarrhythmic agents (AAAs), designed to help control cardiac rhythm disorders, have to be used with extreme caution in heart failure patients. Many AAAs (with the exception of β-blockers) are contraindicated in heart failure patients, such as Class I drugs. A seemingly paradoxical side effect of AAAs is pro-arrhythmia. These drugs, intended to control certain rhythm disorders, may actually make the heart more susceptible to other types of rhythm disorders. Since many HF patients die from rhythm disorders and are vulnerable to arrhythmias, certain AAAs may be particularly dangerous.

In addition, most AAAs are negative inotropes, which means they would have clinically relevant side effects in most HF patients.

Amiodarone is the only AAA that is not a negative inotropic agent and, as such, may be used judiciously in HF patients to suppress ambient ventricular tachyarrhythmias. However, a recent large clinical trial (SCD-HeFT) has shown that amiodarone did only about as well as a placebo (no drug) in terms of reducing mortality in Class II and Class III HF patients with an LVEF of ≤ 35%, while an implantable cardioverter-defibrillator did reduce mortality.[12] Thus, while amiodarone may well prevent some ventricular tachyarrhythmias in HF patients, it clearly does not eliminate all of them. This has given considerable impetus to the notion that device therapy is vitally important to HF patients, since devices in the SCD-HeFT trial did reduce mortality.

Still, many HF patients who receive CRT-D systems may still be prescribed amiodarone, in an effort to minimize the number of life-saving shocks they might need and to prevent many rhythm disorders. However, the notion that amiodarone protects HF patients from arrhythmic death has been shown to be false. At best, it can help control rhythm disorders and might possibly make CRT-D therapy more comfortable by reducing therapy deliveries.

Outside the USA, amiodarone may be prescribed to suppress ambient supraventricular tachyarrhythmias, particularly atrial fibrillation. In the USA, such use would be off-label.

There are a few other drugs that might come into play for HF patients. In 2005, the Food and Drug Administration cleared for market release a new combination drug of hydralazine and isosorbide dinitrate (trade name Bidil®) to slow HF progression in blacks. This is the first drug approval in the USA based on genetic criteria. Hydralazine and isosorbide dinitrate are vasodilators that help dilate peripheral blood vessels and may be prescribed for any HF patient, but clinical evidence has shown it is far more effective in blacks than non-blacks.

New drugs under investigation include endothelin antagonists, vasopeptidase inhibitors and cytokine antagonists. Although there are ongoing studies, it is unlikely that we will see any significant new pharmacological breakthroughs for HF in the next few years.

When considering the role of drugs in HF patients, it is important for clinicians who work with CRT systems to remember that drugs are always required in HF patients. The major clinical trials (MADIT II, CARE-HF, COMPANION, SCD-HeFT) all required patients to be on optimal pharmacological therapy at baseline and drug therapy was carefully monitored throughout the study. This is the gold standard for any HF patient: optimal and constantly monitored drug therapy as the foundation.

Not only can drugs interact with each other, drugs may interact with devices. Some drugs affect defibrillation thresholds (DFTs), the amount of energy the device needs to defibrillate the heart reliably. In particular, amiodarone has been associated with increases in DFTs, which is an important programming consideration for CRT-D therapy. Digoxin and β-blockers can slow the heart and bring on symptomatic bradycardia, which may necessitate bradycardia pacing support. Some of these side effects may occur gradually, so clinicians should monitor such patients and adjust device settings as needed.

References

1 Swedberg K, Cleland J, Dargie H et al. Guidelines for the diagnosis and treatment of chronic heart failure (update 2005). The European Society of Cardiology 2005.

2 Faris R, Flather M, Purcell H et al. Current evidence supporting the role of diuretics in heart failure: a meta analysis of randomized controlled trials. Int J Cardiol 2002; **82**:149–58.

3 Pitt B, Zannad F, Remme WJ et al. The effect of spironolactone on morbidity and mortality in patients with heart failure. JAMA 2000; **283**:1295–302.

4 Garg R, Yusuf F. Overview of randomized trials of angiotensin-converting enzyme inhibitors on mortality and morbidity in patients with heart failure. Collaborative Group on ACE inhibitor trials. JAMA 1995; **273**:1450–6.

5 The CONSENSUS Trial Group. Effects of enalapril on mortality in severe congestive heart failure. Results of the Cooperative North Scandinavian Enalapril Survival Study. N Engl J Med 1987; **316**:1429–35.

6 CIBIS II Investigators. The Cardiac Insufficiency Bisoprolol Study II; a randomised trial. Lancet 1999; **353**:9–13.

7 Krum H, Roecker EB, Mohasci P et al. Effects of initiating carvedilol in patients with severe chronic heart fail-

ure. *JAMA* 2003; **289:**712–18.

8   Hjalmarson A, Goldstein S, Fagerberg B *et al.* Effects of controlled-release metoprolol on total mortality, hospitalizations, and well-being in patients with heart failure. *JAMA* 2000; **283:**1295–302.

9   Packer M, Bristow MR, Cohn JN *et al.* The effect of carvedilol on morbidity and mortality in patients with chronic heart failure. *N Engl J Med* 1996; **334:**1349–55.

10 Poole-Wilson PA, Swedberg K, Cleland JG *et al.* Comparison of carvedilol and metoprolol on clinical outcomes in patients with CHF in the Carvedilol or Metoprolol European Trial (COMET): randomized controlled trial. *Lancet* 2003; **362:**7–13.

11 The Digitalis Investigation Group. The effect of digoxin on mortality and morbidity in patients with heart failure. *N Engl J Med* 1997; **336:**525–33.

12 Bardy GH, Lee KL, Mark DB *et al.* Amiodarone or an implantable cardioverter-defibrillator for congestive heart failure. *N Engl J Med* 2005; **352:**225–37.

The nuts and bolts of heart failure drug therapy

- Drugs remain the foundation of all heart failure (HF) therapy. Even patients who receive cardiac resynchronization therapy systems will continue to need drug therapy.
- HF patients typically end up taking four to six or more medications. Management of this type of polypharmacy requires regular monitoring, adjustments and testing. Many drugs for HF have side effects.
- The main drugs that should be considered for HF patients are diuretics, angiotensin-converting enzyme (ACE) inhibitors, β-blockers, spironolactone, digoxin and amiodarone.
- Many patients do not tolerate ACE inhibitors. If ACE inhibitors do not work, guidelines recommend that the patient try an angiotensin-receptor blocker (ARB). However, ARBs should not be considered equivalent to ACE inhibitors, but rather as a possible alternative.
- Most HF patients receive loop diuretics (the most potent type), but patients with milder symptoms may benefit from milder diuretics such as thiazide or metolazone.
- Loop diuretics work at the loop of Henle, a little sodium pump in the nephron (kidney cell). Loop diuretics provide very rapid symptomatic relief of congestion.
- There are no large randomized clinical studies demonstrating the mortality benefit (if any) of diuretics in HF patients. However, diuretics are one of the most established drugs in the HF medicine chest.
- Loop diuretics can deplete the body's serum potassium, which can lead to hypokalemia. Potassium supplementation should be approached cautiously, since it is also possible for HF patients to become hyperkalemic.
- The main loop diuretics are bumetanide, furosemide and torsemide.
- Spironolactone is an aldosterone blocker which has a diuretic effect. Spironolactone is a potassium-sparing diuretic, so patients taking this drug should not be taking potassium supplements.
- Spironolactone is not a new drug, but is relatively new and promising in HF treatment.
- ACE inhibitors work by inhibiting the angiotensin-converting enzyme, which converts the inactive angiotensin-I into the powerful vasoconstrictor angiotensin-II. The alternative drug, ARBs, block the ability of angiotensin-II to relay its message of vasoconstriction by blocking its receptor cells. Both counteract the negative effects of the body's renin–angiotensin–aldosterone system.
- ACE inhibitor generic drug names end in 'pril', while ARB generic drug names end in 'sartan.'
- Randomized clinical studies have shown a mortality as well as morbidity benefit for HF patients taking ACE inhibitors, which have a 'class effect', meaning these same results apply to all ACE inhibitors.
- Guidelines recommend that all HF patients with systolic dysfunction (low LVEF) should take an ACE inhibitor, even if they have no symptoms.
- The most common side effect of ACE inhibitor is a non-productive cough. If the patient cannot tolerate the cough, they may be switched to an ARB.

Continued.

Continued.

- ARBs are much newer drugs. Guidelines advise that HF patients should be prescribed an ARB only if they do not tolerate the 'gold standard' ACE inhibitor.
- Guidelines recommend that all HF patients, even those without symptoms, be prescribed a β-blocker. HF patients should remain on β-blockers even if they derive no apparent symptomatic benefit from the drug.
- Randomized clinical trials have demonstrated both a morbidity and mortality benefit for HF patients taking β-blockers. β-Blockers do not have a class effect, meaning there are somewhat different results for different types.
- β-Blockers block the body's adrenergic system (epinephrine and norepinephrine) and can increase heart rate, speed conduction velocity in the heart and boost the vigor of cardiac contraction.
- β-Blockers may cause fatigue and fluid retention (they should always be prescribed together with a diuretic), particularly at first. The old saying, 'Start low and go slow', applies to the initial dosing of β-blockers. Often a low initial dose can be ramped up later, as side effects subside.
- β-Blockers are associated with bradycardia and sometimes patients need pacing support to maintain a course of β blockade.
- β-Blocker generic names end in 'olol' and the best known are carvedilol, bisoprolol and metoprolol, although there are many others on the market.
- Digoxin is an old drug with positive inotropic properties (increases the vigor of cardiac contraction). It may also slow the heart rate. Digoxin is not appropriate for patients with AV block unless they already have a pacemaker.
- Digoxin has been clinically proven to reduce morbidity in HF patients, but not mortality.

- It is important to dose digoxin properly, since the drug has a very narrow therapeutic range and high doses can induce digitalis toxicity.
- Most antiarrhythmic agents are contraindicated in HF patients because of their proarrhythmic effects. The one antiarrhythmic drug that HF patients may take is amiodarone, a Class III antiarrhythmic agent with minimal proarrhythmic effects.
- Amiodarone is prescribed to reduce or suppress ventricular tachyarrhythmias and it is sometimes used off-label (in the USA) to suppress supraventricular tachycardias. However, it has not been shown to reduce mortality in HF patients. Amiodarone is also associated with many side effects, including organ damage.
- Drugs not only interact with each other, they can interact with devices. Amiodarone may elevate defibrillation thresholds. Digoxin and β-blockers can cause symptomatic bradycardia.
- New pharmacological advances have shown that drugs sometimes work differently on certain genetic or gender groups. For example, a combination of hydralazine and isosorbide dinitrate is marketed in the USA under the trade name Bidil® as a HF drug for blacks. Approved in 2005, Bidil is the first drug cleared for market in the USA based on genetic characteristics. Hydralazine and isosorbide dinitrate were found to have morbidity and mortality benefits in black HF patients, but not in non-black HF patients.
- Many new drugs are being investigated for HF, including endothelin antagonists, vasopeptidase inhibitors and cytokine antagonists. None of these drugs is likely to join the HF arsenal in the immediate future.

Chapter 7

Ventricular Dyssynchrony

The syndrome of heart failure (HF) begins with an insult or injury to the heart (structural damage) and progresses with compensatory mechanisms that involve the neurohormonal system. Only recently have we come to understand another aspect of HF, namely ventricular dyssynchrony. Not all HF patients have ventricular dyssynchrony and clinicians are still a long way from agreeing how to define and quantify degrees of dyssynchrony. However, for many HF patients a missing piece of the puzzle was found when electrophysiologists began to explore the complex subject of out-of-sync activity.

For the heart, timing is everything. In the healthy heart, the electrical impulse that originates in the sinoatrial node must travel down over the atria to the atrioventricular (AV) node, experience a slight delay, and then conduct downward and outward over the ventricles. If this occurs at the right conduction velocity, the result is a heartbeat that allows for proper atrial filling, the atrial contribution to ventricular filling, closure of the valves, ventricular depolarization and repolarization. The right and left ventricles contract at exactly the same time and the left ventricle contracts coherently, i.e. as one unit.

Thus, there are two forms of dyssynchrony. Electrical dyssynchrony involves conduction delays and disorders, while mechanical dyssynchrony involves the heart's sequence of contraction and relaxation.

Patients with HF frequently develop conduction abnormalities, which can significantly alter the conduction sequence of the healthy heart. The two main types of conduction abnormalities in HF patients are:
- Delayed ventricular activation
- Prolonged atrial-ventricular conduction.

About half of all HF patients will have some form of conduction disorder.[1]

HF patients often develop delayed left-ventricular activation owing to left bundle branch block (LBBB). LBBB is a conduction disorder that may also occur independently of HF, but is common in HF patients. In LBBB, the left-sided network of conduction fibers of the heart blocks or delays electrical signals. The result is that the left ventricle contracts after the right ventricle, instead of at the same time. (A patient without HF and without native LBBB experiences a bit of 'artificial LBBB' when he receives a pacemaker; the pacemaker paces the right side of the heart, which then conducts to the left side.)

When the right ventricle contracts before the left ventricle, the result is a condition known as interventricular dyssynchrony. The right ventricle and left ventricles are out of sync. This type of dyssynchrony generally appears on a surface ECG as a prolonged or widened QRS complex. QRS durations generally > 120 ms have been identified as an independent risk factor for HF,[2] although its value as a risk stratifier remains under debate. To be sure, QRS duration is a simple, straightforward, inexpensive marker which does indeed correlate to some degree with electrical dyssynchrony.

Another conduction disorder that may have even more clinical significance for HF patients is the intraventricular conduction delay. This occurs entirely within the left ventricle. With intraventricular conduction delay, the left ventricle's lateral or outside wall contracts before the inner or septal wall. The result is that the left ventricle contracts in segments or waves rather than as a unified whole. Since the pumping chamber is contracting in sections, much of the blood within the left ventricle will slosh back and forth rather than being effectively pumped outward. Intraventricular conduction disorders significantly reduce cardiac output.

Intraventricular and interventricular conduction delays have both been associated with negative clinical consequences.[3,4]

Added to this is a prolonged natural AV delay common in many HF patients. In this situation, there is a longer-than-normal pause between atrial systole and ventricular systole. This AV conduction delay limits the atrial contribution to ventricular filling, encourages diastolic mitral regurgitation and shortens ventricular filling time (see Fig. 7.1).

The effects of a prolonged AV delay can have dramatic clinical consequences for HF patients. Since ventricles rely on atrial kick for up to 30% of cardiac output, the loss of even part of this 'booster pump' action can be profound. Diastolic mitral regurgitation occurs because the atria contract and relax, then a pause (the prolonged AV delay) follows, during which there is such low atrial pressure that the mitral valve remains open. The low atrial pressure and open mitral valve lead to diastolic mitral regurgitation, a decrease in preload, and, in the end, will decrease cardiac output (see Fig. 7.2).

While electrical (out-of-sync electrical conduction) and mechanical dyssynchrony (out-of-sync contraction sequence) are closely related, it is possible to have one form without the other. Electrical dyssynchrony is best demonstrated by a wide QRS on a surface ECG. Mechanical dyssynchrony is usually demonstrated with an imaging technology, such as echo, tissue Doppler, tagged magnetic

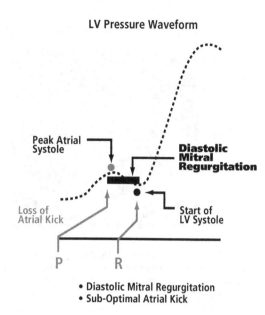

LV Pressure Waveform

- **Diastolic Mitral Regurgitation**
- **Sub-Optimal Atrial Kick**

Fig. 7.2 LV pressure waveform. Prolonged atrioventricular conduction reduces atrial kick, increases mitral regurgitation and has a negative impact on cardiac output.

resonance images (MRI) or pressure–pressure loops (see Fig. 7.3).

Mechanical dyssynchrony is currently recognized as the best predictor of how well a particular patient will respond to cardiac resynchronization therapy (CRT).[5] However, current CRT guidelines use electrical dyssynchrony (QRS duration) for their indications. Thus, there is still no universal agreement as to how clinicians can best quantify dyssynchrony with respect to CRT therapy. Even when physicians attempt to quantify dyssynchrony, there is no standard approach. Physicians may rely on a three-dimensional echo, a two-dimensional echo, a color Doppler flow image, tissue Doppler, or even a tagged MRI.

When mechanical dyssynchrony is present, the right ventricle contracts before the left ventricle. This means the right ventricle is already starting to enter diastole (rest) while the left ventricle is still contracting. The left ventricle relaxes during atrial systole, which virtually eliminates the atrial contribution to ventricular filling. Thus, the cardiac phases of systole and diastole overlap and blur to the point that atria and ventricles are out of sync. Left-ventricular filling time gets truncated and, with the concomitant loss of atrial kick, cardiac output naturally decreases.

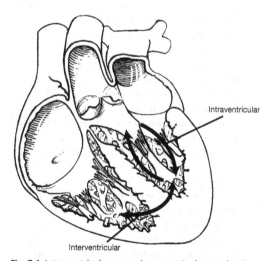

Fig. 7.1 Intraventricular versus interventricular conduction. Interventricular conduction refers to electrical conduction between right and left ventricles, while intraventricular conduction refers to conduction within a single ventricle (indicated here by two arrows forming a circle within the left ventricle).

Echo: Normal and Dilated Cardiomyopathy Patients

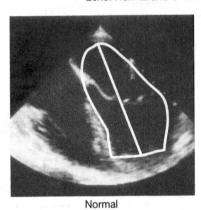
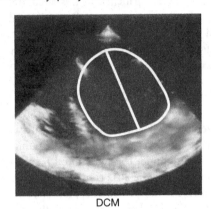

Normal   DCM

Fig. 7.3 Echocardiograms from a patient with a healthy heart and from a patient with dilated cardiomyopathy. An echocardiogram (left) shows a normal left ventricle. A corresponding echo (right) shows ventricles of a patient with dilated cardiomyopathy. When the echo is in motion, the right-side echo image will show disorganized wall motion, characteristic of ventricular dyssynchrony.

CRT is an electrical approach to helping restore synchrony to a failing heart with dyssynchrony. Since not all HF patients have ventricular dyssynchrony, CRT is not a universal treatment that will benefit every HF patient. Furthermore, the 'response' to CRT has been puzzling to clinicians. Some patients with dyssynchrony respond very well to CRT and derive great clinical benefit from this form of device therapy; others with dyssynchrony obtain minimal benefit. (More on CRT optimization and response is contained in Chapter 16.)

HF is a complex syndrome and there are many variables at work that can cause patients with dyssynchrony to have varying degrees of response to CRT. The two main factors considered to play the major role in CRT response are:
- Patient characteristics (type of HF, class)
- Pacing characteristics (sensed and paced AV delay settings, left-ventricular pacing site, interatrial delay, and so on).

Dyssynchrony is an intriguing aspect to HF that affects most patients, either in the electrical form (conduction disorders) or mechanical forms (contraction disorders) or both. In truth, electrical and mechanical dyssynchrony are closely related. CRT was designed to address dyssynchrony by providing an electrical therapy to help manage mechanical dyssynchrony.

References

1   Abraham W on behalf of the MIRACLE study group. Rationale and design of a randomized clinical trial to assess the safety and efficacy of cardiac resynchronization therapy in patients with advanced heart failure: the multicentre InSync Randomized Clinical Evaluation. *J Card Fail* 2000; **6**:369–80.

2   Murkofsky RL, Dangas G, Diamond JA *et al*. A prolonged QRS duration on surface electrocardiogram is a specific indicator of left ventricular dysfunction. *J Am Coll Cardiol* 1998; **32**:476.

3   Xiao C, Roy C, Fujimoto S *et al*. Natural history of abnormal conduction and its relation to prognosis in patients with dilated cardiomyopathy. *Int J Cardiol* 1996; **53**:163–70.

4   Shamim W, Francis D, Yousufuddin M *et al*. Intraventricular conduction delay: a prognostic marker in chronic heart failure. *Int J Cardiol* 1999; **70**:171–80.

5   Yu CM, Fung WH, Lin H *et al*. Predictors of left ventricular remodeling after cardiac resynchronization therapy for heart failure secondary to idiopathic or ischemic cardiomyopathy. *Am J Cardiol* 2003; **91**:684–8.

The nuts and bolts of ventricular dyssynchrony

- Ventricular dyssynchrony can be mechanical (pumping dysfunction) or electrical (conduction disorder) or both.
- Mechanical ventricular dyssynchrony can involve the right and left ventricle beating out-of-sync (interventricular conduction disorder) or the left ventricle not contracting as a unified whole (intraventricular conduction disorder).
- Electrical ventricular dyssynchrony involves a prolonged atrioventricular delay such that there is reduced atrial kick, prolonged diastole and, thus, reduced cardiac output.
- Electrical dyssynchrony is most commonly measured by a prolonged QRS duration (typically > 120 ms) on a surface ECG. Mechanical dyssynchrony is usually evaluated using an imaging technology, such as two-dimensional or three-dimensional echocardiography or, less commonly, a tagged magnetic resonance image.
- Current guidelines use a QRS duration > 120 ms as part of cardiac resynchronization therapy (CRT) device indications, even though CRT devices actually address mechanical dyssynchrony.
- Not all HF patients have ventricular dyssynchrony and patients may have varying degrees of electrical and/or mechanical dyssynchrony.
- When a HF patient has delayed left-ventricular activation, it is usually caused by left bundle branch block. This causes the right ventricle to contract slightly before the left ventricle. In contrast, the right and left ventricles of the healthy heart contract at exactly the same time.
- With intraventricular conduction delay, the left ventricle contracts in sections or waves, rather than as a whole. Typically, the lateral (outside) wall of the left ventricle contracts first, then relaxes as the septal (interior) wall contracts. The result is that much of the blood in the left ventricle sloshes back and forth rather than being pumped outward.
- All forms of ventricular dyssynchrony impair the heart's ability to pump and ultimately lead to reduced cardiac output.
- CRT is a form of electrical cardiac rhythm management that addresses ventricular dyssynchrony. It is appropriate only for those HF patients with ventricular dyssynchrony. Even among HF patients with ventricular dyssynchrony, there are varying degrees of 'response' to CRT that are still unexplained.

Chapter 8

Arrhythmias in Heart Failure Patients

The failing heart is a fertile ground for arrhythmias. Since heart failure (HF) is a complex syndrome of conditions, there may be multiple factors contributing to any given arrhythmia.

As clinicians, it is important to remember that patients with HF are at special risk of rhythm disorders. The three main types of arrhythmias prevalent in HF patients are potentially life-threatening ventricular tachyarrhythmias, bradyarrhythmias, and supraventricular tachyarrhythmias [in particular, atrial fibrillation (AF)]. This exposes HF patients to special risks and may complicate their treatment.

The mechanisms that create arrhythmias in HF patients vary widely and typically create three main types of rhythm disorders: the potentially life-threatening ventricular tachyarrhythmias we associate with sudden cardiac death (SCD), bradycardia, and supraventricular tachyarrhythmias, especially AF. As you might expect with a syndrome as complex as HF, multiple rhythm disorders may be at work in the same patient.

Factors associated with arrhythmogenesis in HF patients include mineral or chemical imbalances in the body, such as low levels of serum potassium (hypokalemia) or low levels of serum magnesium (hypomagnesemia). The increased amount of catecholamines circulating the body may also make a patient more susceptible to arrhythmic events. Patients who have survived a heart attack may have arrhythmic substrates around myocardial lesions.

Many drugs prescribed or recommended for HF may contribute to arrhythmogenesis. β-Blockers and digoxin, in particular, are associated with bradyarrhythmias. Since β blockade confers a clinically proven mortality benefit to HF patients, physicians may prescribe pacing support rather than discontinue the drug in the presence of symptomatic bradycardia. Antiarrhythmic agents, although not commonly prescribed to HF patients, are associated with some pro-arrhythmic risks, including an association of some agents with torsades-de-pointes ventricular tachycardia (Fig. 8.1).

The physical manifestations of HF also play a role in causing arrhythmias. For example, if a HF patient has dilated cardiomyopathy, the heart muscle has stretched to the point that it may shorten its period of refractoriness and set the stage for re-entry tachycardia. Increased sympathetic tone can encourage arrhythmic events. Many HF patients have conduction delay in the His-Purkinje system, which can en-

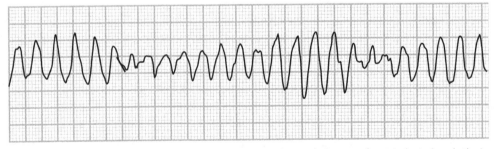

Fig. 8.1 Torsades-de-pointes. Torsades-de-pointes or 'twisting points' is a particular type of ventricular tachyarrhythmia that takes its name from its unusual appearance on the ECG. Torsades-de-pointes is associated with antiarrhythmic drugs. In fact, many antiarrhythmic agents have the curious side effect of being pro-arrhythmic. That is, while they may counteract certain rhythm disorders, they may actually set the stage for other types of arrhythmias to occur.

courage bradycardia events. Finally, patients with a dilated heart have an increase in endocardial surface area, which is believed to play a role in arrhythmogenesis.

Just as HF progresses to a physical form of ventricular remodeling, in which the heart's lower pumping chambers assume a new and distorted shape, there is also a form of electrical remodeling (or 're-wiring') involved in HF. The mechanisms behind electrical remodeling include changes at the cellular and even molecular level in response to chemical and ion-channel transformations during HF. The results of this electrical remodeling include new forms of impulse generation from the sinoatrial (SA) node or the heart's 'natural pacemaker'. The failing heart may experience sinus node dysfunction (leading to symptomatic bradycardia) or generation of ectopic beats. Fibrosis and changes in gap junctions between cardiac cells can lead to distorted impulse conduction, which can result in bradyarrhythmias or form re-entry circuits that can predispose the patient to tachycardia. As ventricular

repolarization changes with remodeling, the QT period extends, which may provoke a ventricular tachyarrhythmia. Changes in ventricular repolarization during electrical remodeling also affect the spatial dispersion of ventricular repolarization, contributing to intraventricular dyssynchrony.

In addition to the dilated or enlarged heart, the ventricular walls of the heart may sometimes thicken with progressive cardiac disease. This reduces the volume the ventricles can hold and can also affect electrical conduction and pumping action (see Fig. 8.2).

Ventricular tachyarrhythmias

The two main culprits in arrhythmias in HF patients remain abnormal impulse formation (ectopic beats, sinus node dysfunction and premature atrial or ventricular contractions) and re-entry. Re-entry is a mechanism at the root of the majority of tachyarrhythmias in all patients (not just HF patients). In re-entry, an impulse gets 'trapped' in an endless

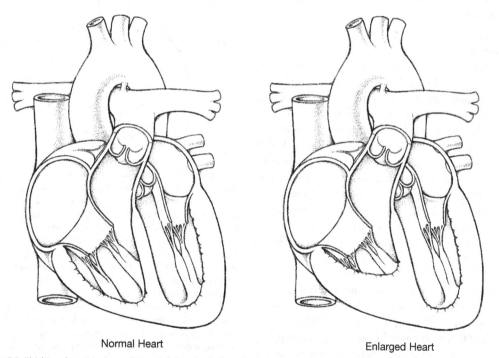

Normal Heart   Enlarged Heart

Fig. 8.2 Thickened ventricular wall. Heart failure can affect the heart's geometry in many different ways. Some patients develop an enlarged or dilated heart, which is rounded and flabby. In this example, the heart develops markedly thickened ventricular walls and maintains a more pointed shape. Any distortion of the physical form of the heart may also impact its ability to conduct electricity properly.

loop. It circulates around and around, causing the heart to try to depolarize and repolarize as fast as the impulse travels the loop.

Re-entry requires several preconditions. First, the patient must have a suitable re-entry pathway, which is a closed loop in which one side conducts electricity faster than the other side. Second, the patient must experience a triggering event, typically a premature ventricular contraction. If that out-of-sync event can enter the loop at the right time, the 'fast' and 'slow' legs of the loop can allow the impulse to travel around the loop, constantly meeting vulnerable rather than refractory tissue (see Fig. 8.3).

Not all patients are physically capable of supporting a re-entry tachycardia, in that not everyone has the substrate (or abnormal conduction pathway) to have such an event. However, myocardial lesions from a prior heart attack or other heart conditions may make such substrates more prevalent in some populations than in others. HF patients, who typically have sustained some degree of myocardial injury and are prone to aberrant impulse formation, are quite likely to experience re-entry-type tachyarrhythmias. This is particularly true since HF patients may experience slowed conduction in some areas of the heart, which helps facilitate the re-entry loop.

Before Holter monitoring became common practice, it was believed that SCD or cardiac arrest was a relatively rare phenomenon. Today, we recognize that SCD is a major killer. It is estimated that 50–60% of all patients with dilated cardiomyopathy experience ventricular tachyarrhythmia and about half of all congestive HF patients die suddenly.[1] Among patients with hypertrophic cardiomyopathy, 90% have been shown to experience some form of ventricular arrhythmic events and 20–30% have episodes of non-sustained ventricular tachycardia.[2]

In New York Heart Association (NYHA) Class II or III, SCD is the main cause of death, i.e. it causes more death than pump failure or other causes. However, it is important to remember that the incidence of SCD increases with NYHA class, although in NYHA IV so many more patients die of pump failure that it obscures the fact that all HF patients are at risk of SCD and that risk increases as HF progresses (see Fig. 8.4).

While HF patients are at increased risk of potentially deadly ventricular tachyarrhythmias, ven-

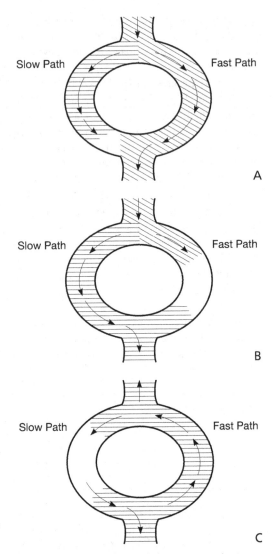

Fig. 8.3 Re-entry diagram. Re-entry requires a conduction pathway that splits into two paths, one of which must conduct electricity faster than the other. When electrical energy enters the 'loop', some of it travels down the fast path, some travels down the slow path. The fast path becomes refractory first (white patch), meaning that electricity traveling down the fast path now hits a 'dead end' in the form of refractory tissue that cannot be stimulated (B). Meanwhile, electrical energy is still traveling down the slow path. The slow path now becomes refractory (white patch) (C). Electrical energy from the slow path that now reaches the bottom of the loop finds that tissue on the fast path is now vulnerable and capable of being stimulated. This means that some of that energy may travel upward along the fast path! This starts the 'endless loop' of energy which enters the circular pathway and then cycles faster and faster around the loop. This electrical energy tries to depolarize the cardiac tissue at increasingly faster rates.

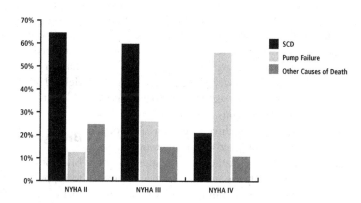

Fig. 8.4 Deaths by New York Heart Association (NYHA) Heart Classification. While more people with advanced NYHA Class IV heart failure (HF) die of pump failure than of sudden cardiac death (SCD), SCD actually increases with advancing HF. While the risk of SCD is eclipsed by the rapidly increasing risk of death by pump failure, the incidence of SCD increases with worsening HF. However, more Class IV patients die of pump failure than any other cause. (Source: Merit-HF Study.)

tricular tachyarrhythmias affect a much broader patient population. Implantable cardioverter-defibrillators (ICDs) have proven effective at helping rescue patients from potentially lethal ventricular tachyarrhythmias, including ventricular fibrillation (VF) (Fig. 8.5). However, even in the context of HF, it is important to understand the difference between what have come to be called secondary-prevention patients and primary-prevention patients.

The secondary-prevention patient is a person who has the good fortune to have either been rescued from a life-threatening ventricular tachyarrhythmic episode or meets standard criteria (specific types of documented ventricular arrhythmic activity), while the primary-prevention patient is one who is deemed to be at high risk of SCD, but who has not experienced any such event to date. In fact, a primary-prevention patient may have no demonstrated clinical evidence of any arrhythmic activity at all.

The distinction between primary-prevention and secondary-prevention patient underscores our growing understanding of the value of implantable defibrillation capability in an expanding patient population. Among HF patients, there are both primary-prevention and secondary-prevention ICD candidates.

Three large randomized clinical trials have demonstrated that HF patients with sustained ventricular tachycardia (VT) (i.e. secondary-prevention patients) have received mortality benefits from ICDs. The AVID,[3] CIDS[4] and CASH[5] studies indicate that an ICD may reduce mortality by as much as 30% in certain HF patients.

Ischemic HF patients (those with coronary artery disease and possibly a history of myocardial infarction) were found to derive significant mortality benefits from ICD therapy. The MADIT[6] and MUSTT[7] studies found that ischemic HF patients with a left-ventricular ejection fraction (LVEF)

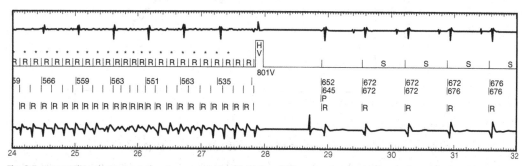

Fig. 8.5 Intracardiac electrogram showing ventricular fibrillation (VF) and rescue shock. The tracing at the bottom left-hand side shows a patient experiencing VF. The strip annotates these rapid, sensed ventricular events with the letter R. When the arrhythmia is diagnosed, the device delivers high-voltage therapy (seen as HV) and, after a pause, a normal sinus rhythm is restored (S notations).

of ≤40% derived a 50% reduced risk of mortality with an ICD. The mortality benefit in the MADIT II study was 30% less in the ICD group compared with the conventional therapy group[8] (Fig. 8.6).

By far the largest primary-prevention ICD trial to date is the SCD-HeFT trial,[9] which enrolled NYHA Class II and III HF patients with an LVEF ≤ 35%. Patients were divided into three groups: an ICD group, an amiodarone group and a control group. All patients received state-of-the-art drug therapy for HF at baseline. Only the amiodarone arm received amiodarone. The study found that basic shock-only ICDs reduced mortality in these patients by 23% (Fig. 8.7). Surprisingly to some, amiodarone did not confer a mortality benefit. In fact, the amiodarone and placebo groups did about the same.

Since amiodarone is frequently prescribed to HF patients in the hopes of managing arrhythmias, the SCD-HeFT trial surprised many clinicians. However, it is important to remember why amiodarone would be prescribed in this setting. Amiodarone reduces the overall number of ambient tachyarrhythmias. This means that an ICD patient taking amiodarone might well experience fewer episodes of VT and be spared some shocks. However, amiodarone cannot prevent every single arrhythmia and it can-

not rescue a patient once an arrhythmia occurred. Thus, the finding that amiodarone does not significantly reduce mortality in HF patients is really not that surprising, nor does it diminish amiodarone's rightful role in overall rhythm management even in ICD patients.

Bradyarrhythmias

Bradycardia is characterized by heart rates too slow to support the patient's metabolic needs. Symptomatic bradycardias can be roughly grouped into two broad categories: sinus node dysfunction and atrioventricular (AV) block. Sinus node dysfunction, sometimes nicknamed sick sinus syndrome, occurs when the SA node or the heart's natural pacemaker is unable to generate stimulating pulses at an adequate or appropriate rate. The heart's conduction system may be intact, but the heart's signals to beat are too slow (Fig. 8.8). Chronotropic incompetence, the inability of the heart to alter rate in response to exertion or stress, is typical in sinus node dysfunction. Although hard statistics are difficult to find, most pacemaker experts would guess that about half of all pacemaker patients have sinus node dysfunction.

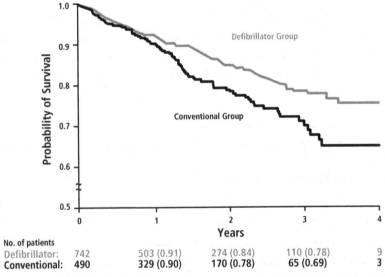

No. of patients				
Defibrillator:	742	503 (0.91)	274 (0.84)	110 (0.78)	9
Conventional:	490	329 (0.90)	170 (0.78)	65 (0.69)	3

Fig. 8.6 Mortality graph from MADIT II. The MADIT II study found that prophylactic implantable cardioverter-defibrillators reduced the risk of death in patients with low ejection fractions even if they had no prior evidence of a ventricular tachyarrhythmia.

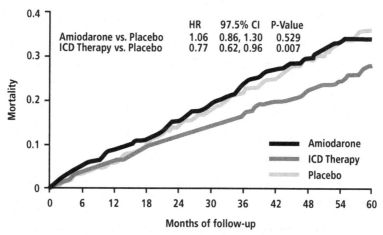

Fig. 8.7 Mortality graph (3 lines) for SCD-HeFT. SCD-HeFT randomized New York Heart Association Class II and III patients with a low ejection fraction into three groups. The placebo group received basic cardiac drug therapy for heart failure (HF). A second group received those drugs plus amiodarone, an antiarrhythmic. The third group took standard HF drugs but with no amiodarone and they were implanted with an implantable cardioverter-defibrillator (ICD). SCD-HeFT found that ICDs reduced mortality but amiodarone did about as well as a placebo in reducing the risk of death in these patients. Note that, like MADIT II patients, the SCD-HeFT patients did not have prior documented evidence of ventricular tachyarrhythmias.

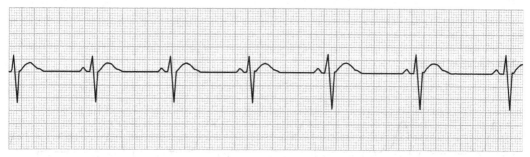

Fig. 8.8. ECG of sinus bradycardia. This ECG shows a textbook example of sinus bradycardia. There are clear atrial and ventricular complexes and 1:1 atrioventricular synchrony (i.e. one atrial beat for each ventricular beat) but the beats fire too slowly. Bradycardia can cause symptoms that range from mild to debilitating. Conventional pacemakers were first designed to address symptomatic bradycardias.

The other half of pacemaker patients has a form of AV block, also called heart block. In this syndrome, the SA node fires stimulating pulses at the right rate but as the electricity conducts over the atria and through the AV node on its way to the ventricles, it is blocked at the AV node. Actually, the term AV 'block' is something of a misnomer, since AV block also occurs when the electrical energy is delayed (not stopped, just slowed down) at the AV node. There are varying degrees of AV block, with the most severe (third-degree AV block or complete heart block) a complete dissociation of atria and ventricles. For these patients, the AV node does in-

deed 'block' all electrical signals from the atria. As a result, the atria have their own rhythm and the ventricles beat at a slower escape rate (Fig. 8.9).

Bradycardia, particularly more advanced forms, usually brings with it a variety of unpleasant and even debilitating symptoms, including fatigue, light-headedness, dizziness, even fainting. People with bradycardia have limited physical endurance and may find themselves prevented from going about their ordinary daily activities.

HF patients may present with concurrent bradycardia (it is not unusual for cardiac patients to have multiple disorders of the heart) or they may develop

Second-degree Type I AV block

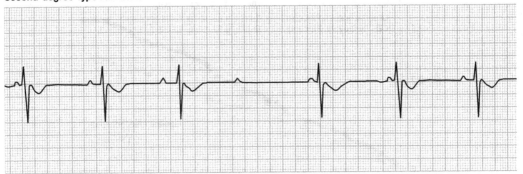

Second-degree Type II AV block

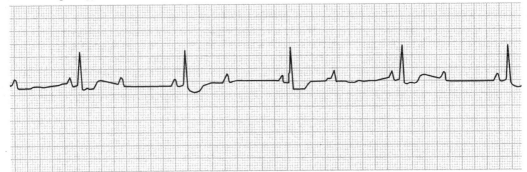

Third-degree AV block

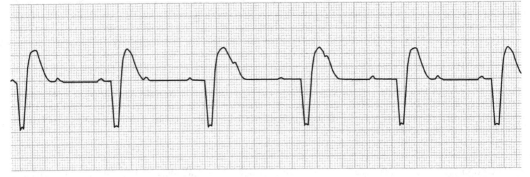

Fig. 8.9 Some types of atrioventricular (AV) block. AV block occurs when the impulse from the atrium gets delayed or perhaps blocked altogether in the AV node and thus does not reach the ventricle at the appropriate time. There are three degrees of AV block, and two types of second-degree AV block. First-degree AV block is relatively mild and may be asymptomatic. In this illustration, the first tracing shows second-degree Type I AV block, which shows a progressively lengthening PR segment until the point that a P-wave appears without an associated QRS complex. Second-degree Type I AV block is also known as Mobitz I or Wenckebach. The second tracing shows second-degree Type II AV block (also known as Mobitz II), which has relatively stable PR intervals, a wider QRS complex and dropped QRS complexes. The bottom tracing is third-degree AV block, the most severe form. In this example, no signals from the atrium conduct to the ventricles, resulting in a complete dissociation of atria and ventricles.

it with disease progression or drug interactions. In particular, β-blockers and digoxin, two drugs commonly taken by HF patients, are associated with bradycardia.

Should a HF patient develop symptomatic bradycardia as a result of β-blockade, the physician may opt to use an implantable device with pacing support to maintain an appropriate rate without having to discontinue the drug. Since β-blockers in particular are associated with a clinically and statistically significant mortality benefit for HF patients, they should be continued if at all possible.

As regards conventional right-ventricular pacing, the DAVID study found that rate-modulated dual-chamber (DDDR) pacing at 70 pulses/min in patients with a standard ICD indication, an LVEF of ≤40%, and no pacing indication resulted in an increase in the combined endpoint of hospitalization for congestive heart failure (CHF) or all-cause mortality.[10] DAVID is a complex study, but it is worth discussing here since it has definitely changed how many clinicians approach conventional pacing therapy in HF patients.

The DAVID study included only patients with a standard ICD indication and without a standard pacing indication. Thus, it is important to remember that a patient with a standard pacing indication (such as symptomatic bradycardia) is not the population that DAVID studied. All DAVID patients had some degree of systolic dysfunction, evidenced by the entrance requirement of an LVEF ≤ 40%. A total of 506 patients were randomized into two groups and each received a dual-chamber conventional ICD. In one group, the ICDs were programmed to VVI backup pacing at 40 pulses/min. In the other group, the ICDs were programmed to DDDR pacing at 70 pulses/min. The study's primary endpoint was all-cause mortality (i.e. death for any reason at all) or hospitalization for congestive heart failure. The primary endpoint was a composite, which means that if a patient met either criterion (death or CHF hospitalization), the endpoint was counted as satisfied. Patients were followed for a mean period of about 8 months (Fig. 8.10).

DAVID is sometimes erroneously described as a study that compared pacing modes (VVI to DDDR) or an ICD study (it did use ICDs, but the study evaluated response to pacing). In actual fact, it compared VVI backup pacing at 40 pulses/min with DDDR pacing at 70 pulses/min. Since no patients actually had a standard pacing indication, these two programming choices meant that the VVI backup group was rarely paced (even at 12 months, the VVI backup group was paced less than 3% of the time), while the DDDR group at 70 pulses/min was frequently paced (over 50% of the time, even at 3 months and up to 61% of the time at 12 months).[11]

Thus, it might be useful to think of the DAVID trial as a study which compared pacing with non-pacing in patients not indicated for pacing in the first place.

There are also other aspects to consider. DAVID compared base rates; the DDDR base rate of 70 pulses/min is quite high, much higher than the base rates of 50 or 60 pulses/min that are usually programmed. In addition, the VVI backup group experienced a natural PR interval, i.e. a natural atrial contraction which conducted to the ventricle and caused a ventricular contraction. The DDDR group, on the other hand, experienced the artificial AV interval caused by pacing.

Regardless of the exact mechanisms, the study found that 26.7% of the DDDR 70 pulses/min group met the composite endpoint (death or CHF hospitalization) at 1 year, versus just 16.1% of the VVI backup group. This difference was significant, but when the two facets of the composite endpoint were separated, the DDDR 70 pulses/min group showed worse scores but the differences did not reach statistical significance (see Table 8.1).

All patients in the DAVID study received a dual-chamber ICD which was then programmed to pace according to the protocol, either VVI 40 pulses/min or DDDR 70 pulses/min. The ICDs were conventional devices, which paced using a right-ventricular (RV) standard pacing lead positioned at or near the RV apex. It appeared that this type of pacing—at least in patients not indicated for pacing—exacerbates LV dysfunction in patients with some degree of LV impairment. In other words, RV pacing seems to make LV dysfunction worse, at least in some patients.

Although this was surprising to the clinical community, there had been some hints that perhaps RV pacing was not ideal for patients with LV dysfunction. In the MADIT II trial, for example, a subgroup analysis suggested that while ICDs and pacing conferred a mortality benefit on heart attack survivors with an LVEF ≤ 30%, it appeared to increase HF hospitalizations.[12] It was easy to be sceptical about that suggestion, in that a substudy, by definition, is on a topic that the clinical trial never set out to study. It is an incidental by-product of the study and cannot withstand serious scrutiny. At most, a subgroup analysis can indicate where clinicians need to do further research.

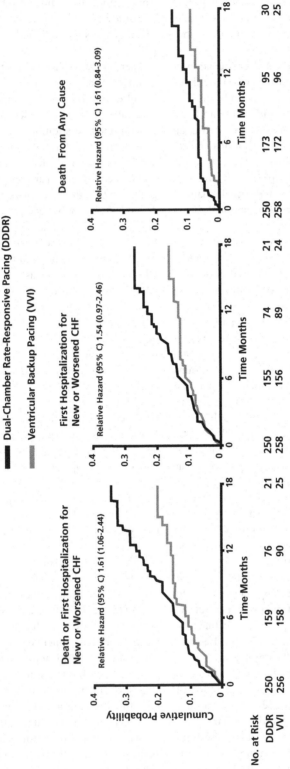

Fig. 8.10 End-points from the DAVID trial. In the DAVID trial, implantable cardioverter-defibrillator patients without a standard pacing indication were randomized into two groups: one received VVI backup pacing at a very low rate (very infrequently paced), while the other group received rate modulated dual-chamber (DDDR) pacing at 70 pulses/min (frequently paced). The DDDR-70 group had a worse outcome than the VVI-backup group, leading some to speculate that conventional right-ventricular pacing can exacerbate heart failure.

Table 8.1 DAVID event rates by arm

One-year event rate	Combined	CHF hospitalization	Death
VVI-backup 40 pulses/min	16.1%	13.3%	6.5%
DDDR-70 pulses/min	26.7%	22.6%	10.1%
P-value	0.03	0.07	0.15

The composite or combined primary end-point [all-cause mortality or hospitalization for congestive heart failure (CHF)] showed a statistically significant difference by study arm, favoring the VVI-40 backup group. While the left-ventricular ejection fraction DDDR-70 group had higher rates of CHF hospitalization and death (taken independently), these differences did not reach statistical significance. Source: The DAVID Trial Investigators. JAMA 2002; 288:3115–23.

However, the MADIT II substudy findings resonated with some clinicians, who were sharing anecdotal reports of the very same thing. Standard RV pacing appeared to worsen LV dysfunction in patients with compromised LV function.

The possible mechanisms behind this are not difficult to understand. When a patient has impaired LV function (evidenced by a low ejection fraction percentage), it indicates that the LV is not able to pump as efficiently as it should. The root of the problem may be structural heart damage, myocardial dysfunction (such as cardiomyopathy), electrical or mechanical dyssynchrony or, most likely, some combination of these conditions.

RV pacing induces what might be called 'artificial left bundle branch block' by stimulating the right ventricle and allowing the electrical energy to radiate across to the left ventricle. This contradicts the normal conduction pathway of the healthy heart, where the electrical energy flows downward from the atria over the AV node and proceeds simultaneously to the right and left ventricles (Fig. 8.11). The RV lead paces the right ventricle first, causing it to contract slightly in advance of the left ventricle. This induces what might be considered a mild form of ventricular dyssynchrony. Although this is conjecture, it appears that patients with good systolic function are able to tolerate this relatively well. Patients with standard bradycardia pacing indications and good systolic function have received RV pacing therapy with good results. There are many long years of positive results in such patients.

Patients with compromised LV function, however, seem at risk during RV pacing for worsening LV function. Another clinical study for a very unusual clinical population may have shed further light on this topic. In late 2005, the PAVE study evaluated the use of biventricular versus RV pacing in patients scheduled to undergo an AV nodal ablation for the management of AF.[13] Since an AV nodal ablation essentially severs the electrical connection between atria and ventricles, it is standard procedure to implant a permanent pacemaker in such patients. These so-called 'ablate-and-pace' patients typically receive single-chamber conventional pacemakers. Although patients who undergo AV nodal ablation for AF are not a large group, the ablate-and-pace procedure has been around for many years and met with overall good results.

PAVE studied 184 of these ablate-and-pace patients and randomized them into two groups: one group received a conventional (RV) pacemaker and the other a biventricular (BV) pacemaker. In this case, the biventricular pacemaker was a low-voltage pulse generator (pacemaker) with three leads. One lead paced the atrium, one lead was placed in the right ventricle and the third lead was placed in the coronary sinus to stimulate the left ventricle. The RV and LV leads paced together (BV pacing), causing the right ventricle and left ventricle to contract together.

PAVE used a functional measurement for its primary endpoint: the distance patients could cover in the 6-min hallway walk test. As secondary endpoints, quality-of-life questionnaire scores were compared and LVEF scores were measured. PAVE did not use mortality as an endpoint. The BV patients did significantly better in the hallway walk

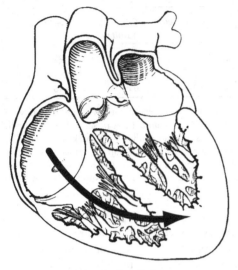
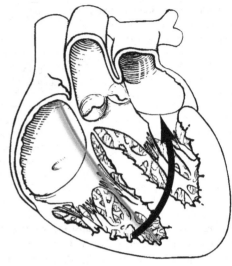

Normal Conduction Pathway   Paced Conduction Pathway

Fig. 8.11 Normal and paced conduction pathways. In the healthy heart, the electrical impulse originates in the high right atrium (sinoatrial or SA node) and then travels outward and downward. A conventionally paced heart has a ventricular lead placed at or near the right ventricular apex. Ventricular conduction then proceeds from the apex upward and outward. This abnormal conduction pathway is thought to contribute to ventricular dyssynchrony in those with some degree of systolic dysfunction to begin with.

test and LVEF scores compared with RV patients, but there was no significant difference in quality-of-life scores. Remarkably, when PAVE data were stratified by LVEF scores, it was found that patients in the BV group who had an LVEF ≤45% showed a significant 73% improvement in the hallway walk test compared with RV patients. Further, when data were stratified by NYHA class, Class II or III patients in the BV group showed a significant 53% improvement in the distance covered in the hallway walk test compared with the RV patients (Fig. 8.12). The stratified results suggest that patients with impaired systolic function (in this case, determined by a low LVEF score or a high NYHA classification) derive greater benefit from BV pacing compared with RV pacing than patients with more normal systolic function. One could turn that statement around and also say that PAVE strongly suggests that RV pacing is worse than BV pacing for patients with LV dysfunction.

Further analysis of the PAVE data also suggests something interesting. The differences in results for the BV pacing group versus the RV pacing group were not due to the fact that the BV pacing group did better. When data were observed closely, the BV

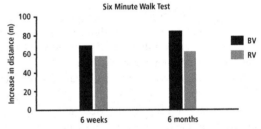

Fig. 8.12 PAVE 6-min walk test. The PAVE trial had functional end-points rather than morbidity and mortality. At the end of 6 months, post-AV-nodal-ablation patients who received a BV (CRT) device covered significantly more distance in the 6-min walk test and had higher left-ventricular ejection fraction scores than patients who received a conventional pacemaker. Note that in the walk test, all patients (BV and RV) improved, but the BV patients improved more.

group was able to maintain much of its functional status over time, while the RV group's status deteriorated. For example, the mean LVEF scores were assessed in both groups. In 6 months, the LVEF scores for the BV patients remained steady at around 46%. However, the LVEF scores for the RV patients decreased by 3.1% in the first 6 weeks and by a total of 3.7% over 6 months. Thus, PAVE suggests that it is

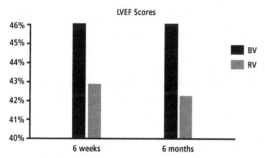

Fig. 8.13 PAVE left-ventricular ejection fraction (LVEF) scores. The PAVE study found that post-AV-nodal-ablation patients who received a BV (CRT) device had significantly better LVEF scores at 6 months compared with those who got a conventional (RV) pacemaker. Note that BV patients maintained their LVEF scores over 6 months, while RV patients' scores deteriorated.

not so much that BV pacing makes patients better, it is just that RV pacing appears to make them worse! (Fig. 8.13).

The PAVE study evaluated only ablate-and-pace patients with chronic AF. The PAVE study had no entrance requirements relating to LVEF score, QRS duration or NYHA classification. (At baseline, the mean LVEF scores were around 46% and roughly half of the patients could be classified as NYHA Class II.) However, such patients have a similar pathology to patients with severe AV nodal or infranodal conduction disorders. Thus, the PAVE study is another piece of the puzzle that suggests RV pacing should be used only with very careful consideration, if at all, in the HF population.

For that reason, cardiac resynchronization therapy (CRT) systems (which are similar to the so-called BV devices used in the PAVE trial) offer an excellent alternative approach to HF patients who need pacing support.

Supraventricular tachycardia

The adjective before tachycardia describes the place in which the tachycardia originates, not necessarily the chamber(s) affected. For example, AF is fibrillation originating in the atria, but which usually involves a characteristic rapid and erratic ventricular response (to which most symptoms can be attributed). Supraventricular tachycardia is a general term for any and all tachyarrhythmias that originate

above the ventricles. For HF patients, this usually means AF, a common comorbidity with HF.

AF and HF form a vicious circle, with one worsening the other. Both AF and HF are progressive and complex disorders.

A patient with HF is susceptible to arrhythmias, including re-entry-type tachyarrhythmias, which can originate in the atria as well as the ventricles. Rapidly beating atria cause the ventricles to beat too quickly, which can lead long term to tachycardia-induced cardiomyopathy and reduced cardiac output. The reduced cardiac output can set off the cascade of compensatory mechanisms which lead to HF.

AF is associated with an increased risk of stroke because blood that pools in the fibrillating atria may clump together to form a clot that may enter the blood stream and lodge in the brain. Patients with AF may suffer from a range of symptoms, from very mild to debilitating. Further, AF is a progressive disorder that ranges from paroxysmal (sudden onset, spontaneous resolution) to persistent (longer lasting, requires medical intervention to resolve) to permanent (refractory to treatment) or chronic (Fig. 8.14).

AF in a HF patient creates a troublesome clinical situation, in that the AF exacerbates the HF and may not be responsive to any treatment. Patients without HF may be given anti-arrhythmic agents to manage AF, but such drugs are generally not used in HF patients because of their negative inotropic qualities and the risk of pro-arrhythmia. Although amiodarone is not cleared by the Food and Drug Administration in the USA for the treatment of supraventricular tachycardia, it is used in other countries in that way and is often given off-label in the USA for that purpose.

AF is a progressive disorder and moves from paroxysmal AF at the outset to persistent and finally to permanent. Paroxysmal AF is, as the name suggests, of sudden onset and usually terminates spontaneously. Patients with paroxysmal AF may be asymptomatic and even unaware there is any rhythm disorder; when symptoms do occur, they can be mild. Paroxysmal AF may be characterized by very brief episodes and no medical intervention is required to resolve the arrhythmia. In fact, even if paroxysmal AF is diagnosed (it often goes undetected), it is tempting to consider it a benign sort of condition.

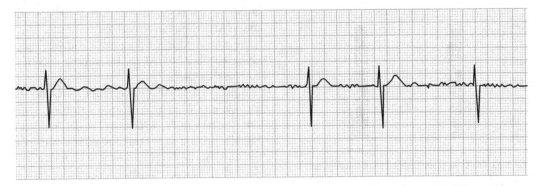

Fig. 8.14 Atrial fibrillation (AF) on ECG. AF is a common and difficult arrhythmia which manifests on the ECG as rapid, seemingly chaotic atrial activity that may or may not involve a rapid, erratic ventricular response.

Specialists in rhythm disorders have a saying about AF: 'AF begets AF'. It gets worse. Paroxysmal AF progresses to persistent AF. In this stage, episodes are of longer duration and some form of medical intervention (chemical or electrical cardioversion, typically) is required to resolve the arrhythmia. Patients start to report symptoms. Persistent AF is treatable, but troublesome.

Interestingly, most of the symptoms associated with AF are not related directly to the high atrial rate but to the abnormally high ventricular rate that AF induces. As the atria beat faster and faster, a heart with normal (or even somewhat normal) conduction capability conducts those fast atrial beats down to the ventricle. The result is that the ventricles beat faster and faster, trying to keep up with the atria. While this rapid ventricular response is not techni-

cally a VT, it may look like VT if you see the ventricular tracing and it certainly feels like VT to the person experiencing it! (Fig. 8.15).

The condition progresses from persistent AF to permanent AF, also known as chronic AF. As the name suggests, permanent AF does not respond to medical intervention at all; it is drug and treatment refractory. It does not go away.

While rapid ventricular response to AF is an important consequence of AF to manage, it must be remembered that a rapid atrial rate can only drive the ventricles up to a certain speed. After ventricular depolarization and contraction, the ventricular myocardial tissue becomes refractory. Further atrial impulses during that refractory period will not cause the ventricles to depolarize and contract. The result is that a patient with AF has a much higher

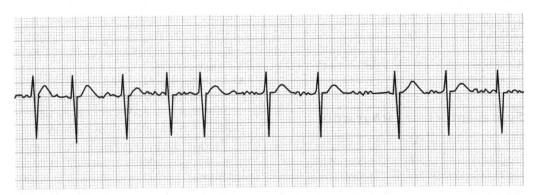

Fig. 8.15 Atrial fibrillation (AF) with rapid ventricular response. This patient probably has some symptoms associated with rapid ventricular activity. However, the rhythm disorder is not truly ventricular in origin, although it may provoke the same symptoms as a ventricular tachyarrhythmia. This is a supraventricular tachycardia, specifically AF (note the rapid atrial beats) with a rapid ventricular response. As is typical with this fairly common rhythm disorder, the ventricular response is erratic.

atrial rate than a ventricular rate, although both rates are above normal.

While AF may well be the most common rhythm disorder in the world, there is a great deal about the condition that is not understood. What is clear is that AF is a progressive, complicated condition and responds to a variety of different therapeutic options. Specialists in this area tend to group their approach to AF into two different camps known as 'rate control' and 'rhythm control'.

Rate control aims to treat AF by controlling the rate of the ventricles and essentially not worrying about the rate of the atria. Probably the best example of a pure 'rate control' approach to AF management is AV-nodal ablation or some other form of atrial ablation. If the source or focus of the AF can be identified (and in patients with AV-nodal re-entry tachycardia, this is more clear-cut than in other types of AF patients) and excised using radiofrequency (RF) ablation, the physician essentially destroys the electrical connection between atria and ventricles. Electrically speaking, atria are fully dissociated from ventricles. The patient remains in permanent AF, but the atrial rate has no way of influencing the ventricular rate. Many patients who get this procedure require permanent pacing (and the PAVE study demonstrated that CRT confers more benefits to these patients than conventional RV pacing,[13] which was once the standard of care) because the ventricles must now beat on their own and the natural ventricular rate (also called the ectopic rate) is often too slow to support most activities.

Other 'rate control' approaches include drugs that do nothing to resolve the AF as a rhythm disorder but can slow the overall heart rate. Rate control is essentially what pacemakers do when they mode switch: when the pacemaker detects a high atrial rate, it switches off atrial tracking so that the atrial rate no longer influences the ventricular paced rate.

The other approach to AF is 'rhythm control', which tries to return the heart to normal sinus rhythm, which, in turn, would resolve the rapid ventricular response. In its early stages and in certain patients, rhythm control with pharmacological therapy may be a desirable strategy. However, not all AF patients respond to rhythm control and AF can progress to the point that rhythm control is no longer viable.

References

1 Galvin JM, Ruskin JN. Ventricular tachycardia in patients with dilated cardiomyopathy. In: Cardiac Electrophysiology from Cell to Bedside. Zipes DP, Jalife J, eds. Philadelphia: Saunders 2004:578.

2 Maron BJ. Ventricular arrhythmias in hypertrophic cardiomyopathy. In: Cardiac Electrophysiology from Cell to Bedside. Zipes DP, Jalife J, eds. Philadelphia: Saunders 2004:601.

3 Domanski MJ, Saksena S, Epstein AE *et al.* Relative effectiveness of the implantable cardioverter-defibrillator and antiarrhythmic drugs in patients with varying degrees of left ventricular dysfunction who have survived malignant ventricular arrhythmias: AVID Investigators—Antiarrhythmics versus Implantable Defibrillators. *J Am Coll Cardiol* 1999; **34**:1090–5.

4 Sheldon R, Connolly S, Krahn A *et al.* Identification of patients most likely to benefit from implantable cardioverter-defibrillator therapy: the Canadian Implantable Defibrillator Study. *Circulation* 2000; **101**:1660–4.

5 Kuck KH, Cappato R, Siebels J, Ruppel R. Randomized comparison of antiarrhythmic drug therapy with implantable defibrillators in patients resuscitated from cardiac rest: The Cardiac Arrest Study Hamburg (CASH) *Circulation* 2000; **102**:748–54.

6 Moss A, Hall W, Cannom D *et al.* Improved survival with an implanted defibrillator in patients with coronary artery disease at high risk for ventricular arrhythmia: Multicenter Automatic Defibrillator Implantation Trial Investigators. *N Engl J Med* 1996; **335**:1933–40.

7 Buxton AE, Lee K, Fisher JD *et al.* A randomized study of the prevention of sudden death in patients with coronary artery disease: Multicenter Unsustained Tachycardia Trial Investigators. *N Engl J Med* 1999; **341**:1882–90.

8 Moss AJ, Zareba W, Hall WJ *et al.* Multicenter Automatic Defibrillator Implantation Trial II Investigators: Prophylactic implantation of a defibrillator in patients with myocardial infarction and reduced ejection fraction. *N Engl J Med* 2002; **346**:877–83.

9 Bardy GH, Lee KL, Mark DB *et al.* Amiodarone or an implantable cardioverter-defibrillator for congestive heart failure. *N Engl J Med* 2005; **352**:225–37.

10 The DAVID trial investigators. Dual-chamber pacing or ventricular backup pacing in patients with an implantable defibrillator. *JAMA* 2002; **288**:3115–23.

11 Wilkoff BL and the DAVID Trial Investigators. The dual chamber and VVI implantable defibrillator (DAVID) trial: rationale, design, results, clinical implications and lessons for future trials. *Card Electrophysiol R* 2003; **7**:468–72.

12 Moss AJ, Wojciech Z, Hall WJ *et al.* Prophylactic implantation of a defibrillator in patients with myocardial infarction and reduced ejection fraction. *N Engl J Med* 2002; **12**:877–83.

13 Doshi RN, Daoud EG, Fellows C *et al.* Left ventricular-based cardiac stimulation post AV nodal ablation evaluation (the PAVE study). *J Cardiovasc Electrophysiol* 2005; **16**:1160–5.

The nuts and bolts of arrhythmias in heart failure patients

- Heart failure (HF) patients are susceptible to many different types of rhythm disorders and many of them will present with multiple arrhythmias. The three main types of rhythm disorders in HF patients are bradyarrhythmias, potentially life-threatening ventricular tachyarrhythmias and supraventricular tachyarrhythmias.
- The main form of supraventricular tachyarrhythmia that afflicts HF patients is atrial fibrillation (AF), which may be the most common rhythm disorder in the world. It complicates HF management and exacerbates the condition.
- Rhythm disorders in HF patients may be caused by mineral imbalances (hypokalemia, hypomagnesemia), increased catecholamines and damage to the myocardium (e.g. lesions from a prior infarction). A damaged heart muscle (from dilated or hypertrophic cardiomyopathy) may have shortened its period of refractoriness and be prone to re-entry tachycardia.
- HF patients not only experience a physical ventricular remodeling, electrical remodeling may also occur at the cellular level, resulting in sinus node dysfunction and generation of ectopic beats, such as premature ventricular contractions. The QT period may extend as a result of this electrical remodeling, which can provoke certain types of ventricular tachycardias.
- Many HF drugs affect the patient's heart rhythm. Digoxin and β-blockers are associated with bradyarrhythmias. Many antiarrhythmic agents have established pro-arrhythmic side effects.
- Sudden cardiac death (SCD), typically from a severe ventricular tachyarrhythmia including ventricular fibrillation, is prevalent in HF patients. The worse the HF according to the New York Heart Association (NYHA) scale, the more SCD cases occur. However, SCD is disproportionately high in the lower NYHA classes (Class II, in particular), since fewer Class II patients die of pump failure. However, SCD is a major cause of death and serious risk for all HF patients.
- Ninety percent (90%) of hypertrophic cardiomyopathy patients experience some form of ventricular arrhythmic events and about 50–60% of patients with dilated cardiomyopathy have ventricular tachycardia.
- ICDs (implantable defibrillators) offer a rescue function: they can defibrillate a heart in a life-threatening ventricular tachyarrhythmia. As such, ICDs have been shown to reduce mortality in certain types of HF patients. The largest and best known of these clinical trials is the SCD-HeFT trial, which found ICDs significantly reduced mortality in HF patients compared with drug therapy alone or compared with drug therapy plus amiodarone.
- SCD-HeFT was a good example of a 'primary-prevention trial'. Primary-prevention patients are those who receive a device although they have not yet experienced a potentially life-threatening ventricular tachyarrhythmia. They can be compared with secondary-prevention patients, who receive a device in response to documented evidence of such a ventricular tachycardia. There has been a great deal of investigation recently in primary-prevention patients, including HF patients.
- Many HF patients have bradyarrhythmias and require pacing support. Conventional pacemakers pace in the right-ventricular (RV) apex. There is growing evidence and much awareness among pacing experts that conventional RV pacing can make HF worse. Although the DAVID study is very complex,

Continued.

Continued.

it is frequently cited in this context. However, DAVID studied ICD patients who were not indicated for permanent pacing; it is unknown how conventional pacing affects HF patients with standard pacing indications. Unnecessary RV pacing appears to exacerbate LV dysfunction.

- RV pacing induces what might be called 'artificial left bundle branch block' (LBBB) by stimulating the right ventricle slightly ahead of the left ventricle and changing the normal conduction pathways. It has been suggested that patients with normal ventricular function tolerate this artificial LBBB well enough, but those with left-ventricular dysfunction do not.
- The PAVE study evaluated 'ablate-and-pace' patients who received an AV nodal ablation for the management of chronic AF. While PAVE did not use mortality as an end-point, patients who received cardiac resynchronization therapy (CRT) devices post-ablation had significantly improved functional scores over those who received conventional RV pacemakers. Conventional RV pacemakers were once the standard of care for 'ablate-and-pace' patients. Today, CRT devices are indicated for this condition.
- A supraventricular tachycardia (SVT) is any tachycardia that originates above the ventricles. The main one of interest in HF patients is AF. AF and HF are co-morbidities; they form a vicious circle where one makes the other worse. Patients with either AF or HF tend to develop the other over time.
- Rhythm disorders are named for the chamber or location in which they originate. Thus, a supraventricular tachycardia may produce a rapid ventricular rate, but it differs from a ventricular tachycardia in that the origin is supraventricular (literally: above the ventricles), whereas a ventricular tachycardia originates in the ventricles. Many atrial tachyarrhythmias provoke a rapid ventricular response, which often causes more symptoms than the rapid atrial rate.
- AF is a progressive disorder that moves from paroxysmal AF (sudden onset, spontaneous termination, minimal or no symptoms) to persistent AF (longer duration, typically symptomatic, requires medical intervention) to permanent or chronic AF (no longer responds to medical intervention and does not go away).
- AF management approaches can be grouped into 'rate control' approaches versus 'rhythm control' approaches. Rate control seeks to manage the rapid ventricular response and does not specifically address the AF; ablation of an AF focus is a form of rate control. Rhythm control (involving pharmacological therapy) seeks to restore normal sinus rhythm, which would, in turn, address the rapid ventricular response.

Chapter 9

Indications for CRT

Heart failure (HF) is a complex syndrome, and its management involves balancing multiple treatment options to meet the specific (and changing) needs of an individual patient. One of the most promising recent developments for HF patients is the emergence of a device-based treatment option known as cardiac resynchronization therapy (CRT). CRT involves using low-voltage stimulating pulses (typically 2 or 3 V output) to cause the failing heart to contract in a more synchronized, coherent, efficient way. CRT systems rely on three leads: one in the right atrium, one fixated on the right-ventricular side of the ventricular septum, and another located in the coronary sinus. While it is not entirely inaccurate to say that a CRT device helps resynchronize the right and left ventricles, its primary therapeutic benefit is that it resynchronizes the contraction of the left ventricle with itself so that the large left ventricle contracts as a single unit, instead of in sections. Thus, the right-ventricular lead and the coronary sinus lead both act to stimulate the left ventricle in such a way that it contracts as one unit. This 'left-ventricular synchronization' provides the major benefit of a CRT system in terms of improving pumping efficiency. The right ventricle is also stimulated in the process, so the right ventricle contraction is also synchronized.

At present, it is thought that patients who have a disorganized left-ventricular contraction are the ones who would most benefit from CRT. For official indications, this type of patient is described as one with a low ejection fraction, New York Heart Association (NYHA) Class III or IV heart failure and a QRS duration of > 120 ms.[1]

The wide QRS is the subject of some controversy, although it is the only marker for ventricular dyssynchrony for which there is some degree of professional consensus. Ventricular dyssynchrony is defined as a ventricular contraction (both right and left) that does not occur as a unified whole. In many HF patients, the left ventricle contracts in segments or sections rather than all at once. The result is that part of the left ventricle is already repolarizing (starting to relax) at the same time as other areas of the left ventricle are depolarizing (starting to contract). Ventricular dyssynchrony within the left ventricle causes a lot of the blood contained in the left ventricle to slosh around, back and forth, rather than being pumped outward. This dyssynchronous ventricular contraction may be evident on the surface ECG as a prolonged QRS complex. The standard definition of 'wide QRS' is > 120 ms, although in some studies a cut-off of 130 ms or even 150 ms was used instead.

There may be other ways to better measure mechanical dyssynchrony. Work is being conducted on echocardiography as a possible measure. Further, there is growing evidence that a so-called 'narrow QRS' can also accompany forms of ventricular dyssynchrony. While it is pretty clear that we do not yet possess the 'perfect' marker for ventricular dyssynchrony, we do know what ventricular dyssynchrony can do. Ventricular dyssynchrony is associated with:

- Less-than-optimal ventricular filling
- Reduced LV dP/dt (rate of rise of ventricular contractile force or pressure)
- Prolonged duration of mitral regurgitation (which makes it more severe)
- Paradoxical septal wall motion (this means that the incoherent left ventricular contraction causes the septum to contract and relax 'out of sync' with the rest of the left ventricle).

Ventricular dyssynchrony is not present in all HF patients, but it exists in a subset of HF patients and can be expected to develop in many HF patients who did not present with it initially. Ventricular dyssynchrony is associated with higher mortality rates among those HF patients who do have it.[2–4]

Cardiac resynchronization therapy addresses mechanical dyssynchrony by creating a unified, coherent and thus efficient ventricular contraction from a segmented, ineffective contraction. By restoring ventricular synchrony, CRT can also reduce secondary mitral regurgitation. Studies have shown functional improvement with CRT systems also. There are suggestions that CRT may be able to reverse ventricular remodeling.

Thousands of HF patients have been studied in large, randomized clinical trials evaluating the effectiveness of CRT devices. But one word of caution about these device trials: some trials use low-voltage CRT systems that could deliver only stimulating output pulses (maximum output around 7.5–10 V), while others evaluated CRT systems with defibrillation capability. These latter devices are actually implantable cardioverter-defibrillators (ICDs), which offer CRT stimulation instead of conventional pacing. Nicknamed CRT-D devices, these ICDs-plus-CRT complicate some of the randomized trials, in that it is unclear in some studies whether the benefits conferred by the devices are attributable to CRT, defibrillation, or some combination of the two therapies. While CRT devices without defibrillation have been studied and will be discussed, clinical practice in the USA at present favors the CRT-D system.

The first important caveat in understanding CRT indications is that CRT devices never replace optimal pharmacological therapy, i.e. HF drugs. Patients should already be on a well-managed regimen of HF drugs before CRT is used. Implanting a CRT system does not change the patient's need to continue their regular HF drugs. As a matter of fact, the leading studies that have evaluated CRT devices always assume an optimal HF drug regimen as baseline.

A meta-analysis of possible mortality benefits of CRT on HF patients found that this benefit emerged after just 3 months of treatment.[5] While there have been numerous CRT studies, there are a few landmark studies that are worth discussing in more detail. These are COMPANION, CARE-HF, SCD-HeFT (which was not specifically a CRT study) and PAVE (which was not specifically a HF study).

The COMPANION study (2000–2002, published in 2004)[6] enrolled 1520 NYHA Class III or IV patients who had had at least one HF hospitalization in the 12 months prior to enrolment. COMPANION patients also had to have a QRS duration > 120 ms, a left ventricular ejection fraction (LVEF) score of ≤35% and be receiving optimal pharmacological therapy for their condition. COMPANION excluded patients with a standard indication for a pacemaker or ICD. Patients were randomized into three arms: drug therapy alone, drug therapy plus CRT and drug therapy plus CRT-D (Fig. 9.1).

COMPANION used a composite primary endpoint of all-cause mortality or first hospitalization for any reason. As a composite end-point, the end-point was considered fulfilled if a patient met either criterion (all-cause mortality or first hospitalization for any reason). COMPANION found that CRT and

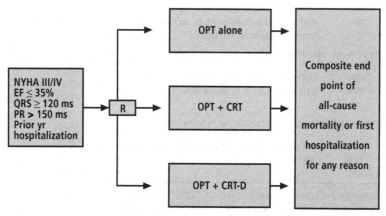

Fig. 9.1 COMPANION study design. COMPANION evaluated the effects of both CRT-P and CRT-D [cardiac resynchronization therapy (CRT) pacing and CRT pacing plus defibrillation] on New York Heart Association Class III and IV patients with a low ejection fraction and a wide QRS complex who were already on optimal pharmacological therapy (OPT). The study randomized patients into three groups.

CRT-D devices significantly reduced the risk of a patient reaching the composite primary end-point by about 20%. Further, CRT reduced the risk of all-cause mortality by 24% ($P=0.059$) and CRT-D reduced the risk of all-cause mortality by 36% ($P=0.003$) compared with drugs alone (see Table 9.1).

COMPANION remains the largest CRT trial to date and it demonstrated that CRT and CRT-D devices reduced morbidity and mortality in the most symptomatic HF patients. However, since COMPANION used both CRT and CRT-D devices, it was hard to know if the mortality benefits were due to CRT or the rescue function of defibrillation or a combination. In short, sceptics wondered if the benefits in the COMPANION study might not be the already established mortality benefits of ordinary ICD therapy.

Results from COMPANION showed that CRT and CRT-D did about equally well in terms of the primary end-point, i.e. defibrillation did not seem to play much of a role. When mortality was viewed in isolation, CRT-D performed better than CRT. CRT systems reduced the risk of mortality by 24%, which was actually not significant ($P=0.059$). (In most large, randomized clinical trials a P-value of ≤ 0.05 is considered significant. This could be expressed another way, in that it means there is a 95% probability that the results were due to the study variable and only 5% probability the observed results occurred by chance. A P-value of 0.059 is sometimes called 'borderline significant', but, in fact, most serious analysts would say it is 'NS' or not significant. To be fair, however, it can be said that a P-value of 0.059 'trends toward significance'.)

Since COMPANION patients with CRT or CRT-D devices had fewer hospitalizations as well as fewer deaths, it appeared that the devices were having a beneficial effect on HF itself. Even more encouraging for CRT advocates is the fact that CRT and CRT-D were achieving these results in the most symptomatic HF patients, namely those of Class III and Class IV. Up to that time, there was some sense in the HF community that the most severe patients were likely to derive little or no benefit from device-based therapy.

The CRT study with the most impact to date involved a total of 813 patients from 2001 to 2003:

Table 9.1 Summary of COMPANION results

Twelve-month rate of death or hospitalization for any reason (primary end-point)

Drugs alone	68%	Either type of CRT significantly reduced the risk of the primary end-point by about 20%
Drugs plus CRT	56%	
Drugs plus CRT-D	56%	

Twelve-month rate of death from any cause (secondary end-point)

Drugs alone	19%	CRT-D reduced the risk by a significant 36%
Drugs plus CRT	15%	(CRT alone reduced the risk by an amount that
Drugs plus CRT-D	12%	tended towards significance)

Twelve-month rate of death from or hospitalization for a CV cause

Drugs alone	60%	CRT reduced the risk by about 25% while CRT-D reduced the risk by about 28%
Drugs plus CRT	45%	
Drugs plus CRT-D	44%	

Twelve-month rate of death from or hospitalization for heart failure

Drugs alone	45%	CRT reduced risk by 34% while CRT-D reduced risk by 40%
Drugs plus CRT	31%	
Drugs plus CRT-D	29%	

COMPANION found that both cardiac resynchronization therapy (CRT) and CRT-D (CRT without and with defibrillation) reduced morbidity and mortality in patients with advanced heart failure. Because the COMPANION study involved both CRT and CRT-D devices, it was unclear what benefits could be ascribed specifically to CRT. Yet COMPANION strongly suggested that CRT stimulation in and of itself conferred benefits.

CARE-HF.[7] Conducted in the UK and USA, CARE-HF enrolled NYHA Class III and IV HF patients with an LVEF of ≤35%, a wide QRS (≥120 ms) and who had no standard pacemaker indication and no atrial arrhythmias. In many ways, the CARE-HF patient population was the same group studied by COMPANION and, like the COMPANION study, CARE-HF required all patients to be on optimal drug therapy for HF at baseline. However, unlike COMPANION, CARE-HF only used one type of device, the CRT system without defibrillation. Patients were randomized into two groups, drugs alone and drugs plus CRT (Fig. 9.2).

The primary composite end-point in the CARE-HF study was all-cause mortality or first hospitalization for a major cardiovascular cause. Patients in the CRT group showed a 37% reduction in meeting the composite end-point compared with the drugs-alone group. The secondary end-point was all-cause mortality and the CRT group showed a 36% reduction in that versus the drugs-alone group. CARE-HF investigators published in their report that for every nine CRT devices implanted, one death and three hospitalizations for a major cardiovascular cause could be avoided (Fig. 9.3).

The CARE-HF study established the morbidity and mortality benefits of CRT therapy, totally apart from the known benefits of defibrillation. Some observers thought that CRT might possibly confer a morbidity benefit on HF patients, but CARE-HF showed that CRT—without any defibrillation capability—also reduced mortality. The CARE-HF in-

vestigators found that CRT systems lowered the rate of sudden cardiac death (SCD); just 7% of patients in the CRT group succumbed to SCD during the study. It is possible that the use of a CRT-D system would have reduced this number even further.

So if CRT alone reduces morbidity and mortality, how does it do it? CARE-HF investigators wrote in their study that they believed CRT reduced cardiac dyssynchrony, which, in turn, improved left-ventricular function. That reduced mitral regurgitation, which caused perfusion pressure to rise, cardiac filling pressure to fall, and then brought about favorable left-ventricular remodeling. Just as the progressive worsening of HF involves a cascade of events starting with ventricular dyssynchrony, the CARE-HF investigators were suggesting that undoing the damage of HF might involve restoring ventricular synchrony.

The CRT patients in the CARE-HF study experienced this cascade of events as reduced symptoms, an improved feeling of well-being, and a lower risk of hospitalization and death. In fact, no other study at this time better reflects the positive benefits of CRT on advanced HF patients.

The PAVE study also used CRT devices exclusively to establish a new indication for CRT devices, but it did not implant the systems in HF patients.[8] Instead, PAVE studied the relatively small group of patients undergoing an elective atrioventricular (AV) nodal ablation for the management of permanent atrial fibrillation (AF). An AV nodal ablation of this sort dissociates the atria from the ventricles

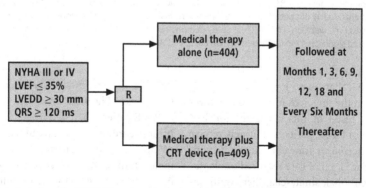

Fig. 9.2 CARE-HF study design. The CARE-HF study evaluated advanced heart failure patients (Class II or IV) with low ejection fractions and a wide QRS receiving optimal medical therapy into two groups. One group received a cardiac resynchronization therapy (CRT-P) device, the other did not. No patients received a CRT-D device. The CARE-HF study was designed to evaluate the specific morbidity and mortality benefits of CRT stimulation in a CRT-P system, apart from any rescue function that defibrillation might have offered (in a CRT-D device).

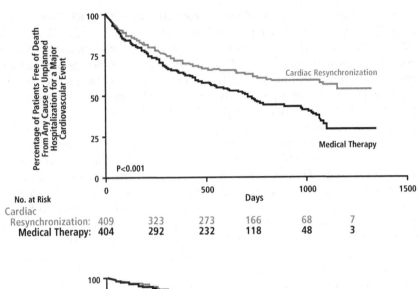

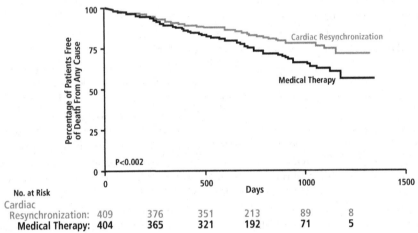

Fig. 9.3 CARE-HF survival graphs. The primary end-point of the CARE-HF study was a composite of death from any cause or unplanned hospitalization for a major cardiovascular event. Results are captured in the top graph, which shows that cardiac resynchronization therapy (CRT) patients and medical-therapy-only patients started out with similar rates, but, over time, CRT patients clearly did better. When all-cause mortality was viewed in isolation, the CRT patients also did better, particularly as time went on. The CARE-HF study demonstrated that CRT devices—even without defibrillation capability—conferred significant mortality benefits on advanced HF patients.

in such a way that there is no longer any electrical conduction from the upper chambers to the lower chambers. As a result of this iatrogenic form of third-degree heart block, patients routinely receive a permanent pacemaker for ventricular rate support. The standard level of care required implantation of a conventional, single-chamber (ventricular) pacemaker with a single lead fixated in or near the right-ventricular (RV) apex. PAVE randomized these so-called 'ablate-and-pace' patients into two groups: one received a conventional RV pacemaker,

the other got a so-called 'biventricular system,' i.e. a CRT device (Fig. 9.4).

PAVE patients had to have AF for at least 30 days prior to enrolment and have undergone a successful AV nodal implantation to be included. As with other major studies, PAVE patients were expected to be on optimal drug therapy for their condition at baseline. In addition, PAVE patients could not be able to walk more than 450 m in the 6-min hallway walk test.

PAVE patients did not have to have HF to enroll; in fact, NYHA Class IV HF was a specific exclusion

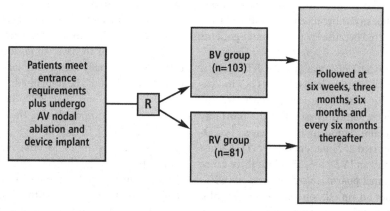

Fig. 9.4 PAVE study design. The PAVE study evaluated patients indicated for an elective atrioventricular nodal ablation to manage atrial fibrillation. These patients typically receive a permanent pacemaker after the ablation ('ablate-and-pace'). In the PAVE trial, patients were randomized into two groups, with one receiving a conventional (RV) pacemaker and the other receiving biventricular stimulation (CRT-P).

criterion. An ICD indication also excluded potential patients. However, there were no criteria to deal with issues such as systolic dysfunction (the mean LVEF score at baseline for PAVE patients was about 46%) or cardiac dyssynchrony (there was no QRS duration requirement).

PAVE found that CRT patients had significantly higher scores in the 6-min walk test and LVEF scores compared with the RV pacemaker group in the study and, when data were stratified, it was found that CRT patients with a lower LVEF to begin with scored a significant 73% improvement in the 6-min walk test versus RV patients with the same LVEF scores. While PAVE did not evaluate mortality at all and demonstrated some functional improvement in only a small subset of patients, it created some news.

First, PAVE opened a new indication for CRT: the post-AV-nodal ablate-and-pace patient. Second, it showed that CRT was offering benefits, particularly in patients with some degree of systolic dysfunction (as evidenced by a low LVEF score).

In 2003, about 30 000 AV nodal ablations were performed in America[9] and the procedure is widely viewed as safe and effective. CRT systems are now indicated for such 'ablate-and-pace' candidates and the PAVE study showed that CRT benefits may actually be applicable to a wider group of patients than HF patients alone. On the other hand, the PAVE results also seem to bolster what the other

studies were showing, namely that CRT was particularly valuable in patients with some degree of LV dysfunction.

PAVE also offered a new clue in the puzzle. One of the study's secondary end-points looked at LVEF scores at baseline, then at 6 weeks and finally at 6 months. At 6 months, the CRT patients had significantly better scores than the RV pacemaker patients. However, careful scrutiny of the study results shows that what really happened was that the CRT patients were able to maintain their LVEF scores over the 6 months post-implant (see Fig. 9.5), while

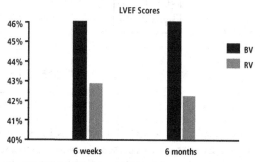

Fig. 9.5 PAVE left ventricular ejection fraction (LVEF) scores. Patients who received a biventricular (BV) device in the PAVE trial had significantly better LVEF scores at 6 months after the procedure compared with patients who received a conventional (RV) pacemaker. As the graph shows, BV patients maintained their LVEF scores, while RV patients lost ground with their LVEF scores over time.

the RV pacemaker patients got worse. Thus, the difference did not occur because CRT made patients better; it occurred because RV pacing made patients worse!

Although SCD-HeFT was not a CRT study, it deserves special mention in discussing CRT indications because it was a landmark primary-prevention trial which helped to establish the mortality benefits of defibrillation in HF patients.[10] SCD-HeFT randomized 2521 patients with NYHA Class II or III HF and an LVEF of ≤ 35% into three arms: those on optimal pharmacological therapy (OPT) for HF but not on amiodarone, those on OPT plus amiodarone, and those on OPT without amiodarone but with an ICD. SCD-HeFT used single-chamber ICDs that were conservatively programmed; in other words, the main benefit the ICD patient derived from the device was rescue defibrillation (see Fig. 9.6).

As usual, all patients were on state-of-the-art drug therapy for their heart failure. The primary end-point in SCD-HeFT was all-cause mortality. The theory behind the SCD-HeFT study was that HF patients were at risk of SCD and there were two main ways to address this risk: with a drug (amiodarone) or with an ICD. At the time, ICDs were not routinely prescribed for prophylactic implantation, i.e. a patient had to have some documented evidence of potentially dangerous tachyarrhythmias before an ICD would be implanted.

SCD-HeFT found that ICDs decreased mortality by 23% compared with the control group (HF drugs alone). In fact, in the SCD-HeFT study, amiodarone was about as effective in reducing mortality as the placebo (Fig. 9.7). This not only demonstrated that ICDs reduce mortality in primary-prevention patients with Class II or III HF and systolic dysfunction (LVEF ≤ 35%), it also made many in the clinical community question the value of amiodarone. Actually, amiodarone remains an important part of the medicine cabinet for HF patients, but it is just that SCD-HeFT found it did not confer mortality benefits. Amiodarone does work well at suppressing what could be called 'ambient arrhythmias', those background tachycardic events that many HF patients experience. As such, it is very possible that amiodarone did indeed reduce the total number of tachyarrhythmias

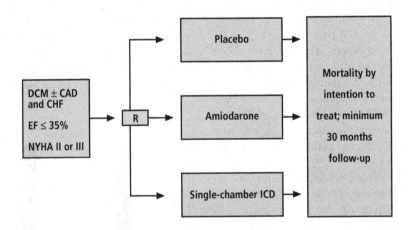

DCM = dilated cardiomyopathy, CAD = coronary artery disease, EF = ejection fraction

Fig. 9.6 SCD-HeFT study design. SCD-HeFT evaluated New York Heart Association Class II or III patients with dilated cardiomyopathy and low ejection fractions and randomized them into three groups. All groups received state-of-the-art medication for their heart failure. One group was the control or placebo group; they received medications only. The second group received state-of-the-art medical therapy plus amiodarone, an antiarrhythmic agent. The third group received state-of-the-art medications and a single-chamber implantable cardioverter-defibrillator (ICD). The third group did not receive amiodarone. The idea was to compare the two main approaches to ventricular tachyarrhythmias with the control: drug therapy with amiodarone and the rescue therapy of ICD devices.

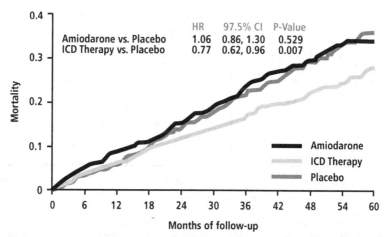

Fig. 9.7 SCD-HeFT survival graph. Although SCD-HeFT was not a cardiac resynchronization therapy study, it is one of the most important clinical trials in device history because it clearly established the mortality benefits of device therapy in New York Heart Association Class II and III patients. It surprised many that amiodarone did only about as well as the placebo in this trial. However, it must be recognized that while amiodarone is recognized for suppressing ventricular tachyarrhythmias, nobody ever claimed that the drug could successfully prevent every single possible ventricular arrhythmia. Thus, SCD-HeFT clearly established the mortality benefits of rescue defibrillation from an implantable cardioverter-defibrillator.

experienced by patients who took the drug. In fact, many clinicians think that amiodarone and an ICD are a good combination: amiodarone can reduce the overall number of tachyarrhythmias and the ICD can rescue from any life-threatening tachyarrhythmia that manages to break through. This suggests that an ICD patient taking amiodarone might experience fewer shocks and, for patients, the fewer shocks the better.

SCD-HeFT was the first large-scale study that 'exploded' ICD indications to include a large number of primary-prevention patients. Thus, SCD-HeFT established that many HF patients need defibrillation.

SCD-HeFT patients received only backup cardiac pacing. However, what if a SCD-HeFT type of patient (a primary-prevention patient, NYHA Class II or III, LVEF ≤ 35%) also needed permanent pacing? This is not such a far-fetched scenario. Many HF patients have rhythm disorders, including symptomatic bradycardia. In addition, some of the drugs routinely administered to HF patients can provoke symptomatic bradyarrhythmias (notable among these are β-blockers and digoxin). If such a patient were given the same type of device used in the SCD-HeFT study, that patient would receive conventional RV pacing.

Yet there is evidence to suggest that conventional RV pacing induces a form of artificial left bundle-branch block that can exacerbate systolic dysfunction. The DAVID study actually compared pacing modalities in two groups of ICD patients who had conventional ICD indications but no pacing indication.[11] Frequent RV pacing in DAVID patients resulted in an increased risk that the patients would meet the combined primary end-point of all-cause mortality or CHF hospitalization. In other words, the main message from DAVID was that unnecessary RV pacing makes LV dysfunction worse (see Fig. 9.8).

Our understanding of HF is by no means complete. These major studies give insight, but no final answers. Yet they can help clinicians understand why CRT-D systems are increasingly prescribed for HF patients. CRT has demonstrated benefits in even the most severe HF patients. Defibrillation has been shown to reduce mortality in Class II and III HF patients and most clinicians today would certainly use caution about prescribing RV pacing in any patient with compromised systolic function. Thus, these findings contribute to current industry trends, which involve more and more CRT-D systems in use in HF patients.

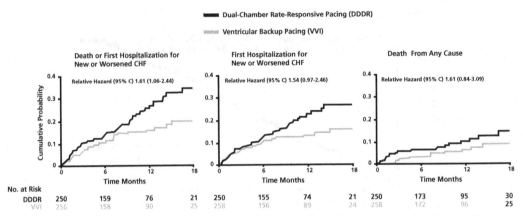

Fig. 9.8 DAVID results. The DAVID study is one of the most intriguing device studies in recent memory. Implantable cardioverter-defibrillator patients without a standard pacing indication who were frequently paced (DDDR, 70 pulses/min) had significantly higher rates of death and hospitalization for congestive heart failure than similar patients who were programmed to very infrequent pacing in the form of VVI-backup pacing at a low rate. The DAVID study added weight to growing evidence that conventional right-ventricular pacing seems to exacerbate heart failure. However, the mechanisms involved are still unknown. A DAVID II study is underway.

References

1   Hunt SA, Abraham WT, Chin MH *et al*. ACC/AHA 2005 Guideline Update for the Diagnosis and Management of Chronic Heart Failure in the Adult. Available at www.Circulation.org Accessed July 5, 2006.

2   Xiao HB, Roy C, Fujimoto S, Gibson DG. Natural history of abnormal conduction and its relation to prognosis in patients with dilated cardiomyopathy. *Int J Cardiol* 1996; **53:**163–70.

3   Shamim W, Francis DP, Yousufuddin M *et al*. Intraventricular conduction delay: a prognostic marker in chronic heart failure. *Int J Cardiol* 1999; **70:**171–8.

4   Unverferth DV, Magorien RD, Moeschberger ML. Factors influencing the one-year mortality of dilated cardiomyopathy. *Am J Cardiol* 1984; **54:**147–52.

5   McAlister F, Ezekowitz J, Wiebe N *et al*. Cardiac resynchronization therapy for congestive heart failure. *Evid Rep Technol Assess (Summ)* 2004; **106:**1–8.

6   Bristow MR, Saxon LA, Boehmer J *et al*. Cardiac-resynchronization therapy with or without an implantable defibrillator in advanced chronic heart failure. *N Engl J Med* 2004; **350:**2140–50.

7   Cleland JGF, Daubert JC, Erdmann E *et al*. The effect of cardiac resynchronization on morbidity and mortality in heart failure. *N Engl J Med* 2005; **252:**1539–49.

8   Doshi RN, Daoud EG, Fellows C *et al*. Left ventricular-based cardiac stimulation post AV nodal ablation evaluation (the PAVE study). *J Cardiovasc Electrophysiol* 2005; **16:**1160–5.

9   Stambler B. New nonpharmacological treatment option for ventricular rate control in permanent AF demonstrated effective: results of the Post AV-Nodal Ablation Evaluation (PAVE) trial. Available at http://www.medscape.com/viewprogram/3047_pnt Accessed April 21, 2005.

10 Bardy GH, Lee KL, Mark DB. Amiodarone or an implantable cardioverter-defibrillator for congestive heart failure. *N Engl J Med* 2005; **352:**225–37.

11 The DAVID Trial Investigators. Dual-chamber pacing or ventricular backup pacing in patients with an implantable defibrillator. *JAMA* 2002; **288:**3115–23.

The nuts and bolts of cardiac resynchronization therapy indications

- Cardiac resynchronization therapy (CRT) is a type of low-voltage stimulation involving three leads: one in the right atrium, one in the right ventricle against the septum, and one in the coronary sinus.
- CRT devices can be low-voltage pacemakers (CRT or CRT-P systems) or incorporate defibrillation (CRT-D devices).
- CRT works to combat ventricular dyssynchrony, which refers to an inefficient ventricular contraction. Ventricular dyssynchrony may involve an out-of-sync right and left ventricle, but more typically involves a left ventricle which contracts in sections rather than as a unified whole. The real power of CRT may be to synchronize the left-ventricular contraction as a coherent unit rather than to synchronize left and right ventricles.
- A wide QRS (> 120 ms) is generally used as a marker for ventricular dyssynchrony, although not all of those with ventricular dyssynchrony have a wide QRS.
- Ventricular dyssynchrony is associated with suboptimal ventricular filling, reduced rate of rise of ventricular contractile force, prolonged time for mitral regurgitation and paradoxical septal wall motion of the left ventricle.
- CRT addresses ventricular dyssynchrony, a condition present in many but not all HF patients.
- The two largest CRT clinical trials to date are COMPANION (CRT-P and CRT-D systems) and CARE-HF (CRT-P only). Both established morbidity and mortality benefits for CRT patients compared with patients on heart failure (HF) drugs alone.
- The largest device trial to date is SCD-HeFT, which established the prophylactic benefits of implantable cardioverter-defibrillator (ICD) therapy in Class II and III HF patients. ICD therapies reduced mortality in HF patients even if they had no prior evidence of rhythm disorders.
- The PAVE trial showed that CRT-P improved functional capacity of post-AV-nodal ablation patients compared with similar 'ablate-and-pace' patients who received conventional right-ventricular (RV) pacemakers.
- The DAVID trial suggests that frequent RV pacing in patients not indicated for pacing can exacerbate HF. The theory is that RV pacing induces a form of artificial left bundle-branch block or pacemaker-induced ventricular dyssynchrony. Patients with normal ventricular function may tolerate this well, but those with impaired ventricular function do not.
- While formal indications for CRT are still being sorted out, clinical preference is shifting toward CRT-D devices, which offer the benefits of pacing support without the apparent risks of RV pacing plus the life-saving rescue function of defibrillation.

Chapter 10

Types of CRT Systems

Cardiac resynchronization therapy (CRT) is a low-voltage stimulation therapy. In terms of the stimulating pulses generated by the device, CRT systems use the same kind of output pulse as a conventional pacemaker. These output pulses are generally about 1–3V at about 0.4ms duration. In fact, most CRT systems, like most conventional pacemakers, have a maximum output of about 7.5–10V. CRT always involves stimulation via three leads.

When it comes to cardiac rhythm management devices, there has always been a kind of 'Swiss Army knife' mentality among the engineers who design them. An implantable device represents a long-term commitment to a specific technology for the patient who wears it. For that reason, manufacturers like to add all potentially useful features into a device, providing they can work together well. With electronic and technological advances, today's cardiac rhythm management devices do more, last longer, and are smaller than ever before.

In conventional pacemakers, almost all modern devices today offer the auto mode switch algorithm, although not all patients who receive a pacemaker have high atrial rate activity. The concept is that the feature is potentially useful. After all, just because a patient does not have an atrial rhythm disorder today does not mean he will not develop one over time, i.e. before his pacemaker needs replacement. If the feature is not needed, it is simply inactive. If it should be required, it is available without any need for a device revision.

The same thinking applies to CRT systems, which most commonly incorporate defibrillation capability. These devices are sometimes called CRT-D systems or even implantable cardioverter-defibrillators (ICDs) with CRT. In terms of design, they are an ICD with a built-in CRT device instead of a built-in pacemaker (see Fig. 10.1).

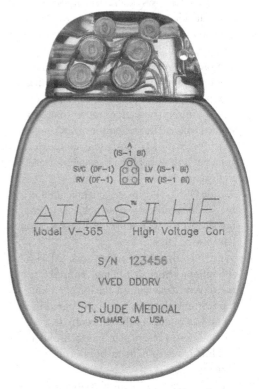

Fig. 10.1 CRT-D device. This typical CRT-D device has the rounded contours and relatively small footprint characteristic of modern implantable devices. It is not larger than a conventional implantable cardioverter-defibrillator, although the clear epoxy header is taller, since it needs to be able to accommodate three leads.

CRT devices may also be simpler units without the built-in defibrillator. In this case, they more closely resemble pacemakers and may even be called CRT-P or CRT pacemakers. They can deliver only low-voltage stimulation (see Fig. 10.2).

Regardless of whether the system is CRT-D or CRT-P, all CRT devices incorporate a pulse genera-

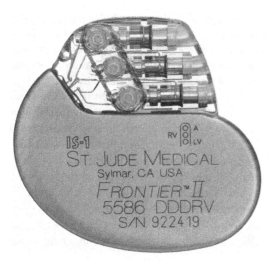

Fig. 10.2 CRT-P device. This is a CRT-P system, a stimulation device which allows three leads to plug into the clear epoxy connector. This device delivers cardiac resynchronization therapy (biventricular pacing) and atrial pacing, but does not offer defibrillation.

tor (nicknamed 'can') and three leads or insulated wires which plug into a clear plastic epoxy connector (nicknamed 'header') at the top of the pulse generator.

The pulse generator

The pulse generator is a marvel of engineering design. Incorporated in the hermetically sealed titanium case are complex electronic circuitry and memory chips that rival a computer. Most of the pulse generator's 'brains' are incorporated on a small circuit board called the 'hybrid' (because it incorporates different types of electronic circuitry). Foremost among the components is a precise timing mechanism (crystal oscillator) on which the pulse generator relies for its split-second timing. The circuits include sensing circuitry (to receive, filter, amplify, rectify and then interpret incoming signals from the heart) and output circuits which deliver exactly timed output pulses at programmed parameter settings (pulse amplitude or voltage and pulse width or duration in ms). Advanced counters allow the pulse generator to keep an ongoing record of cardiac activity. Memory chips store up not only counts of cardiac activity, but can even save intracardiac electrograms for subsequent downloading and evaluation.

The entire CRT system is powered by a battery, which occupies the largest area of real estate within the pulse generator housing. The battery technology in implantable cardiac rhythm management devices is remarkable: small-sized batteries can generate enough energy to keep an implantable system going for years. The battery chemicals used in these devices are known for a reliable discharge curve, meaning the batteries wear out very gradually and in highly predictable patterns. That provides many years of safe service and plenty of time to plan for a foreseeable end-of-service.

If the pulse generator also contains a defibrillator, there will be a larger battery and specialized components called capacitors. A defibrillator has to be able to deliver a very powerful output pulse; measured in volts, a defibrillating shock from an ICD can measure 700 V or more. Capacitors are the components that allow a less than 700-V battery to deliver a 700-V shock.

The best way to think of a capacitor is to imagine a bucket. When the ICD decides to deliver a shock, it starts a process known as 'charging'. Electrical energy is delivered and keeps flowing into the capacitors, like water being continuously poured into a bucket or a holding tank. When the capacitors are charged to the capacity necessary to deliver the appropriate shock, the ICD delivers the energy all at once, in one giant bolus.

One of the greatest technological challenges to building the first ICDs was figuring out how to let a small, implantable device with a modest battery deliver a massive jolt of energy to the heart. Capacitors (which actually come from the same technology that created the flash bulb in photography) enabled that. The earliest ICDs used bulky capacitors, which contributed to the thickness and weight of those first devices. Advances in capacitor technology, including the ability to build the so-called 'flat capacitors' (nicknamed 'flat caps') helped radically downsize ICD systems.

'Charge time' in a CRT-D device refers to the length of time it takes from the point at which the device decides to deliver a shock and the point at which the device is charged to the point that it can actually do so. In general, new devices have shorter charge times than older ones.

Although capacitors work like buckets for holding a charge and then delivering it, unlike a bucket, they do not ever completely empty out on their own. Within the capacitors, even after therapy delivery, there frequently remains what is known as a residual charge. In addition, in non-committed CRT-D systems, it is possible for the device to launch a charging sequence but then abort the shock delivery (this would happen, for example, if an arrhythmia was diagnosed but resolved spontaneously before the device was fully charged). In such a situation, there is a charge in the capacitors that is not required. In the case of an aborted shock, the device gradually 'bleeds off' the energy in a painless way which allows the capacitors to empty. In addition, modern devices have automatic mechanisms to clean out residual charge that builds up over time. This process is called 'reforming' or 'capacitor maintenance' and may be done manually, if needed. During reforming, the dielectric component within the capacitor is cleaned by charging the capacitors to capacity and then allowing the charge to dissipate painlessly. It is more typical to rely on the automatic reforming process of the device. Since the process is painless, patients are not aware when automatic capacitor maintenance occurs.

All of the electronics and battery of the device are encased in a titanium housing which is laser-welded to create a hermetic seal. The only point of entry into or out of the pulse generator are some 'feed through' connections contained at the top of the device and protected by a clear epoxy connector. When a lead is plugged into one of the connector ports, it establishes an electrical connection with the feed-throughs and can receive energy from (and transmit signals from the heart to) the pulse generator's interior.

Leads

Leads are thin insulated wires that are meant to function for many years in the most hostile environment on earth: the human body. All leads consist of one or more wires in the middle (called a 'conductor'), insulation (polyurethane 55D or silicone), and metal tips on each end. On the proximal end of the lead, the metal tip or pin plugs into the pulse generator's connector port. On the distal end, the lead will have one or more electrodes.

A CRT system requires three leads: one in the right atrium, one in the right ventricle fixated on the ventricular septum (the wall between the right and left ventricles) and another in the coronary sinus (see Fig. 10.3). All three leads have certain things in common: configuration, insulation and fundamental structure. Each lead also has certain special characteristics for its particular objective.

All leads have a configuration or polarity; they are either unipolar or bipolar. Actually, that is rather confusing, since any electrical circuit has to have to poles in order to work. The difference between a unipolar (one pole) or bipolar (two poles) lead is how many of these poles are located on the lead itself. A unipolar lead has one electrode at the distal tip. It forms its electrical circuit from distal electrode to the pulse generator can, creating a wide antenna. This accounts for two particular traits of the unipo-

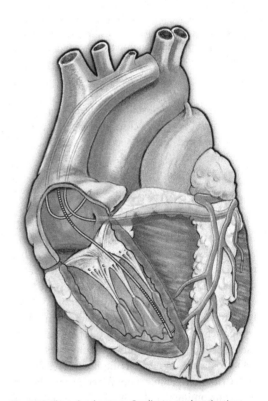

Fig. 10.3 Three-lead system. Cardiac resynchronization therapy (CRT) devices typically rely on three leads to deliver therapy. There is one lead in the right atrium for atrial pacing, another lead affixed at or near the septum within the right ventricle and a third lead placed in one of the coronary veins in such a way that it can stimulate the left ventricle. Although technically not in the left ventricle, this third lead is often called the LV lead. If the device is a CRT-D system, the lead in the right ventricle is the one that delivers defibrillation energy.

lar lead: it leaves a big artefact or 'spike' on a surface ECG (because it has a big antenna) and it is more often associated with muscle stimulation than the bipolar configuration.

A bipolar lead has two electrodes at the distal end: one at the tip and a second ring electrode a short distance away. It has a very compact antenna. As a result, bipolar leads have small pacing spikes on a surface ECG, but are less likely to be associated with muscle stimulation. However, because a bipolar lead requires two conductors (one for each electrode), it is bulkier and has a larger diameter than a comparable unipolar lead.

In a CRT or CRT-D system, leads can be unipolar or bipolar. Furthermore, it is possible to use unipolar leads and bipolar leads in combination with each other, e.g. a unipolar atrial lead and bipolar ventricular leads. The decision as to the type of lead to use is left to the implanting physician and may depend on a number of factors, including the patient's anatomy, the likelihood of muscle or diaphragmatic stimulation, and physician preference. It should also be noted that a bipolar lead can be reprogrammed (using the device programmer) to function as a unipolar lead, but the opposite is not true. (This is because a unipolar lead only has one electrode and one conductor and thus cannot act as a lead with two electrodes and two conductors.)

All leads have an outer layer of insulation to protect the body from the conductor wires (and vice versa!). There are two insulation materials in widespread use in implantable devices: polyurethane and silicone. Both have long track records of safety and reliability for use in the body. Polyurethane (leads today use exclusively the 55D type of polyurethane, but many years ago other types of polyurethane were also used) is a relatively thick and somewhat rigid material. Polyurethane leads are easy to implant and generally receive high marks in terms of handling characteristics. However, they may be prone to environmental stress cracking (ESC), a type of crazing or thin cracking that can develop over time. If ESC is severe enough, bodily fluids can seep into the lead and cause a short circuit.

Silicone is a much softer material and is not associated with ESC. However, as a material, silicone tends to be a bit tackier or stickier than polyurethane, which can make the leads harder to maneuver or manipulate, particularly when two or more leads

are being implanted at the same time. In addition, the very softness of the silicone (which gives it great flexibility) makes it more prone to nicks, which can also damage the lead.

Both types of insulation materials are widely available; in fact, many manufacturers offer leads using both types of insulation. Both silicone and polyurethane can be regarded as safe and reliable insulation; the decision to use one type over the other is largely a matter of physician preference.

The basic structure of every lead is a conductor (one for unipolar leads, two for bipolar leads) wrapped in insulation with a connector pin at the proximal end and an electrode (or two for bipolar leads) at the distal end. The electrodes are especially designed to provide optimal electrical characteristics, so they often have a textured surface which gives them a relatively large surface area (improved electrical characteristics) in a relatively small footprint.

Although all leads share these characteristics, there are special features of leads depending on their application.

Atrial leads

A CRT system requires a lead to be placed in the right atrium. This lead can be the exact same lead that would be used in the right atrium by a conventional pacemaker. For improved placement in the right atrium, atrial leads are available in a preformed J shape (see Fig. 10.4). These so-called atrial J leads are maneuvered into the heart using a straight stylet (which temporarily straightens the preformed J shape). When they are in place near the right atrial appendage, the stylet is withdrawn and the lead takes the J shape, which pops it into place.

Atrial leads have a fixation mechanism on the distal end to help anchor the lead. There are active-fixation mechanisms (such as a corkscrew or screw-in helix) and passive-fixation mechanisms (small flexible tines or fins that protrude from the end of the lead). An active-fixation lead is literally screwed into place into the myocardium, while a passive-fixation lead is lodged into the trabeculae of the myocardium (see Fig. 10.5). The choice between an active-fixation and a passive-fixation lead depends on the lead location (many, but not all, implanting physicians seem to favor an active-fixation lead for the thin and relatively smooth walls of the

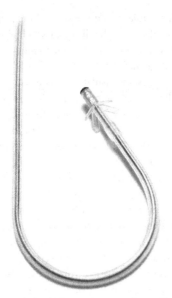

Fig. 10.4 Atrial J lead. The most commonly used lead in the right atrium is the so-called 'atrial J' lead, named for the preformed J-shaped curve at the distal end of the lead. The lead is temporarily straightened by insertion of a straight stylet during lead implantation. When the stylet is withdrawn, the lead resumes its J-shape, which helps it take the proper position in the right atrium.

right atrium), the patient's anatomy and physician preference. Active-fixation leads may take slightly longer to place in the heart, but they are also easier to remove in the acute phase.

The ventricular lead

The lead implanted in the right ventricle in a CRT system will vary depending on whether the system is a CRT-P device (low-voltage) or a CRT-D (CRT with ICD) system. A low-voltage device requires a right-ventricular (RV) pacing lead, the same type of the lead that would be used in a conventional RV pace-

maker. These leads are 'straight' and are implanted in the ventricle using a straight stylet. Like an atrial lead, they can have either an active-fixation mechanism or a passive-fixation mechanism. Passive-fixation mechanisms can work quite well in the trabeculated regions of the right ventricle (see Fig. 10.6).

In a conventional pacing system, the RV lead would normally be implanted at the apex (the far tip) of the chamber or even in the right-ventricular outflow tract (RVOT), which is the area just beyond the apex. For CRT pacing, the same lead is now implanted so that the distal electrode interfaces with the ventricular septum. The ideal position is about midway on the right ventricular side of the septum or inner wall between right and left ventricles (see Fig. 10.7)

The reason for a septal wall placement of the RV lead in CRT systems versus the conventional pacemaker RV lead position in the RV apex involves the nature of CRT. It has been observed that CRT stimulation is most effective when the RV lead and the left-ventricular (LV) lead are separated by the most physical distance. The LV lead is somewhat restricted in terms of where it can be permanently placed, so by moving the RV lead to a higher, septal position, this 'geographical distance' is preserved in a way that enhances CRT stimulation.

If the CRT system is a CRT-D device, then the RV lead has to be a defibrillation or tachycardia lead, capable of delivering a high-energy shock to the heart. A conventional pacing lead cannot withstand this amount of energy. A defibrillation lead is basically the same as a pacing lead, except that it has more robust physical characteristics which enable it to deliver high-energy therapy. The shock is delivered through a coil rather than a conventional pacing-type electrode. However, a defibrillation lead can do everything that a conventional pacing lead can do:

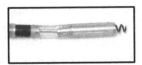

Active Fixation

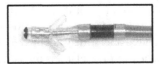

Passive Fixation

Fig. 10.5 Active- and passive-fixation mechanisms. Leads in the right atrium or right ventricle are affixed to the myocardium using two main types of mechanisms. The active-fixation mechanism usually involves a corkscrew or helix which is twisted into the heart muscle. Passive-fixation mechanisms rely on small projections (typically tines or fins) to help the lead embed itself into the trabeculae inside the heart.

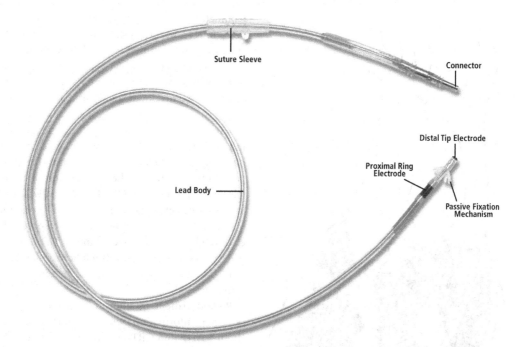

Fig. 10.6 Anatomy of a right-ventricular (RV) lead. This is a typical RV passive-fixation pacing lead. It has two electrodes (a proximal ring electrode and a distal tip electrode), making it a bipolar lead. The metal connector plugs into the clear epoxy header on the pulse generator. The suture sleeve is used to help secure the lead in place near the pocket during the implantation procedure. By stitching carefully through the loop on the suture sleeve, the lead can be held safely in proper position without damaging the lead insulation.

it can also pace and sense the heart. It has the same active-fixation or passive-fixation mechanisms for placement. Septal wall placement of a defibrillation lead does not impair its ability to defibrillate the heart, although all lead placement requires testing.

The left-ventricular lead

The lead unique to CRT systems is the lead intended for placement in the coronary sinus (CS), which is sometimes called the LV or left-heart lead. Actually, that is something of a misnomer, since this lead is actually not placed literally in the left ventricle. Its location in the CS or in one of the other cardiac veins branching off the CS (the great cardiac vein, the lateral vein, posterior vein, etc.) has been shown to allow for stable implant and to stimulate the outside of the left ventricle. Like the RV lead in a CRT system, the lead's primary intention is to pace the left ventricle.

While the LV lead has the same conductor, insulation, electrode(s) and configuration as the other leads, it has a distinctive and unusual shape. Because

it must be maneuvered into the CS and placed in one of the cardiac veins, most LV leads have specific shapes aimed at allowing secure placement. These shapes may be an S-curve or an angle (see Fig. 10.8). The LV lead relies on its shape rather than a fixation mechanism for reliable position.

Programmer and monitoring systems

One component of the CRT system which is often overlooked is the device programmer. A programmer is essentially a tabletop computer that works with proprietary software so that it can communicate with an implanted device. The bidirectional telemetry required to allow this back-and-forth flow of information and commands seems commonplace to most clinicians today who work with implanted devices, but it actually traces back to the space program. It is based on the same communications technologies that allow satellites in space to communicate back-and-forth with stations on earth.

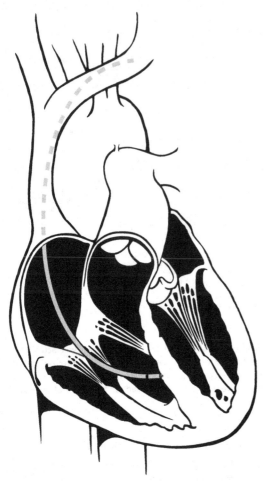

Fig. 10.7 Right-ventricular (RV) lead on septum. In cardiac resynchronization therapy systems, the RV lead is ideally fixated about midway on the ventricular septum, the interior wall that separates the right from left ventricles.

Programmers today are used to program the device, download diagnostic information, adjust parameter settings and provide information on everything from battery status to lead integrity. The same programmers that are used with pacemakers and ICDs are used with CRT systems, so there is not much of a learning curve with CRT devices for the clinician used to conventional pacemakers or ICDs.

Of growing interest are so-called 'remote patient monitoring systems' or ways for the patient to permit bidirectional telemetry from the comfort of his own home. Remote patient monitoring dates back to the 1980s with the proliferation of 'transtelephonic monitoring' (TTM), a system which allowed a pacemaker patient to transmit information via wrist electrodes from their implanted pacemaker through normal telephone lines. TTM is still in widespread use today, but its application has been limited to downloading some basic pacemaker information.

Remote patient monitoring systems today can download information from ICDs and CRT devices (both CRT-P and CRT-D). While not offering the full programmability of a conventional programmer, remote patient monitoring systems can allow patients to check in with the clinic periodically, to evaluate battery status and device integrity, and to download diagnostics. For example, remote patient monitoring can be used when an ICD patient receives a shock. Instead of making an appointment to see the physician the next day or rushing to the local emergency room, a patient can download information via a remote patient monitoring system (from home) and learn if they need to see the doctor.

There are a variety of remote patient monitoring systems (see Fig. 10.9) in use today, and further refinements to these systems may be expected in coming years. They have transmitters or small units that the patient keeps at home which relay information

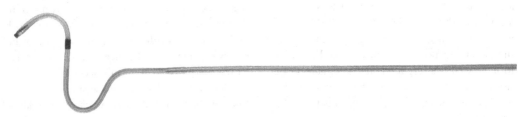

Fig. 10.8 Left-ventricular (LV) lead. The lead that travels through the coronary sinus and gets permanently placed in one of the coronary veins typically has an unusual shape to help facilitate the challenges of navigating and finding a secure placement in this environment. This LV lead has a characteristic S-shape to meet this objective. Other types of LV leads may have different distal configurations.

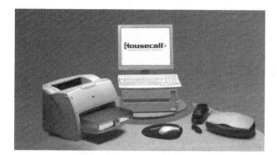

Fig. 10.9 Housecall Plus System. This remote patient-monitoring system allows patients with cardiac resynchronization therapy (CRT-D) devices to check their devices and even download diagnostic or other data to a clinic using normal telephone landlines. Remote patient monitoring is of increasing importance as more and more device patients enter an already overburdened healthcare system.

either by conventional phone lines or via a wireless connection through the internet to a receiving station. The receiver may be located in a physician's office or it may be in the office of a special service which receives, evaluates and forwards these reports.

Remote patient monitoring has not yet even begun to replace the routine follow-up visit. Only a visit to the clinic can adjust parameter settings or provide a thorough evaluation of all aspects of device therapy. However, for patients for whom traveling to the clinic represents a hardship (either because of geography or their own infirmity), remote patient follow-up is a viable alternative to some follow-up visits. In addition, it is a great aid for post-shock care of defibrillation patients and it may be used periodically to replace one or two routine follow-ups a year.

The nuts and bolts of types of CRT systems

- Cardiac resynchronization therapy (CRT) is a type of low-voltage stimulation therapy and may exist in a pacemaker-like device (CRT-P system) or an implantable cardioverter-defibrillator (ICD) (CRT-D system). While both devices are approved for use and will be seen in clinical practice, physicians are already expressing a clear preference for CRT-D devices.
- All CRT systems consist of a pulse generator plus three leads: one for the right atrium, one placed in the right ventricle against the septum and one placed in the coronary sinus (CS) to stimulate the left ventricle.
- The right-ventricular (RV) lead of a CRT system is typically placed about midway on the right ventricular septum, in such a way as to maximize the distance between its pacing electrodes and those of the left-ventricular (LV) lead, which is placed through the CS and into one of the coronary veins.
- CRT devices use the same kind of right atrial lead that a conventional pacemaker or ICD would use. A CRT-D system uses an RV defibrillation lead (the same as an ICD would use), whereas a CRT-P system uses the same

kind of RV lead that a conventional pacemaker would use.
- The LV lead is unique to CRT systems. It is used in both a CRT-P and CRT-D system. It has the characteristics of an ordinary lead, but it does not have a fixation mechanism. It anchors in place because of a unique distal geometry (often an S-shape or an angle).
- The biggest component inside a CRT or CRT-D system is the battery, which can last many years and discharges reliably and predictably over time.
- CRT-D systems use capacitors to deliver the high-energy outputs required to defibrillate the heart.
- All CRT devices can be followed and checked using programmers, similar to how pacemakers and ICDs are checked.
- Remote patient monitoring is now allowing CRT-D and CRT-P systems to be checked from the patient's home. These systems do not offer all of the features (and no device programmability) of an in-clinic follow-up using a programmer, but they can be used to check a CRT-D patient post-shock or as an alternative to a check-up in certain cases.

Chapter 11

Implant Procedures

While pacemaker and implantable cardioverter-de-fibrillator (ICD) implantation procedures have become virtually routine (and sometimes out-patient) procedures at many hospitals around the world, cardiac resynchronization therapy (CRT) system implantation poses unique and specific challenges to the implanting team. While device implantation and right-ventricular (RV) and right-atrial (RA) lead placement is fairly straightforward by decades of established practice, placing the left-ventricular (LV) lead can be difficult. At the time this book was written, there was actually no established consensus among device implanters as to 'preferred' techniques, although many successful implanting physicians recommend specific tips and methods. As a result, this chapter will attempt to sketch out briefly what goes on during a CRT device implant, with the caveat that implanting techniques may differ by physician. In fact, some of what is described here may not be common clinical practice in a few years!

In many ways, CRT device implant is similar to implanting a pacemaker or ICD, with the notable addition of the LV lead. In any device implant procedure, the order of implant is as follows:
- The pocket is formed
- Venous access is obtained
- The leads are placed and tested
- Leads are plugged into the device
- The system is tested
- The device with leads securely plugged in is placed in the pocket and the pocket is closed.

Pocket formation

Although I have no statistics on this subject, it appears that most ICDs and CRT-D systems are implanted in a pocket on the left side of the patient's body. For pacemakers, the prevailing thought was to implant the device on the patient's non-dominant side (which is the left side for the majority of us). However, it seems as if defibrillating-type devices (and most CRT devices implanted are CRT-D devices) tend to be left-sided implants regardless of the patient's dominant hand or other factors. Only when the patient's anatomy, in particular the vascular system, precludes a left-sided implant is the right side considered.

The pocket is formed between the fascia and the muscle in the upper pectoral region. The patient is anesthetized and an incision is made using blunt and sharp dissection. The goal is to create a pocket that is big enough to accommodate the pulse generator but not big enough to allow the device to shift around or migrate. The pocket is formed between the fascia and the muscle. Most implanting physicians will place a sponge soaked in antibiotic solution in the pocket while the rest of the procedure occurs.

Venous access

The leads are placed in and around the heart by introducing the lead into a vein, maneuvering it carefully through the vein into its final location and then assuring its fixation. For implanting just about any device, the two predominant paths of venous access are known as the cephalic cutdown or the subclavian stick. To be sure, other routes of venous access can also be used: the internal or external jugular veins, the axillary vein or the iliofemoral vein. However, most implanters prefer to use the cephalic or subclavian approaches unless there is a compelling reason to avoid them.

Subclavian stick is sometimes called the Seldinger technique. An 18-G needle attached to a 10-ml syringe containing anesthetic is introduced through the pocket incision. With the needle bevel-side-down, the implanting physician advances it carefully along the tissue plane at the level of the junction of the medial and middle third of the clavicle; the implanter then advances it toward a point just above the notch in the sternum. When the clavicle is reached, the needle's angle of entry is increased, allowing the tip to slide under the bone. Once under the clavicle, the needle should be maneuvered carefully at the same angle; the implanter can use negative pressure on the syringe to check for blood aspiration (which verifies that the cephalic vein has been punctured). If an artery is punctured, bright red blood will appear. If this occurs, remove the needle quickly and apply pressure on the puncture until it is adequately closed.

The subclavian stick method is sometimes called the 'blind' subclavian stick method, for good reason: the implanting physician is locating the subclavian vein using the needle! There is a risk of injury with this method, but it has been used safely and effectively for many years. It seems to have the best track record with patients with normal subclavian veins. If repeated attempts at the subclavian stick method fail, it is probably because the vein is partially or totally occluded or in an abnormal location.

The cephalic approach requires a traditional venous cutdown. In normal anatomy, the cephalic vein is located in the deltopectoral groove (between the deltoid and pectoral muscles). Once the vein is located, it should be gently exposed, lifted, and a small incision made. Cephalic cutdown is more of a true surgical approach, although advanced surgical skills are not necessary to incise the vein. All things being equal, the cephalic approach is probably more challenging than the subclavian approach, but the clinical judgment of the implanting physician should prevail. Reasons for selecting one point of venous entry over others include: location of the vein, whether or not the vein is twisted and makes sharp bends (tortuous vasculature), diameter of the vein, quality of the vein (occlusion) and preference of the implanting physician.

Implanting the leads

Most CRT devices require the implantation of three leads (one in the right atrium, one in the right ventricle and one LV lead). Most implanting physicians will first implant the RV lead, because having a viable RV pacing lead in place assures that the patient can receive emergency pacing in the event that asystole occurs. This is actually not a far-fetched scenario. As the implanting physician starts to introduce hardware into the venous system (guide wires, introducers, leads), trauma to the right bundle branch in a patient with pre-existing left bundle branch block (LBBB) has been known to induce temporary high-degree atrioventricular (AV) block or even asystole. While this is rare, it is a very sensible precaution to assure that an RV lead is properly in place before attempting to implant the other leads.

In order to get the RV lead into the vein and on its proper way, most implanters will use an introducer, which allows passage of a thin guide wire into the vein to the heart. A guide wire does just what its name implies: it guides the lead into the heart.

When just taken out of the box, the RV lead is just a very thin, insulated wire and is too floppy to pass through the vein. A thin wire called a stylet can be inserted into the lead. The stylet gives the lead enough rigidity to facilitate its passage through the vein without making it overly stiff. (Stylets are available in a variety of thicknesses.) Once the RV lead is securely on its way, the guide wire may be removed. The stylet remains in place until the lead is properly fixated.

Carefully maneuvering the RV lead under fluoroscopic observation, the implanting physician guides the lead through the vein, into the right atrium, over the tricuspid valve and into the right ventricle. The ideal fixation point for the lead tip is about midway on the ventricular septum, the wall inside the heart that separates the right and left ventricles. The lead tip attaches to the interior of the heart using an active-fixation mechanism (a corkscrew or helix twists into the myocardium) or a passive-fixation mechanism (tines or fins lodge in the trabeculae).

Once the lead is fixated, it is tested. Using a pacing system analyzer (a handheld device) or the programmer, the implant team checks to see whether the lead can pick up intrinsic cardiac signals of adequate size from this location and whether or not an output pulse through the lead to this point of the myocardium is adequate to cause a cardiac depolarization and contraction. These measurements are sensing and pacing threshold values, and they are covered in more depth in the next chapter.

It is not unusual in any device implant to have to reposition the leads to obtain more favorable threshold values. In the myocardium, a tiny shift in location can have a marked effect on pacing and sensing characteristics of the lead. Once acceptable thresholds are obtained and recorded, the lead is permanently fixated (if it has not been already) and the implanter proceeds to the next lead.

The RA lead can technically be implanted before or after the LV lead, but many implanters prefer to place the RA lead before the LV because if the LV lead implant fails and has to be re-attempted via a thoracotomy, the RA and RV leads will already be in place. On the other hand, there is no particular medical necessity to implant the RA lead ahead of the LV lead.

The RA lead can be inserted at the same point of venous access as the RV lead, or the implanting physician may decide to gain access from a separate site. If the RV and RA leads use the same entry point, the guide wire can be kept in place in a method known as the 'retained guide wire technique'. If two points of entry are used, two guide wires are likely to be required.

Atrial leads usually have a preformed J-shape configuration at the distal end. Before the atrial J-lead is inserted into the vein, a straight stylet is inserted, temporarily straightening the lead and giving it the necessary rigidity to navigate the venous system. Like the RV lead, it is carefully maneuvered into place under fluoroscopy. When it enters the right atrium, ideally near the right atrial appendage, the stylet is withdrawn, causing the lead to spring back into its preformed J shape. That motion should put the tip of the atrial lead near an atrial wall close to the right atrial appendage. The lead can then be fixated using an active- or passive-fixation mechanism.

Just like the RV lead, the RA lead should be tested for acceptable threshold values in sensing and pacing. Like other leads, the RA lead may exhibit markedly different pacing and sensing characteristics in different locations. For that reason, it is not unusual during device implantation for the implanting physician to try more than one atrial lead position before deciding on the appropriate placement of the RA lead.

Once the RA and RV leads are properly placed, the guide wires are removed.

The final lead to be placed is usually the most challenging: the LV lead. This requires cannulation of the coronary sinus, i.e. the insertion of a small tube (cannula) into the coronary sinus opening (os) which can be accessed from the right atrium. To accomplish this, the implanting physician needs to have a good idea about both normal coronary sinus anatomy and the coronary venous system, but also specific information about the individual patient's veins.

In a classic 'textbook' heart, blood is fed into the right atrium via the coronary veins that wrap around the exterior of the heart. The great cardiac vein (GCV) feeds into the coronary sinus (CS), which, despite its name, is actually a vein. The CS has a tiny outlet which delivers the deoxygenated blood directly into the right atrium; it is called the ostium or os. In a normal heart, the os of the CS is located at the bottom or floor of the RA, fairly close to the annulus of the tricuspid valve. The goal of LV lead implant is to introduce a small tube (cannula) or sheath into the CS in such a way that the LV lead can be passed successfully through the vein, into the right atrium and then out the os of the CS into the coronary venous system.

The first major challenge to CS cannulation involves locating the os of the coronary sinus (see Fig. 11.1).

There is considerable anatomic variation in os location among individuals, even those without heart failure (HF) or other cardiac conditions that may have altered cardiac structure. While the 'textbook' os should be in the inferior right atrium, it may be higher. In patients with dilated hearts (which includes many HF patients) or those with atrial fibrillation (AF), the right atrium may be enlarged and have folds or pouches that can obscure the os of the CS. Further compounding the difficulty is the fact that the os is often partially covered by a little flap known as the Thebesian valve.

The coronary sinus itself is quite short, usually about 3 or 4 cm. It is located posterior-inferior in the A-V groove, and it empties into the GCV, which, in turn, branches into a variety of veins of variable accessibility.

Cannulation of the CS requires specialized tools, but there is no clear consensus among implanters as to which tools are the 'best' or preferred. To some degree, the choice of tools depends on the patient's

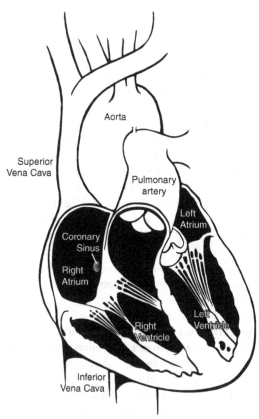

Fig. 11.1 The os of the coronary sinus. The os of the coronary sinus is located at the bottom of the right atrium behind a ridge-like structure.

anatomy as well as the physician's preference. In most cases, the implanting physician will need:

- A fixed-curve or steerable curve EP catheter
- An obdurator
- An LV sheath
- An angiography catheter with or without a guide wire
- The lead itself, with stylet in place.

While these tools are available separately, many manufacturers also package them into delivery systems (see Fig. 11.2). There will no doubt be considerable innovation and advances in these tools in the coming years.

The delivery system is flushed with heparinized saline solution and a hemostatic valve is attached to prevent the backflow of blood. The delivery catheter or sheath should be introduced into the vein, maneuvered under fluoroscopy into the right atrium and then directed toward the os of the coronary

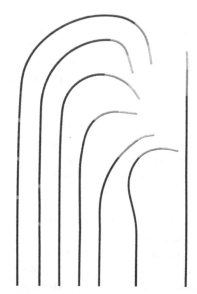

Fig. 11.2 Left-ventricular (LV) lead delivery system. Special tools are required to access and cannulate the os of the coronary sinus. This is an example of some LV lead delivery tools.

sinus. Gentle counter-clockwise torque should be applied and the sheath withdrawn to engage the os.

To verify proper location, an occlusive balloon catheter can be used to inject a puff of contrast medium. If the balloon can effectively block the ostium of the CS so that no blood from the CS flows into the heart, the contrast medium will fill the CS and make it clearly visible on fluoroscopy. Furthermore, the dye will reveal the anatomy of the various branches of the coronary venous system.

This view of the coronary venous network helps the implanting physician determine the best course of the LV lead. The object is to maneuver the LV lead through the os of the CS, through the CS and then lodge it in a coronary vein in such a way that there is maximal distance between the tip electrodes of the LV and RV leads. The coronary venous anatomy of patients differs widely, so it is very important for the implant team to study the individual patient's veins before proceeding.

After contrast and analysis of the venous system, the LV lead is introduced and passed through the cannula into the coronary sinus. In order to facilitate lead passage, a stylet is required. A recent advance in LV lead technology has involved the creation of the so-called 'over-the-wire' (OTW) stylet. A conventional stylet inserts into the interior or lumen of the lead. An OTW stylet works like a guide wire in that it is inserted first and then the lead is passed 'over the wire'. The choice of using a stylet-driven LV lead (i.e. a stylet in the lumen) or an OTW LV lead is usually one of physician preference. However, LV lead placement is so challenging that the OTW method has gained considerable popularity.

The lead is then gently maneuvered through the coronary venous system into its desired location. Unlike RV and RA leads, which may be relocated with relative ease, the LV lead is far more limited in its possible placement locations. In fact, there may be only one viable location for the LV lead in a given patient. The LV lead lacks a conventional fixation method because it does not affix to the coronary vein. Instead, most LV leads today have a unique distal configuration (an S-shape, a hooked shape, or an angular shape), which is designed to help anchor the lead firmly within the vein.

The implant team should first confirm the LV lead's anatomical position on fluoroscopy. The lead should be in a coronary vein on the outside of the left ventricle, ideally at a good distance from the tip of the RV lead (on the inside of the heart against the septum). Placement often occurs in the GCV or one of the lateral veins. Placement in the anterior vein is not recommended. The implanting physician should also confirm that the lead is stable in the vein.

The LV lead, like other leads, requires perioperative testing to confirm proper placement. Testing should be performed before the delivery system or sheath is removed, in case repositioning is required. A stimulus delivered from the pacing system analyzer (PSA) through the LV lead should cause a cardiac contraction. Low thresholds are ideal (a pacing threshold < 1V should be considered outstanding), but LV stimulation typically requires more energy than RV pacing. In fact, it is not unusual for an implanting physician to accept a relatively high pacing threshold from the LV lead, such as 3V and 0.5ms. Lower thresholds are clearly preferable, but the limited opportunities of LV lead placement may cause the implanting physician to accept higher thresholds. Some physicians have observed that increasing the pulse duration of the output pulse can have a more favorable impact on capture in the LV than the RV, so it may help to increase the millisecond setting to help manage high LV thresholds.[1]

Note that many CRT systems sense only from the RA and RV leads and not the LV lead, so there is usually no sensing threshold test to perform.

The phrenic nerve is located on the exterior of the heart and may sometimes be affected by LV stimulation. Phrenic nerve stimulation may produce diaphragmatic stimulation. Even intermittent phrenic nerve stimulation during implant is reason to reposition the LV lead. Phrenic nerve stimulation is one of the more common complications of CRT device implantation and postoperative attempts to 'program around' this problem usually do not work. To test for possible phrenic nerve stimulation, a maximum (usually 10V) output pulse should be delivered to the LV to see if it affects the phrenic nerve. If phrenic nerve stimulation occurs during perioperative testing, the lead should be repositioned. Diaphragmatic stimulation post-implant typically requires surgical revision to correct.

Once the LV lead is properly placed, the delivery system should be carefully removed without dislodging the LV lead. This usually involves gently removing the catheter or sheath without pulling or placing undue stress on the LV lead. Many products on the market today facilitate removal by allowing the sheath to be pulled apart (so-called 'peelable' products) or cut apart ('slittable' sheaths) along the longitudinal axis. Removal of the delivery system and other hardware should be done with extreme care, gentleness, and under fluoroscopic observation.

Leads in the device

At this point, the leads can be plugged into the ports of the pulse generator. The ports are located in the clear epoxy connector ('header') of the device. Note that the ports are specific to the lead. For example, the RA lead must plug into the RA port, and so on. Consult the technical manual or other product literature with the device for more information. Most CRT devices will have some sort of marking on the metal housing of the device itself to designate which leads plug into which ports.

To plug in a lead, insert the metal pin of the lead into the appropriate port. A connection mechanism is usually required to secure the lead firmly in place. In many cases, this involves some sort of setscrew, which can be tightened using a small tool (torque wrench or similar screwdriver-like tool). The setscrew should be tightened to hold the lead in place; follow the manufacturer's instructions. A loose lead will not only perform suboptimally, it may require surgical revision!

All leads should be plugged and secured into the pulse generator connector. A gentle tug on a lead should confirm that it is properly in place.

Testing the system

The leads are tested before they are plugged into the pulse generator to confirm proper placement and functional characteristics. Now that the leads are plugged into the actual pulse generator, it may be useful to observe the device stimulating the heart to confirm that leads are properly secured in the header.

If the CRT system has defibrillation capability, the clinician may want to perform defibrillation threshold (DFT) testing. The concept behind DFT testing is to find the lowest amount of energy that will reliably defibrillate the heart. In actual fact, most DFT testing finds an approximation of that value, since testing defibrillation efficacy involves inducing ventricular fibrillation (VF) and resuscitating the patient. (Patients should not be made to endure repeated tests of this nature!)

In some cases, device-based testing is used. In a device-based test, VF is induced and then the device is allowed to charge and deliver high-voltage therapy. The test is successful if the device performs properly and defibrillates the patient. This test should be conducted only when an adequate number of trained personnel are present and external defibrillation equipment is immediately available. For more information on DFT and device-based testing at implant, please refer to *The Nuts and Bolts of ICD Therapy*.

Closure

Once the device is tested and leads are secured, the device is ready to be inserted into the pocket. The antibiotic-soaked sponge in the pocket is removed and the device is gently inserted into the pocket. If there is excessive length of leads, it is tucked neatly behind the pulse generator in such a way that a subsequent incision to the pocket (for later pulse generator replacement) would not inadvertently nick or cut the leads. The pocket is then sutured closed. The patient may require an overnight or longer stay in the hospital.

Reference

1 Worley S, Leon A, Wilkoff BL. Anatomy and implantation techniques for biventricular devices. In: Device Therapy for Congestive Heart Failure. Ellenbogen KA, Kay GN, Wilkoff BL, eds. Philadelphia: Saunders 2004:198.

The nuts and bolts of implant procedures

- Cardiac resynchronization therapy (CRT) device implantation is similar to pacemaker or implantable cardioverter-defibrillator (ICD) implant, with one challenging exception: the left-ventricular (LV) lead.
- The LV lead should probably be implanted last. The right-ventricular (RV) lead should be inserted first, since it can provide backup or safety pacing in the event that the patient experiences temporary trauma-induced high-degree atrioventricular block or asystole. The right atrial (RA) lead can be implanted before or after the LV lead, although implanting it before the LV lead means that even if the LV lead cannot be implanted, a subsequent thoracotomy to place the LV lead is all that is required to get the system operational.
- Venous access is typically gained using the 'blind' subclavian stick procedure or the cephalic venous cutdown. An introducer is used and a guide wire is inserted first. A stylet is inserted into the lead to give it necessary rigidity for maneuvering through the venous system into the heart. All lead placement should be done under fluoroscopic observation.
- Two leads may be passed through a single entry point, but sometimes multiple access points are required. The LV lead should be inserted via a separate stick, if at all possible.

Continued p. 78.

Continued.

- The RV lead should be affixed somewhere along the middle of the ventricular septum. The LV lead is placed in one of the coronary veins that wrap around the outside of the heart. When placed in optimal locations, the RV lead tip and the LV lead tip should be as far apart spatially as possible.
- The RA lead is typically a preformed J-lead, which is placed in the right atrium. When the stylet is withdrawn, the lead pops into its J shape and can be fixated against the atrial wall.
- In order to place the LV lead, the coronary sinus (which is actually a vein) must be cannulated. To accomplish this, an introducer or special tool is passed through the venous system into the heart and into the right atrium. At that point, a sheath or cannula must be inserted into the ostium (or os) of the coronary sinus. The os is a small inlet, usually located near the floor of the right atrium relatively close to the tricuspid valve. It can be difficult to locate the os when the heart is dilated or anatomically abnormal. Furthermore, access to the os of the coronary sinus can be made more complicated by the anatomical features around the area, including a ridge-like structure (Eustachian ridge) and a flap that may partially obscure the opening.
- Once the coronary sinus is cannulated, the LV lead can be introduced, maneuvered gently through the os and into the coronary sinus and, from there, advanced carefully into the coronary veins.
- It is useful during LV lead implant to use contrast venography to help visualize the coronary sinus (which is only about 3 or 4 cm long) and the venous pathways of the individual patient.
- The LV lead is maneuvered under fluoroscopy into a viable position and tested. The LV lead has no classic fixation mechanism; an unusual shape at the lead's distal end (S shape, angle, curve) helps to anchor it in place.

- Leads should be tested for proper threshold values before they are plugged into the pulse generator. This usually involves the use of a pacing system analyzer. Right-sided leads (RA, RV) should be tested for sensing thresholds (can they reliably sense the heart's intrinsic signals?) and pacing thresholds (can a small amount of energy reliably capture the heart?), while the LV lead should be tested for pacing threshold and also to verify that no phrenic nerve stimulation is occurring. Most LV leads are not used to sense cardiac activity.
- If good threshold values cannot be obtained, the implanting physician may elect to reposition the lead and try again. RA and RV leads generally lend themselves better to repositioning. In the left heart, there may be fewer options to move the lead around.
- As a rule of thumb, it is common to find higher thresholds in the LV than in the RV. While lower pacing thresholds are desirable, higher LV thresholds can still be viable. Sometimes prolonging the pulse width (milliseconds) of the output pulse can be of more benefit in LV stimulation than in RV stimulation.
- Once the leads are properly in place, they are plugged into the connector portion of the pulse generator. Note that a lead should be inserted in the proper port (i.e. there is an LV port for the LV lead, an RV port for the RV lead, and so on). A setscrew and torque wrench are used to tighten the leads in the connector.
- Devices with defibrillation capability may require defibrillation threshold (DFT) testing or device-based testing to be sure the system can reliably defibrillate the patient when he or she is in ventricular fibrillation.
- The pulse generator is placed in a pocket in the upper pectoral region. If there is excess lead, it is neatly tucked behind the pulse generator. The pocket is then sutured closed.

Chapter 12

Basic Programming

While the cardiac resynchronization therapy (CRT) system is indeed leading-edge technology, much of the routine programming of the device relies on basic stimulation parameters familiar to many clinicians from pacemakers. The CRT system's objective is stimulation of the heart. This relies on two basic functions: pacing and sensing. Many of the parameters used are similar to pacing parameters and rely on pacemaker timing cycles. However, one fundamental consideration in CRT systems should be mentioned which differs tremendously from conventional systems: the goal of a CRT device is to pace the ventricles as much as possible, ideally 100% of the time. This is quite the opposite goal of the conventional pacemaker, which tries to pace the ventricles only when absolutely necessary.

All stimulation devices – whether pacemakers, implantable cardioverter-defibrillators (ICDs) with pacing capability, or CRT systems – really only do two things when it comes to stimulating the heart: they pace and they sense. Pacing refers to the ability of an output pulse or stimulus from the pulse generator to cause the cardiac tissue to depolarize and contract. This action is called 'capture'. One of the first parameters to be programmed (this is done at implant and should be checked at every follow-up) is the output pulse. The output pulse is a specific amount of energy governed by two parameters: the pulse amplitude (measured in volts) and the pulse duration or pulse width (measured in milliseconds).

In older CRT systems, the ventricular outputs were tied together, i.e. the clinician could adjust only one set of ventricular settings which governed both the right-ventricular (RV) and left-ventricular (LV) outputs. In particular, 'off-label' use of devices for CRT required this (in such cases, a dual-chamber ICD was equipped with three leads but offered programmability only for atrial and ventricular outputs). Today, advanced CRT systems offer the obvious benefits of independent programmability for RV and LV outputs. This can be particularly useful since the RV and LV pacing thresholds can often differ considerably.

At implant and during follow-up, a capture test should be performed to assess the capture threshold (or pacing threshold) of the patient. The capture threshold is the smallest amount of energy (defined as voltage and milliseconds) required to capture the heart reliably. Each chamber (right atrium, right ventricle, left ventricle) will have its own capture threshold. Capture thresholds change over the course of the day and also over time, particularly with drug interactions and disease progression. Thus, clinicians program the permanent pulse output settings by using a safety margin on top of the capture threshold. As a general rule, the safety margin is 2:1 or 3:1. For example, if the patient's capture threshold is 1 V at 0.4 ms, the permanent settings would be programmed to 2 V at 0.4 ms (2:1 safety margin) or 3 V at 0.4 ms (3:1 safety margin).

Capture testing may be done semi-automatically by the programmer or it can be done manually. Capture testing is the 'step-down' test. A relatively large pacing output pulse is delivered to the chamber of the heart and monitored on the surface ECG or intracardiac electrogram (see Fig. 12.1). If each pacing output (seen on an ECG as a spike) causes a cardiac depolarization and contraction, then capture is confirmed. The output pulse is then decreased in small steps. At each step, capture is noted. As long as capture is confirmed, the test proceeds to the next step down. When capture is lost, the output pulse is increased (so that the patient does not suffer from loss of capture for several beats) and the last output pulse that captured the heart is recorded as the capture threshold.

Conducting a capture threshold test is routine in clinics that manage device patients. The same basic

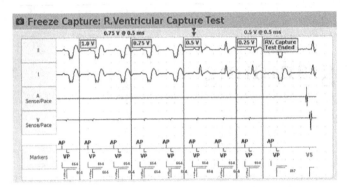

Fig. 12.1 Annotated RV capture test. In this example, RV capture was lost as 0.5V. Annotations show a ventricular pace event (VP) occurred but the ECG shows a sensed rather than paced event.

approach is used in pacemakers, ICDs and CRT devices. Some programmers allow the step-down sequence to proceed automatically, loss of capture to be annotated on screen, and an 'official' on-screen threshold value to be stored by the programmer and printed out for patient records.

The one aspect of capture threshold testing which is sometimes tricky involves what could be called 'forced pacing'. Capture can only be tested if the system is pacing; as soon as intrinsic activity inhibits the device, capture tests cannot be conducted. In the ventricles, a high base rate can often overcome this problem. For CRT patients, the main problem in capture testing will occur in the atrium. If the patient has atrial tachyarrhythmias, it may be impossible to overdrive them with pacing or to find an acceptable base rate (even for a temporary value just for testing purposes). While every effort should be made to test for capture, the fact of the matter is that sometimes in CRT patients, atrial capture testing may not be possible.

When programming a CRT system, great care should be taken to be sure the device can always reliably capture and pace the ventricles, since the goal is 100% ventricular pacing. This can mean programming a CRT system to higher output settings than the same clinicians might use in a conventional pacemaker. In particular, the LV pacing threshold and output settings can be much higher than conventional RV settings. This is because a pacing electrode placed directly on excitable myocardial tissue (e.g. in the right ventricle) can depolarize the heart with far less energy than a pacing

electrode on the LV lead placed in a vein on the exterior of the heart!

It is also important that the CRT system can sense incoming signals. Sensing may be done in the right atrium and right ventricle only (the LV lead in some systems does not sense). The sensitivity setting (mV setting) defines the size signals the device can 'see' and to which it will respond. Some clinicians find sensitivity programming a bit counter-intuitive, so think of the sensitivity setting as a wall at a particular height, described in mV. For example, let us say the patient has intrinsic ventricular signals (measured at implant and later in follow-up) of around 4 mV. If the sensitivity 'wall' is set to 4 mV, then only signals 'taller' than 4 mV (in other words, larger than 4 mV) could be seen by the device. Since the patient's ventricular signals were around 4 mV, the CRT system would not be able to see all of the patient's intrinsic ventricular signals! But if the sensitivity of the CRT system was increased by making the wall lower and setting it to 2 mV, then any signal taller than 2 mV could be seen and sensed. Thus, increasing the mV setting decreases sensitivity and vice versa (see Fig. 12.2).

Some clinicians are initially puzzled by the fact that pacing occurs in all three chambers of a CRT system [in dual-chamber (DDD) mode], while sensing may occur only in the right atrium and right ventricle. (Note that some CRT systems offer LV sensing, but this is not true of all CRT devices.) The purpose of the CRT device is to force the ventricles to act in concert, even in a heart with mechanical dyssynchrony. Thus, sensing in the right ventricle

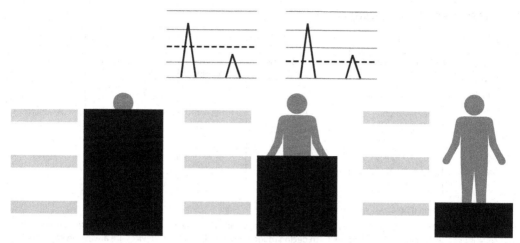

Fig. 12.2 The sensing 'wall'. When a sensitivity setting is programmed, it can be thought of as a wall. Any signal that is tall enough to peek over that wall can be 'seen' by the device, while signals that are too short to be seen over the wall are missed by the device. Thus, setting a sensitivity value of 4 mV means that signals > 4 mV can be seen, but signals < 4 mV will be missed. (A 4-mV sensitivity setting will sense an intrinsic 6-mV signal, but not an intrinsic 3-mV signal.)

can provide sufficient input about intrinsic activity.

Furthermore, if a CRT system does its job well and paces the ventricle 100% of the time, the device will not need to do much sensing!

Basic parameters

Most basic parameters have default or nominal settings that are active in the device as shipped. These so-called shipped settings are values that are typical and might work well in most patients. However, optimal device performance requires a familiarity with parameters and the ability to make subtle adjustments, as required. When programming or adjusting a CRT system, bear in mind that tiny changes can have a large effect on the patient. Do not overcompensate by making big jumps in settings without testing the effect of a small incremental change.

The base rate (also called the pacing rate, paced rate, lower rate limit or basic rate) is the number of pulses the device will deliver to the heart in the absence of intrinsic activity. Typical base rate settings might be 60 or 70 pulses/min. Some CRT systems offer an optional rest rate feature which allows the clinician to program an interim rate, which goes into effect when the activity sensor in the device senses that the patient is inactive and presumed asleep. (Some CRT systems offer a rest rate that is tied to clock time, also.) The idea is that the CRT device can imitate the body's natural heart rate slowdown during sleep.

The mode of the device refers to how the device stimulates the heart (see Fig. 12.3). In the DDD mode, the CRT device paces in 'dual' manner: both atrium and ventricles (think of the right and left ventricles as one unit). It senses in 'dual' manner: both the atrium and ventricle (CRT systems sense only in the right atrium and right ventricle). Its response to an intrinsic event is also 'dual' in that sometimes it is inhibited and sometimes it is triggered. The device can also be programmed to VVI, which would pace and sense the ventricles only (never the atrium) and would respond to intrinsic activity by inhibiting the output pulse.

When the device senses an intrinsic cardiac signal, it can have one of two responses. The first is inhibition, i.e. it withholds or inhibits the next output pulse. For example, a DDD device that senses an intrinsic ventricular contraction in the proper timing will withhold the ventricular output pulse.

Triggering refers to the fact that when an intrinsic event is sensed, it causes the device to deliver an output pulse. Triggered modes are typically used for brief periods of time in tests (VVT, for example).

The NASPE/BPEG Generic (NBG) Code

Position	I	II	III	IV	V
Category	Chamber(s) Paced	Chamber(s) Sensed	Response to Sensing	Rate Modulation	Multisite Pacing
Letters Used	O-None	O-None	O-None	O-None	O-None
	A-Atrium	A-Atrium	T-Triggered	R-Rate Modulation	A-Atrium
	V-Ventricle	V-Ventricle	I-Inhibited		V-Ventricle
	D-Dual (A+V)	D-Dual (A+V)	D-Dual (T+I)		D-Dual (A+V)
	S-Single* (A or V)	S-Single* (A or V)			

Manufacturer's Designation Only

Fig. 12.3 North American Society of Pacing and Electrophysiology and British Pacing and Electrophysiology Group Code. This code is used all over the world to define both pacing modes and describe devices (devices are always described by the highest mode of which they are capable). A cardiac resynchronization therapy device with rate response (also called rate modulation) would be described as DDDRV.

However, a DDD system is also triggered, in that when an intrinsic atrial event is sensed, it triggers the device to deliver an output pulse to the ventricle. This process of matching an intrinsic atrial beat to a ventricular paced event (if the ventricle fails to beat on its own in a timely fashion) is also called 'tracking' or 'atrial tracking'. Pacemakers and CRT devices try to allow for atrial tracking because it provides 1 : 1 atrioventricular (AV) synchrony, i.e. the pairing of atrial events to ventricular events. When every atrial beat is followed by a ventricular beat, the patient receives the benefits of 'atrial kick' and better pumping efficiency.

The problem then arises: what happens if the atria start beating too fast? Atrial tracking is fine if the native atrial rate is a reasonable 60 or 70 beats/min. When high-rate atrial activity occurs, the DDD mode device will try to match atrial sensed events with ventricular paced events, which can lead to uncomfortably high ventricular rates. Since many heart failure (HF) patients have atrial tachyarrhythmias, this scenario is not uncommon with CRT systems in the DDD mode. Since DDD offers considerable benefits to the patient, there is a way to program the device that allows 1 : 1 AV synchrony, but within certain boundaries. The parameter is called the maximum tracking rate (MTR) (sometimes Max Track) and it is essentially a ventricular speed limit. It specifies the highest rate the CRT device will ever pace the ventricle in response to sensed atrial activity. For example, an MTR of 100 beats/min will allow the device to track atrial activity up to 100 beats/min, but after that, it will resort to something called 'pacemaker Wenckebach' or other type of upper-rate response to keep the ventricular paced rate < 100 pulses/min. Of course, that means the patient loses 1 : 1 AV synchrony, but the payoff is that the patient does not have to endure high-rate ventricular pacing.

It is also important to understand the paced and sensed AV delay and the rate-responsive AV delay. In the healthy heart, the atria contract first, there is then a pause, and finally the ventricles contract. A dual-chamber pacemaker or CRT system tries to mimic that normal physiologic sequence by pacing the atrium, allowing for a pause and then pacing the ventricles. This artificially imposed pause between atrial-paced beat and ventricular-paced beat is the paced AV delay. It is a programmable function, with a typical setting of about 200 or 250 ms.

What happens if the atria beat on their own and then the device paces? Once again, the device imposes a pause to allow for the atrial contraction to complete before pacing the ventricle. This is called the sensed AV delay. In many devices, the sensed and paced AV delays are tied together and share the same value, but advanced systems may allow clinicians to program independent settings for the sensed and paced AV delays. The main reason to do so is to accommodate the fraction of a second of time it takes the device to recognize an intrinsic atrial signal. For example, in the paced AV delay, the instant the atrial output is delivered, the paced AV delay timer starts; when it expires, the ventricular output is delivered. If the paced AV delay is set to 250 ms, then 250 ms after the atrial output is fired, the ventricular output is sent. But in the case of an intrinsic atrial event, it may take the device 25 ms or so to sense the intrinsic signal (see Fig. 12.4). Thus, 25 ms pass before the sensed AV delay timer starts, so it is 275 ms after the atrial event commences that the ventricle is paced. Thus, many clinicians like to program a sensed AV delay that is about 25 ms shorter than the paced AV delay.

CRT devices should be programmed to relatively short AV delay values, although the sensed AV delay ought to be slightly shorter than the paced AV delay. The reason for tightening the paced AV delay in a CRT system is simple: it encourages more ventricular pacing. If the AV delay is brief, there is less opportunity for the ventricles to contract spontaneously.

In the healthy heart, there is considerable rate variation over the course of the day. The heart beats slowly when we are asleep or watching TV, but speeds up when we climb stairs, exercise on a treadmill or work around the yard. When the heart beats faster, the healthy heart naturally decreases the pause between atrial contraction and ventricular contraction. When the heart beats slowly, the healthy heart naturally increases that pause. Device manufacturers can imitate that variation in AV delay with a parameter called rate-responsive AV delay. This is a feature that should be activated (no specific setting is required) in patients likely to have a variety of heart rates over the course of the day. Despite its name, rate-responsive AV delay does not involve an activity sensor or rate modulation in response to perceived metabolic need.

On the other hand, some CRT devices do offer an activity sensor and rate response. This parameter is useful for patients who are active or require more rate support during physical activities. This is not likely to be of interest to the severely symptomatic HF patient.

The post-ventricular atrial refractory period (PVARP) is a special timing cycle on the atrial channel which makes it unresponsive to incoming signals immediately following the delivery of a ventricular output pulse. While clinicians like to think

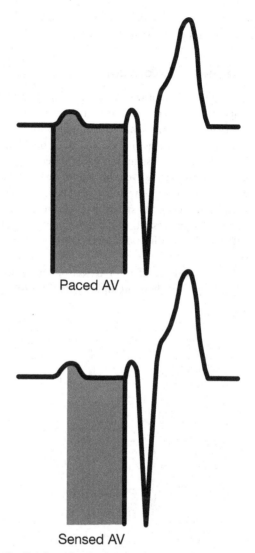

Paced AV

Sensed AV

Fig. 12.4 Sensed and paced atrioventricular (AV) delays. The paced AV delay defines the time from a paced atrial event to the next ventricular event, while the sensed AV delay defines the time from a sensed atrial event to the next ventricular event. When programming AV delay times, it is often useful to program the sensed AV delay slightly shorter (e.g. 25 ms) than the paced AV delay. The reason for this is that the device starts the paced AV delay timer at exactly the moment it delivers an atrial output pulse (see top of figure), while the sensed AV delay requires the device to sense the atrial event and then initiate the timer (bottom figure).

of the right atrium and right ventricle as being quite distinct from each other, in actuality, they are very close together and it sometimes happens that a ventricular output pulse is sensed by the atrial channel of the device. The PVARP timing cycle helps prevent this sort of inappropriate sensing.

Diagnostic information

CRT systems offer a wide range of downloadable diagnostic counters and data to help evaluate the device function. An event histogram can show how much paced and sensed activity is going on. Since the goal of a CRT system is to pace the ventricle as much as possible, the event histogram can provide valuable clues to see how close to that desired 100% ventricular pacing the system has achieved. Atrial pacing is not necessarily of the same interest; good CRT function may include a lot or a little atrial pacing (see Fig. 12.5).

Most devices also offer stored electrograms. Since most HF patients have multiple rhythm disorders,

these stored electrograms can be of great value in case the patient experiences remarkable episodes or spells.

Other features

Some CRT devices offer auto mode switching (AMS), a special feature designed to prevent atrial tracking at high rates. AMS is useful for patients who experience even short runs of atrial tachyarrhythmias, and since many HF patients have atrial fibrillation (AF) or other high-rate atrial activity, it is important to understand how this feature works. Essentially, the CRT system in a DDD or DDDR mode senses atrial activity and tries to pace the ventricle in response in such a way that 1:1 AV synchrony is preserved. The MTR is a good 'speed limit' for this, but when the MTR is imposed, the

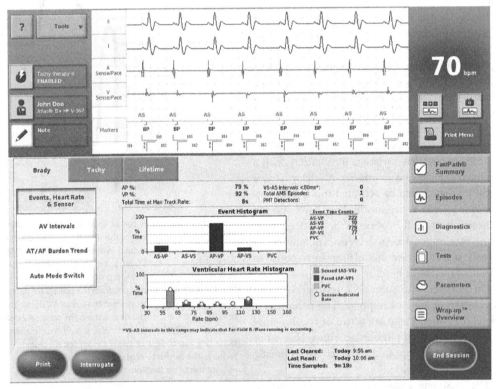

Fig. 12.5 Event histogram. The event and heart rate histograms provide a detailed, easy-to-read report on cardiac activity. The event rate groups cardiac activity by pacing state. In this example, the patient received ventricular pacing (VP) 92% of the time and most events were atrial paced events followed by ventricular paced events (AP–VP). Event histograms can help clinicians determine if they are meeting their CRT objective of 100% ventricular pacing. The heart rate histogram groups cardiac activity by ventricular rate ranges and also color-codes the bar charts for paced versus sensed activity.

device can start to function in 'upper-rate behavior' modes, including a form of pacemaker-induced Wenckebach or heart block.

AMS is a good alternative solution for some patients. In this case, the clinician can program an atrial rate cut-off value, i.e. the highest native atrial rate at which the device will still sense the atrium. As an example, say that high atrial rate value was 120 beats/min. If the patient's atrial rate exceeded 120 beats/min, the device would switch modes, either by switching to a non-tracking mode (DDD to DDI) or by turning off the atrial channel altogether (DDD to VVI). True, the patient loses the benefits of 1 : 1 AV synchrony, but those benefits cannot be preserved during an episode of atrial tachyarrhythmia anyway. During the AMS episode, the device continues to sense the atrium (but not respond to its signals). When it senses the atrial rate has come back within the normal range, it restores the originally programmed mode.

AMS has been particularly useful for patients who experience intermittent but severe atrial tachyarrhythmias. AMS data are recorded in device diagnostics, so that during follow-up, the clinician can determine how many AMS episodes occurred, the rates involved, and the duration of the episodes. Electrograms of the AMS episodes may also be recorded.

Patients with chronic AF should not use AMS, since it would be 'on' all of the time in the face of permanent AF! Such patients should not be programmed to atrial tracking modes.

A few programming considerations

If the patient has normal atrial function, it is a good idea to try to allow for intrinsic atrial activity to prevail as much as possible. (While a CRT system has the goal of pacing the ventricles all of the time, a patient with normal atria should be encouraged to have intrinsic atrial activity along with 100% ventricular pacing.) One way to encourage atrial activity is to program a relatively low base rate. For example, if a CRT device is programmed to a base rate of 40 pulses/min, then any atrial activity > 40 beats/min will inhibit the atrial output. If the patient's atria reliably beat at around 60 beats/min and the device is in a tracking mode (DDD), the ventricles will be paced at the intrinsic atrial rate. Should the atria not beat on their own, the ventricles would still be paced at 40 beats/min.

Patients with intermittent atrial tachyarrhythmias should use a mode-switching algorithm to prevent rapid ventricular pacing in response to high intrinsic atrial rates. Even short runs of this can be uncomfortable for the patient. Ironically, it is usually the rapid ventricular pacing which provokes symptoms in these instances, not the atrial tachyarrhythmia!

Patients with chronic atrial tachyarrhythmias or permanent AF should not be programmed to a dual-chamber tracking mode. A patient with chronic AF may be programmed to a VVI mode, while another with more intermittent atrial arrhythmias might benefit from DDI (dual-chamber mode without atrial tracking).

The nuts and bolts of basic programming

- Much of the programming of a cardiac resynchronization therapy (CRT) system relies on similar terms and timing cycles as conventional pacemakers, with one major difference. A conventional pacemaker tries to encourage intrinsic activity. The objective of a CRT device is to get as close to 100% ventricular pacing as possible!
- CRT systems use the same basic parameter settings as conventional pacemakers: base rate, mode, atrioventricular (AV) delay, rate-responsive AV delay, and post-ventricular atrial refractory period. Special features may include rate response and mode switching.
- CRT systems rely on the same functions as conventional pacemakers: the devices sense (pick up intrinsic cardiac signals) and pace (cause the heart to depolarize and contract by delivering an electrical stimulus).
- The ability of an electrical stimulus to depolarize and cause contraction of the heart is called capture. The minimum amount of energy required to do that consistently defines the capture threshold.
- Output pulse energy is defined by two parameters: the pulse amplitude (in voltage) and the pulse width or pulse duration (in milliseconds).
- Capture thresholds should be taken at implant and then at every follow-up visit. Capture thresholds vary over the course of the day and are known to vary considerably over time, in particular with disease progression and drug interactions.
- The permanent output parameters are programmed based on the capture threshold plus a safety margin. The typical capture safety margin is 2:1 or 3:1.
- All three leads in a CRT system have a capture threshold and require output settings. If a capture threshold is 1V at 0.4 ms, permanent values should be programmed to 2V at 0.4 ms or even 3V at 0.4 ms. Note that the right-atrial output settings will typically be lower than the right-ventricular settings and both will usually be lower than the left-ventricular settings.
- Sensing is defined by the sensitivity value (in mV). If the intrinsic cardiac signal in the right ventricle is 2 mV, then sensitivity must be < 2 mV in order for the CRT device to 'see' those signals. Lowering the mV setting increases sensitivity and vice versa.
- The left-ventricular (LV) lead may not sense. Sensing from the right-ventricular (RV) lead alone is adequate for 'ventricular' sensing. Note that some, but not all, CRT systems have RV and LV sensing.
- Many CRT patients suffer from atrial tachyarrhythmias. To prevent tracking high-rate atrial activity, a maximum tracking limit sets the brakes on how fast the ventricles can be paced in response to atrial activity (i.e. 1:1 AV synchrony may be abandoned in order not to pace the ventricles too quickly). Another approach is mode switching, which either turns off atrial tracking (DDD mode switches temporarily to DDI) or turns off the atrial channel (DDD mode switches temporarily to VVI).
- Diagnostic data from the CRT system include stored electrograms, event histograms and other counters. These data provide important information on the one key objective of CRT stimulation: is the device pacing the ventricles 100%?
- Atrial pacing is not a key objective of a CRT system! In fact, if the patient has relatively intact atria, native atrial activity should be encouraged.
- Although rate-responsive CRT systems are available, the role of rate response in advanced heart failure (HF) remains unclear. Many symptomatic HF patients have limited heart rate variability to begin with and may be extremely restricted in terms of physical activities.

Chapter 13

Advanced Programming

Clinicians used to programming conventional pacemakers and implantable cardioverter-defibrillators (ICDs) have an advantage over novices, in that much of the programming uses familiar terms and equipment. However, there is a fundamental shift that can make cardiac resynchronization therapy (CRT) programming challenging for clinicians with extensive device experience. Conventional pacing involves using parameter settings intended to minimize electrical stimulation to the heart and to keep the device on standby as much as possible. CRT is just the opposite. With CRT, the patient derives therapeutic benefit from the device only as long as it is pacing. Thus, the goal of CRT programming is to achieve 100% ventricular pacing.

In order to achieve maximum ventricular pacing, it is imperative to reduce the number of impulses that originate in the atrium (whether paced or sensed) that conduct down to the ventricles, causing a sensed ventricular event. In terms of 'pacing states', these would be AP–VP or AS–VS events. The four states of dual-chamber pacing are AP–VP (atrial paced event followed by ventricular paced event), AP–VS (atrial paced event followed by ventricular sensed event), AS–VP (atrial sensed event followed by ventricular paced event) and AS–VS (atrial sensed event followed by ventricular sensed event). In a conventional pacemaker, an atrial event that conducts naturally to the ventricles is not something you try to avoid! However, for CRT systems, we want to program the device to minimize the chance that an atrial event can conduct.

One way to do this is with basic programming of the AV delay. The rate-responsive AV delay should also be activated, which automatically shortens the paced or sensed AV delay as the patient's intrinsic atrial rate increases. These are basic programming steps which may not be adequate to achieve the goal of 100% ventricular pacing.

Negative AV hysteresis

Negative AV hysteresis is a very valuable feature for CRT patients, but would almost never be used in patients with standard bradycardia pacing indications. In a conventional pacemaker, hysteresis is programmed to encourage intrinsic activity. Negative hysteresis is set up to do precisely the opposite. When activated, the CRT device will look for intrinsic ventricular beats that occur during the AV delay. When the device detects a VS event (intrinsic ventricular event) during the AV delay, it subtracts a programmed value from the measured AP–VS or AS–VS interval. It then maintains that shortened AV delay for the next 32 cycles. If no additional VS events are detected, the device restores the originally programmed AV delay (see Fig.13.1). Negative AV hysteresis frees the clinician from the need to impose permanently an extremely short AV delay on the patient. Thus, a hemodynamically appropriate AV delay can be programmed, rate-responsive AV delay activated (to help manage high native atrial rates), and finally negative AV hysteresis for those instances when high-rate intrinsic ventricular activity may break through.

Refractory periods: PVAB and PVARP

Lead placement in a CRT system can be challenging, and sometimes the implanting physician is forced to accept less than ideal lead positions. This can result in an atrial lead that is placed in such a way that it senses the ventricular output pulses and inappropriately 'thinks' they are intrinsic atrial events. Counting them as sensed atrial events, the CRT device will try to synchronize ventricular paced beats to them. There are two reasons why CRT patients are more susceptible to this phenomenon (some-

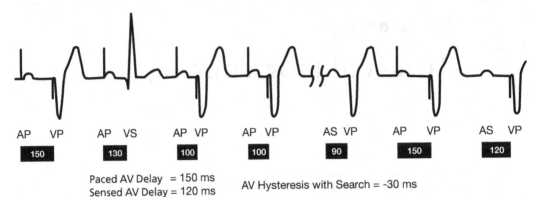

Paced AV Delay   = 150 ms
Sensed AV Delay = 120 ms

AV Hysteresis with Search = -30 ms

Fig. 13.1 Negative AV hysteresis. When the system detects an R-wave, it automatically shortens the AV delay by a programmable value (in this example, 30 ms). If no further sensed ventricular events occur, the device restores the original AV delay after 32 cycles.

times called 'far-field R-wave sensing' or just 'far-R' and also known by an older term, 'crosstalk') than conventional device patients. First, CRT patients are more likely to be frequently paced in the ventricle (more ventricular outputs occur) and second, lead placement may encourage far-R sensing. Fortunately, there is a good way to manage this with a special programming technique.

The parameter PVAB, pre-VAB or pre-ventricular blanking period should be used to minimize far-field R-wave sensing. This parameter 'blanks' the atrial channel for a programmable amount of time just before a ventricular output pulse is delivered. By blanking the atrial channel, the CRT device will not respond to any incoming signals, even if they are strong enough to be detected. A typical pre-VAB

setting might be as brief as 16 ms, but the pre-VAB, combined with the normal post-ventricular atrial refractory period (PVARP) creates enough 'blanking' of the atrial sensing circuits for the ventricular output pulse to be ignored (see Fig. 13.2).

The PVARP is a basic pacemaker parameter which is familiar to most clinicians who work with pacemakers. It refers to the time that the atrial channel is 'blanked' following a ventricular output pulse. In theory, programming the PVARP is easy. But what if the patient has a high intrinsic atrial rate? A high native atrial rate and a long PVARP can result in some atrial sensed events falling into the PVARP, which means they are ignored. For a CRT patient, this means that a native atrial event is not 'tracked' with a paced ventricular event. An intrinsic

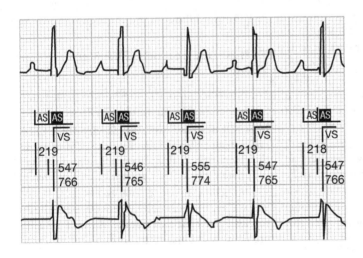

Fig. 13.2 Pre-ventricular atrial blanking (PVAB). The R-waves (sensed ventricular events) are ignored by the atrial channel during PVAB and thus do not affect the rhythm.

ventricular event may follow before the ventricular output pulse can pre-empt it. Thus, programming an appropriate PVARP value requires special consideration. While the PVARP should be long enough to prevent possible far-field R-wave sensing, it must be short enough so that a reasonably timed intrinsic atrial event is still sensed (and can be followed by a ventricular output pulse).

If CRT patients had constant intrinsic atrial rates, this would not be as much of a challenge as it is in real-life clinical practice. CRT patients (like other patients) often have very variable intrinsic atrial rates. With CRT patients, it can be even more severe, since so many heart failure patients have or are in the process of developing atrial fibrillation. For this reason, the notion of a dynamic refractory period came about. To create a refractory period on the atrial channel that could vary with the patient's own intrinsic atrial rates, the rate-responsive PVARP can be programmed. (Do not be confused by the term 'rate-responsive' in this case, which has nothing to do with the activity sensor.) When the patient's native atrial rate exceeds 90 beats/min, the rate-responsive PVARP parameter will automatically reduce the PVARP (shorten the refractory period on the atrial channel). A good programming guideline might be to program rate-responsive PVARP to 'low' to start out. The 'low' setting reduces the PVARP by 1 ms per beat/min > 90. Thus, if the patient suddenly experienced an intrinsic atrial rate of 120 beats/min, the rate-responsive PVARP 'low' setting would automatically reduce the PVARP by 30 ms (120 – 90 is 30). More aggressive settings may be warranted if this is not sufficient.

With all parameter settings, a balancing act is necessary. The danger of going overboard with a very short PVARP setting is that it can open the door to pacemaker-mediated tachycardia (PMT). A PMT is a tachycardia that is actually facilitated by the device.

A PMT requires that the patient has intact retrograde conduction and some sort of triggering event, most commonly a premature ventricular contraction (PVC), atrial undersensing, or loss of atrial capture. Basically, an AS event and its associated ventricular event become dissociated. This dissociated AS event travels backward (retrograde) rather than forward through the heart. The retrograde P-wave is sensed by the atrial sense amplifier, triggering a ven-

tricular event. This starts a vicious circle: cardiac activity now moves forward from atrium to ventricle, then backward from ventricle to atrium. The signals are sensed on the atrial channel and cause pacing. On top of this, the patient may also be experiencing some intrinsic conduction as well. The result is an endless loop tachycardia.

Not all patients have the physiology required to sustain a PMT, but many do. In order for a PMT to occur, the patient needs to have retrograde conduction. This means that conduction in their heart must be able to travel backward from ventricle to atrium. While retrograde conduction is most common in patients with intact AV conduction, there is no reason to assume that just because an impulse cannot travel forward through the heart's conduction pathways it cannot travel backward. There are even patients with complete heart block who have some degree of retrograde conduction!

PMTs involve inappropriate atrial sensing (the atrial channel is sensing real signals, but they are not antegrade atrial events). For conventional pacemaker patients, programming a sufficiently long PVARP is usually a good way to minimize or even prevent PMTs. Unfortunately, for CRT patients, a short PVARP may be more appropriate to help manage high atrial rates. For that reason, the rate-responsive PVARP works well to balance the situation: it shortens the PVARP when the atrial rates are high but does not permanently maintain a PVARP setting that may be too short for the patient over the long term.

There are a few advanced functions in conventional pacemakers which may be of equal value for a CRT patient. These include rate response, rest rate, and a special programmable feature of the auto mode switch algorithm called AMS base rate.

Rate response

Rate response in a cardiac rhythm management system involves some sort of sensor that helps the device assess the patient's perceived metabolic need; this input is used by the device's 'brains' to calculate and then automatically adjust the pacing rate. For example, if the sensor senses that the patient is active, it will automatically increase the base rate. As the patient's activity decreases, the rate slows down accordingly.

By far the most commonly used rate-responsive sensor is the activity sensor, which may be an accelerometer or a piezoelectric crystal. The accelerometer measures forward motion (acceleration) while the piezoelectric crystal measures vibration. Both tie to the patient's activity level. The sensor is contained in the pulse generator; no special leads are required. While there is no such thing as the perfect sensor, these sensors work reasonably well in most patients. Rate-responsive parameters are generally programmed to match the patient's activity level. Very fit, active patients require more aggressive settings than sedentary patients.

Some devices (St Jude Medical systems) offer a rate-responsive parameter option called PASSIVE, which allows the clinician to see how the sensor would have controlled the pacing rate without actually allowing the sensor to drive the rate. The PASSIVE setting is useful in cases where it is unclear if rate response will benefit the patient or what settings are appropriate for that particular patient. When programming rate response is ON, it is important to program a value for the maximum sensor rate parameter (sometimes called Max Sensor or MSR). The MSR defines the highest rate to which the device will stimulate the heart in response to sensor input. For example, if the patient is only somewhat active and does not tolerate paced rates >120 well, an MSR setting could be programmed to 110 pulses/min.

Note that the maximum tracking rate (MTR) and MSR are two different things and go into effect under different conditions. For example, if the MTR is programmed to 130 pulses/min, the ventricle will never be paced over 130 in response to intrinsic atrial activity, even if the native atrial rate exceeds 130 beats/min. If the MSR is programmed to 110 pulses/min, the ventricle will never be paced over 110 pulses/min in response to the activity sensor. This means that the clinician might see ventricular pacing at 125 pulses/min in that patient, but only in response to intrinsic atrial activity (in other words, the MSR 110 pulses/min 'speed limit' would not impact ventricular pacing in response to atrial tracking).

Rest rate

Rest rate may also be useful to enhance the comfort of CRT patients. The theory behind rest rate is to mimic the heart's natural rate slowdown during sleep or periods of profound inactivity. Since CRT patients are frequently stimulated, they may be exposed to 'daytime' or activity-type pacing rates even when they go to sleep. For some patients, this can be very disturbing or at least uncomfortable. Thus, the CRT system is equipped to allow the pacing rate to slow appropriately when the patient goes to sleep.

In some systems, the rest rate is tied to clock time, which is kept by the pulse generator. This method is quite precise; unfortunately, most of us are not quite so precise about the minute we go to bed at night and the minute we wake up. For patients with even slightly erratic schedules or those who travel (time zones can present a problem), this type of rest rate may require frequent modification.

Some devices offer a rest rate feature that is associated with the activity sensor. When the sensor determines that the patient is very inactive (i.e. virtually no sensor input), the device then imposes a preprogrammed rest rate setting, which is low enough to provide patient comfort but not so low that ventricular activity breaks through.

AMS base rate

Another advanced parameter setting involves the AMS base rate. Auto mode switch (see Chapter 12) essentially turns off atrial tracking in the presence of high-rate intrinsic atrial activity. The clinician defines what 'high-rate intrinsic activity' is for the patient by programming an atrial cut-off rate. One problem is that when the system switches mode, it goes back to the programmed base rate. Since the high atrial rate probably increased the ventricular pacing rate (atrial tracking), this can be experienced by the patient as a 'bump' or an unpleasant, sudden rate drop. For that reason, it is often useful to program a different base rate for AMS episodes. This rate should be slightly higher than the normal base rate, but not so high that the patient experiences it as uncomfortable.

For example, if the CRT device was programmed to mode switch at 180 beats/min (atrial rate), the ventricular rate was very close to 180 beats/min at the point of the mode switch. If the normal base rate was programmed to 70 pulses/min, then the patient would switch from near 180 pulses/min ventricular pacing to 70 pulses/min ventricular pacing in a single beat. An AMS base rate of 100 pulses/min could be programmed so that when a mode switch episode occurs, the patient goes from near 180 pulses/min rate to 100 pulses/min. When the atrial rate returns to normal, the base rate will go back to the original 70 pulses/min (see Fig. 13.3).

Diagnostic data

Following a CRT patient involves checking to see how much CRT stimulation is occurring. There are many diagnostic features that can make follow-up more effective. In the previous chapter, we talked about the event histogram. Another useful, but more advanced diagnostic function is the AV interval histogram. This counter tabulates the length of the paced or sensed AV delay in milliseconds and then groups them by ranges. If rate-responsive AV delay is programmed on, expect to see some variation in the AV delay values. The histogram shows which values occur most frequently; this information can help with future programming decisions. The clinician should also be on the lookout for AV delay values that change over time, as this may indicate the need to adjust some programmed values.

If rate response is active and the activity sensor is programmed to ON or PASSIVE, diagnostic data are captured in the sensor-indicated rate histogram. This graph and counter histogram shows how the sensor actually controlled the rate (if the sensor is ON) or would have controlled the rate (if the sensor is PASSIVE). It captures paced activity by rate ranges under sensor drive. The sensor-indicated rate histogram provides clinicians with input on how to best program the sensor settings.

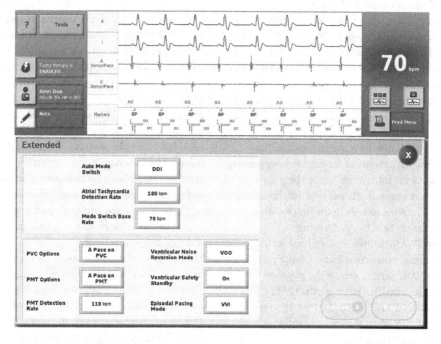

Fig. 13.3 Auto mode switch parameters. The clinician can program the mode desired in the presence of high-rate intrinsic atrial activity (auto mode switch), the cut off atrial rate (atrial tachycardia detection rate), and an interim mode switch base rate. In this example, if the patient's atrial rate exceeds 180 beats/min, the device will switch to DDI pacing at 70 pulses/min.

The nuts and bolts of advanced programming

- Cardiac resynchronization therapy (CRT) programming is intended to encourage 100% ventricular pacing; in this way, it is a different approach from programming a conventional pacemaker.
- Negative AV hysteresis encourages maximal ventricular pacing by automatically shortening the AV delay in the presence of a sensed ventricular event.
- Rate-responsive AV delay automatically shortens the AV delay when the patient's intrinsic atrial rate increases. This mimics healthy cardiac behavior. Note that 'rate-responsive' in this sense does not refer to the activity sensor.
- The pre-ventricular atrial blanking (PVAB) period allows the atrial channel to be blanked for a very short period immediately before a ventricular output pulse is delivered; this along with the post-ventricular atrial refractory period (PVARP) helps prevent far-field R-wave sensing. Far-field R-wave sensing occurs when the atrial sense amplifier picks up the ventricular output pulse and inappropriately 'thinks' it is an intrinsic atrial event.
- CRT patients may be more susceptible than conventional patients to far-field R-wave sensing in that pacing leads often have to be placed where it is anatomically possible and beneficial for CRT, not necessarily in the best location to minimize far-field R-wave sensing.
- A short PVARP setting is often beneficial to maximize ventricular pacing, but a very short PVARP setting can set the stage for pacemaker-mediated tachycardia (PMT). Rate-responsive PVARP allows the PVARP to shorten automatically when the patient's intrinsic atrial rate exceeds 90 beats/min.
- PMTs can occur only in patients with intact retrograde conduction. Not all patients have this. Although unusual, some patients with poor or even non-existent antegrade (forward) conduction may have viable retrograde conduction pathways!
- Some CRT patients will benefit from sensor-driven rate response, which relies on an activity sensor to help drive the pacing rate. If the sensor detects that the patient is active, the pacing rate will automatically increase.
- The maximum sensor rate (MSR) is the highest rate at which the device will pace the ventricles in response to activity sensor input. It is programmed and functions independently of the maximum tracking rate (MTR). In other words, a CRT device can have different MSR and MTR settings.
- A special function called rest rate can automatically lower the pacing rate during sleep or rest. Rest rate may be controlled by the pulse generator's internal clock (which sets specific, clock-based sleep and wake times) or it may be controlled by the activity sensor. When the activity sensor tells the pulse generator that the patient is inactive, the rest rate takes over.
- Auto mode switching (AMS) can employ a programmable AMS base rate, which allows an interim base rate to take over during mode switch episodes. The AMS base rate prevents large rate bumps when the device goes from tracking a high atrial rate back down to the regular base rate (for example, it might go from tracking an atrial rate of 120 beats/min and pacing around 120 pulses/min in the ventricle down to the base rate of 60 beats/min in one beat).
- Diagnostic data can help assess CRT function and assist the clinician in future programming choices. The event histogram shows the cardiac events and the percentage paced (100% ventricular pacing is the goal). The AV interval histogram shows the AV delay values and can also be useful. The sensor-indicated rate histogram shows how the sensor controls the rate (if the sensor is ON) or would have controlled the rate (if the sensor is PASSIVE).

Chapter 14

Basic ECG Interpretation for CRT Systems

All device therapy relies on the surface ECG for quick, reliable assessment of system function. For any device, an ECG test should be done in the acute phase, to verify proper capture and sensing, and further ECG evaluations should occur during regular follow-up sessions. However, the cardiac resynchronization therapy (CRT) device presents some challenges in ECG interpretation, even for those experienced in analyzing ECGs from conventional pacemakers and implantable cardioverter-defibrillators (ICDs).

A surface ECG measures electrical activity between two poles on the body. The standard three-lead ECG configuration (which is suitable for most CRT systems) places the poles as shown in Table 14.1. This may also be seen in Eintoven's triangle (see Fig. 14.1).

Any cardiac rhythm management device provides electrical stimulation to the heart which travels in a certain direction or vector. How that energy gets translated to the ECG tracing depends on how the depolarization front (the energy of the waveform) hits the positive pole of the ECG lead (see Fig. 14.2). When the depolarization front moves toward the positive pole, the ECG will show a positive inflection. When the depolarization front moves away from the positive pole, the ECG will show a negative deflection (see Fig. 14.3).

The fundamentals of ECG interpretation for CRT patients involve understanding these vectors (movements) and their relationship to lead placement. In a healthy, unpaced heart, the main vector of the depolarization front proceeds from atrium downward through the ventricles. This appears on a Lead I ECG as a positive R-wave but on a Lead III ECG as a slightly negative R-wave. This is because the vector of the depolarization front is traveling more positively with respect to Lead I (see Fig. 14.4).

In conventional or right-ventricular (RV) pacing, the vector of depolarization travels upward from the ventricle. Depending on where the stimulating electrode of the RV pacing lead is located, the vector may be neutral or isoelectric with respect to Lead I, or it may be somewhat positive or somewhat nega-

Table 14.1

Lead	Positive pole	Negative pole
I	Left arm (black)	Right arm (white)
II	Right leg (green)	Right arm (white)
III	Left leg (red)	Left arm (black)

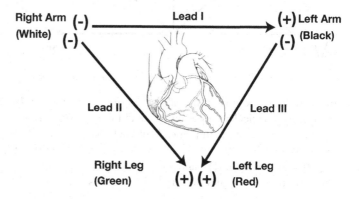

Fig. 14.1 Einthoven's triangle. This is a good visual representation of the leads, poles and direction of current flow in a standard three-lead ECG.

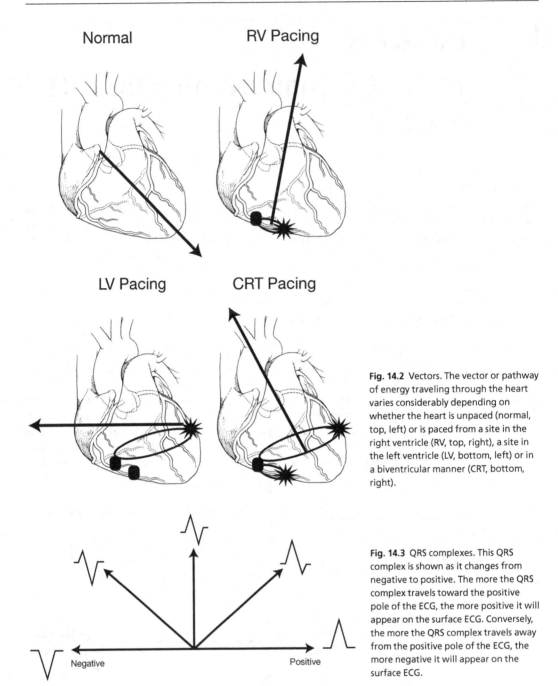

Fig. 14.2 Vectors. The vector or pathway of energy traveling through the heart varies considerably depending on whether the heart is unpaced (normal, top, left) or is paced from a site in the right ventricle (RV, top, right), a site in the left ventricle (LV, bottom, left) or in a biventricular manner (CRT, bottom, right).

Fig. 14.3 QRS complexes. This QRS complex is shown as it changes from negative to positive. The more the QRS complex travels toward the positive pole of the ECG, the more positive it will appear on the surface ECG. Conversely, the more the QRS complex travels away from the positive pole of the ECG, the more negative it will appear on the surface ECG.

tive. (An isoelectric or neutral Lead I tracing would occur if the ventricular output hit the Lead I positive-to-negative continuum perpendicularly.) (See Fig. 14.5)

With left-ventricular (LV) and no RV pacing, the depolarization vector goes from right to left. This vector of depolarization will show up on Lead I as strongly negative, since it is heading almost directly toward the negative pole of Lead I (see Fig. 14.6). Biventricular pacing or CRT creates an overall pattern of energy flow that originates from the RV and LV regions and proceeds upward. The flow of en-

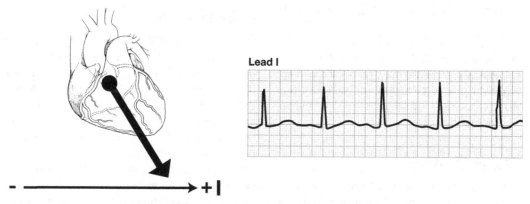

Fig. 14.4 Lead I in an unpaced heart. The poles of Lead I are indicated with respect to the vector of the depolarization front. Note that the resulting ECG tracings show a positive R-wave. This particular rhythm is a normal, unpaced beat.

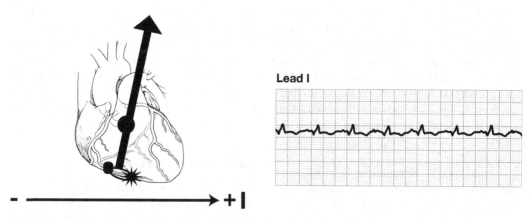

Fig. 14.5 Lead I during right-ventricular (RV) pacing. In RV pacing, the depolarization front moves from the ventricles upward. Depending on where it hits the Lead I line, the R-wave on Lead I may appear slightly positive, slightly negative or even neutral (isoelectric) if it hits perpendicularly. Note that the exact placement of the stimulating electrodes can have considerable impact on the surface ECGs.

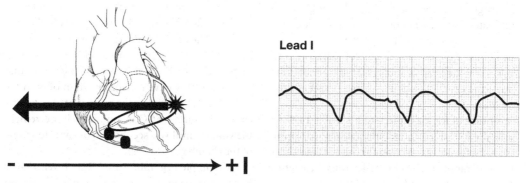

Fig. 14.6 Lead I during left-ventricular (LV) pacing. This heart is paced only from the left ventricle, meaning that the depolarization front is traveling from left to right. This will often show up on Lead I as a negative R-wave.

ergy affects ECG morphology in Lead I as somewhat isoelectric or negative.

These basic depolarization vectors are good examples of 'textbook' ECGs you are unlikely to encounter in real clinical practice. A CRT system is a combination of RV and LV pacing, which commences about midway down the ventricles and proceeds upward.

Capture testing

Most CRT devices available today have independent outputs, i.e. the LV and RV pulse amplitudes and pulse durations may be programmed separately. When assessing capture during the acute or follow-up phase, capture loss is determined independently for each ventricle.

For modern devices with independent outputs, a separate capture test is done for each chamber, that is, there is an atrial capture test, an RV capture test, and an LV capture test. The ventricular capture tests can be conducted in the DDD mode, which maintains the benefits of AV synchrony throughout the test. One disadvantage to threshold testing in the DDD mode is that merely reducing the pacing rate is not always enough to guarantee loss of capture.

Capture tests can be conducted semi-automatically with the programmer device, which follows a step-down protocol. The clinician sets up the test by specifying chamber, mode, and other information on the programmer (see Fig. 14.7). The device runs through the test automatically and provides the capture threshold information. Note that the test can be observed on Lead I and II surface ECGs as well as on atrial and ventricular channel electrograms. Below the tracings, the programmer annotates events. Annotations always reveal how the device 'sees' events, not what the events truly are. Thus, the clinician should compare the tracings (what the heart is doing) with the annotations (what the device 'thinks' it is doing) to see if there are mismatches.

A printout for the capture test (see Fig. 14.8) reveals the four tracings and annotations. The printout is useful documentation for the patient's chart. The programmer may also make available capture data in a trend format (see Fig. 14.9)

Unipolar LV leads

A unipolar LV lead is one that has one distal (tip) electrode. In a CRT-D system, this means the lead paces by forming an electrical circuit from the LV tip to the RV ring electrode or from the LV tip to the RV coil, depending on the device and the type of lead in place. A CRT-D device with a unipolar LV lead will not form an electrical circuit from LV tip to can, because the device functions as an ICD.

While pacing from a unipolar LV lead in a CRT system does not normally pose a problem, there are instances of anodal stimulation. Anodal stimulation occurs when pacing from the LV tip (negative pole or cathode) to the RV ring (positive pole or anode) can actually cause the anode (RV ring electrode) to capture the tissue surrounding it. This may make it difficult to conduct an LV capture test, because LV pacing with anodal RV stimulation can cause both ventricles to contract, even though only LV pacing is going on. Anodal stimulation is usually seen at higher output settings and poses no threat to the patient. However, anodal pacing should be considered, particularly in cases where the device is programmed to pace the LV before the RV (see Fig. 14.10).

Tied output devices

While CRT systems manufactured today offer independent RV and LV outputs, in clinical practice, you may encounter older 'tied output' devices. A tied output occurs when the LV lead and RV lead share the same pacing pulse and sensing circuit. A tied output system may be the result of hardwiring in the device itself or it may be that LV and RV leads were connected together using a special adapter.

In a tied output device, the pacing output travels from the device to both LV and RV leads simultaneously. The output is the same for both leads (for example, a 5-V pulse amplitude setting means both leads receive a 5-V output pulse). It also means that the measured R wave is a combination of both the LV and RV. To determine the capture of each ventricle, use the surface ECG as you gradually decrement the voltage until you see the loss of capture in one of the chambers.

For example, beginning with CRT or biventricular (BV) pacing, step-down the output until the device

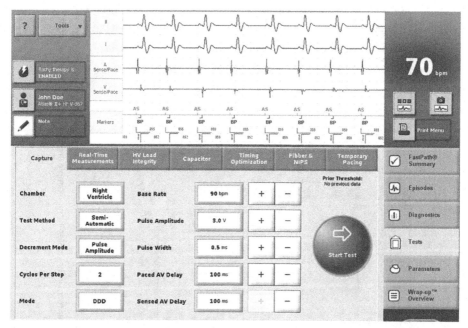

Fig. 14.7 Right-ventricular (RV) threshold test in a cardiac resynchronization therapy (CRT) system. The clinician specifies capture test information on the programmer which conducts the test semi-automatically. The programmer provides Lead I and Lead II surface ECG tracings, as well as atrial and ventricular channel electrograms.

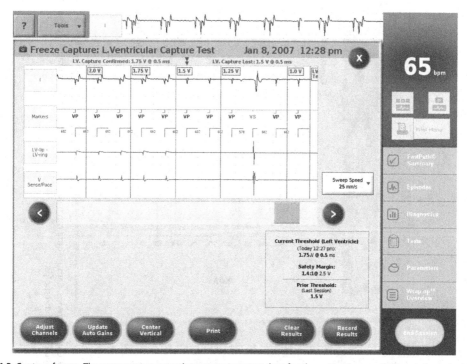

Fig. 14.8 Capture freeze. The programmer can print out capture test data for the patient's record. The printout provides four tracings (Lead I and II surface ECGs and atrial plus ventricular electrograms) and detailed annotations.

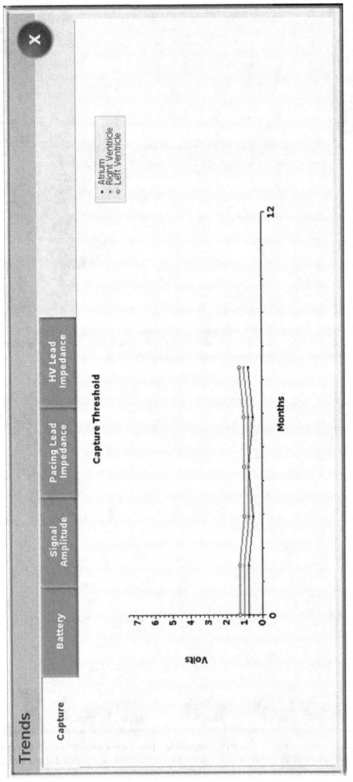

Fig. 14.9 Capture trends. Capture data can be viewed as trends over time in graphic format. Note that left ventricular thresholds in this example are consistently higher than right ventricular or atrial thresholds.

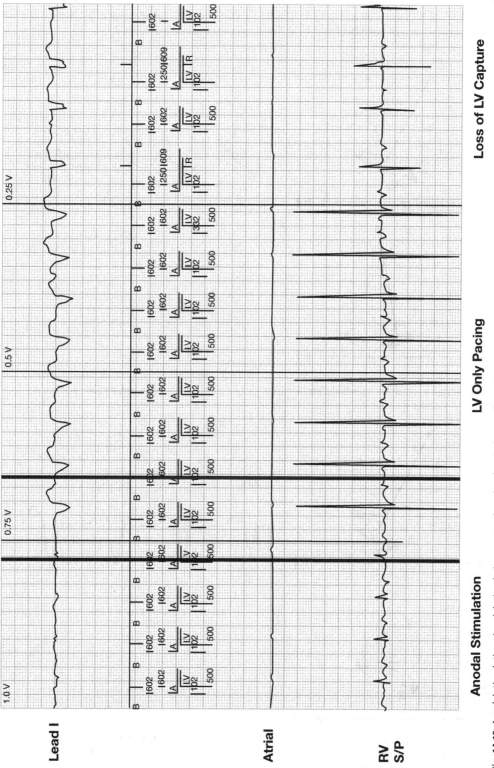

Fig. 14.10 Anodal stimulation. Anodal stimulation occurs when the electrical circuit formed by a unipolar left-ventricular (LV) lead causes anodal tissue (around the right-ventricular (RV) ring electrode) to depolarize, leading to an RV contraction. In this example, anodal stimulation appears, followed by LV-only pacing and then a loss of LV capture.

transitions from BV to single-chamber ventricular pacing, e.g. BV to RV pacing only (Fig. 14.11). Since the capture thresholds of chambers may be differ-ent, it may be that the RV loses capture first. In such a case, the clinician would see BV pacing transition to LV pacing only (Fig. 14.12).

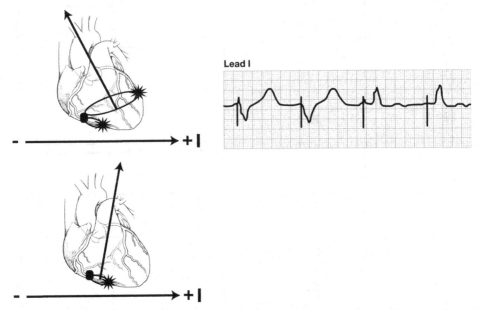

Fig. 14.11 Biventricular (BV) to right-ventricular (RV) pacing. In this example, the tied-output device begins with BV pacing but, as outputs are stepped down gradually, left-ventricular capture is lost. At that point, only RV pacing occurs.

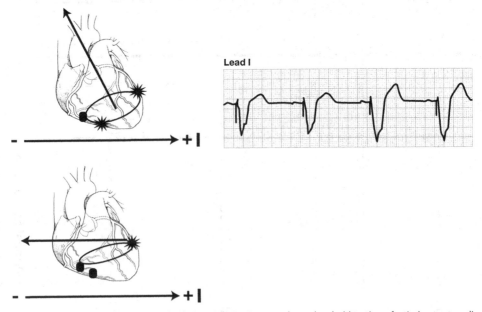

Fig. 14.12 Biventricular (BV) to left-ventricular (LV) pacing. During step-down threshold testing of a tied output cardiac resynchronization therapy device, it may be that right-ventricular capture is lost first. In this example, the device transitions from BV to LV pacing only.

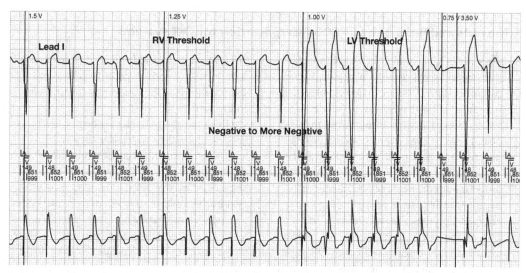

Fig. 14.13 Morphology changes during capture testing. A tied-output cardiac resynchronization therapy (CRT) system with the ECG set up as Lead I goes from negative to more negative, indicating that biventricular (true CRT) pacing was lost as the right-ventricular (RV) lead lost capture. All capture was lost at 0.75 V, meaning that the left-ventricular (LV) threshold was 1.0 V. Typically, the RV threshold is lower than the LV threshold, but this is not always the case!

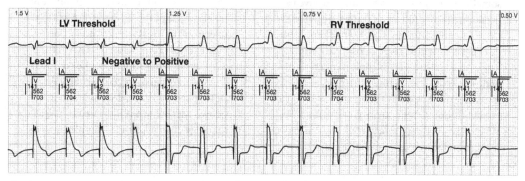

Fig. 14.14 Capture test. In this capture test, the ECG is set up as Lead I; the bottom tracing shows the intracardiac electrogram (IEGM). The annotations show just A and V markers, since this is an older tied-ouput system and both ventricles respond as one unit. The morphology change in Lead I at 1.25 V shows that there was some sort of significant change. Since the morphology of the QRS went from negative to positive, stimulation went from cardiac resynchronization therapy to right-ventricular (RV) only. This means left-ventricular capture was lost at 1.25 V. Pacing continues, meaning that there was still viable RV pacing at 1.25 V. In fact, RV pacing continues until all pacing is lost at 0.50 V, meaning that the RV threshold is 0.75 V

Capture threshold test tracings for tied output systems may look like those shown in Figs 14.13 and 14.14.

Although distinctly different than ECG analysis for conventional pacemakers and ICDs, analysis of CRT tracings relies on the same fundamentals: a good knowledge of basic electrocardiography, an ability to see morphologies and discern patterns, and a sense of depolarization movement. Devic-es with tied outputs offer ECGs that may show a couple of changes in waveforms as capture is lost in one chamber before the other. Today's devices with independently programmable LV and RV outputs allow clinicians to conduct separate capture threshold tests. When analyzing CRT tracings or any tracing, it is important to remember that devices can really only do two things: pace and sense.

The nuts and bolts of basic ECG interpretation for CRT systems

- A surface ECG measures electrical conduction from a positive pole to a negative pole. The ECG or intracardiac electrogram captures the movement of the depolarization wavefront (vector) toward or away from the positive pole. The more the vector moves in a positive direction, the more positive the deflections on the tracing. Conversely, the more the vector moves toward the negative pole, the more negative the deflections on the tracing.
- For most purposes, a Lead I and Lead III ECG or a surface ECG set up as Lead I and an intracardiac electrogram suffice for CRT ECG evaluation. Sometimes other leads are required; a 12-lead ECG may even be needed for more precise evaluations.
- When looking at an ECG from a cardiac resynchronization therapy (CRT) system, sometimes changes in the tracing (positive to negative; positive to more positive; negative to more negative) indicate significant changes in device performance, such as loss of capture.
- The actual vectors seen in clinical practice vary with where the stimulating electrodes are placed in the heart. Thus, every CRT patient's ECG can be slightly different in polarity.
- When true CRT pacing occurs, the vector moves upward and shows up as negative deflections of the QRS on both Lead I and Lead III tracings. The degree of negativity in these deflections will depend on where the lead electrodes are located in the heart.
- CRT devices may have independently programmable left-ventricular (LV) and right-ventricular (RV) outputs which allow for individual LV and RV threshold tests, or they may have 'tied' ventricular outputs which require the clinician to program (and test) both ventricular leads as one unit. As a general rule, older devices offer tied ventricular outputs while newer systems offer independent LV and RV outputs.
- RV and LV pacing thresholds may be the same but are often different, with the LV threshold typically higher than the RV threshold.
- Unipolar LV leads may produce anodal pacing, which occurs when the electrical circuit from the tip electrode of the LV lead connects to the ring electrode of the RV lead. Anodal pacing may sometimes occur before loss of capture in a CRT system, but should not be confused with true CRT pacing. In general, the shift from true CRT pacing to anodal stimulation in a step-down capture test is indicated by a QRS morphology change prior to complete loss of capture.

Chapter 15

CRT System Optimization

Cardiac resynchronization therapy (CRT) uses electrical energy to try to synchronize the mechanical contractions of the heart. The art and science of adjusting the electrical timing parameters in such a way that it improves the mechanical performance of the heart is called timing optimization. For patients who fail to respond to CRT or who derive some, but not maximal, benefit from their CRT device, timing optimization may be the best solution.

CRT systems impact the intricate split-second timing of atrial and ventricular systole and diastole. In a healthy heart, there is a sufficiently long period of ventricular diastole to allow for the atrial contribution to ventricular filling. Ventricular systole should occur promptly, but not so soon that it cuts off diastole. In fact, some experts are advancing the notion that, for certain patients, a CRT device's primary benefit is improving diastolic function![1]

Furthermore, left and right ventricles should contract together (interventricular contraction) and the left ventricle should contract as a unified whole rather than in segments or waves (intraventricular contraction). These are mechanical processes which are controlled in the CRT patient by some seemingly simple parameters: the atrioventricular (AV) delay and the ventricular-ventricular (VV) timing.

Echocardiography is often used to help clinicians better visualize how CRT timing maps onto the physical activities of the heart. Echocardiography relies on a transducer which shoots sound waves that penetrate soft tissue and then return (or 'echo') to the imaging platform at different speeds. The echo image is a visual representation of how these sound waves bounced back, which helps clinicians visualize what's going on with soft tissue.

One common type of echo used on CRT patients is called two-dimensional (2-D) or 'real-time' echo. Although 2-D echos generate individual images, they can be created so quickly that the clinician can see a 'real-time' impression of how the heart is beating. While 2-D imaging is very commonly used, it gives a flat, two-dimensional image that takes a bit of practice to interpret. The 2-D image will reveal the main landmarks of the heart (e.g. the chambers, septum, and valves). The 'real-time' flow of images will show how the ventricles contract (together or independently), when the valves open and close.

The ideal mechanical sequence is for the onset of the left-ventrivular (LV) contraction to occur precisely at the peak of the left-atrial (LA) systolic event. In systole, the mitral valve should be closed; in diastole, the mitral valve should open. Conversely, the aortic valve should be closed during diastole but open in systole.

Another type of echocardiography involves motion mode or M-mode. M-mode uses just a single sector of the 2-D image to display cardiac motion more rapidly. M-mode is oriented around a 'sampling line' (which may appear as a dotted white line on the echo) and the movement of all cardiac structures along the sampling line are displayed. M-mode gives a sense of depth as well as motion.

Color-flow Doppler assigns color codes to help illustrate the flow of blood within a sampled area, based on both blood flow direction and speed. The standard color scale shows blood traveling toward the transducer as red, while blood flowing away from the transducer is blue. The color is more extreme the faster the blood is traveling. Color-flow Doppler can be extremely useful in identifying mitral regurgitation.

Spectral Doppler, sometimes called pulsed wave Doppler, also measures blood flow velocity but at specific points in the heart. For instance, a clinician might use a pulsed wave Doppler to determine how fast blood is flowing through the mitral valve.

Echocardiography can be very useful in assessing systolic function, including determining ejection fraction values and stroke volumes. Echo is also a useful tool in optimizing AV delay timing in a CRT system using what is known as the iterative method.

The ideal AV delay for a CRT patient is one that allows for complete atrial kick, that is, for the atria to fully contract (and contribute optimally to the filling of the ventricles) before the onset of ventricular systole. On Doppler echo, these events show up as E waves and A waves. The E wave describes the passive filling of the ventricles, that is, this is the time period during which blood pours into the relaxed ventricles (ventricular diastole). The A wave describes the physical contraction of the atria, that is, atrial systole. Thus, the E wave occurs first, followed by the A wave (atrial kick) and then the ventricular contraction. This ventricular contraction is sometimes called an isovolumetric contraction because the volume of blood within the ventricles remains static; no more new blood flows into the ventricles during the isovolumetric contraction. Likewise, the isovolumetric relaxation of the ventricles describes the time when the ventricles relax prior to any new inflow of blood (see Fig. 15.1).

The E and A waves may fuse on the echo, which occurs when the atrial contribution to ventricular filling is inappropriately reduced. A fused A and E wave also increases the chance that mitral regurgitation might occur during the ventricular diastole. Last but not least, when the E and A wave bump into each other, diastolic filling time is reduced (see Fig. 15.2). When there is E and A fusion on a Doppler echo, changing the AV delay can help to separate them and improve cardiac function.

When optimizing the AV delay with Doppler echo, the goal is to set the sensed and paced AV delay intervals to the shortest time possible that allows for complete active filling of the ventricles, that is, the shortest sensed and paced AV delays that permit a complete and distinct E and A wave to appear. The iterative test uses a step-down protocol from a relatively high value (typically around 220ms), decreasing in 10 or 20ms steps, until the A wave changes visibly.

At 200 or 220ms, the E and A wave should be fused. As the AV delay times are decreased, the E and A wave will start to separate. Since the goal is to find the shortest possible AV delay settings, the step-down protocol continues. It should stop when the A wave undergoes a change in morphology called 'truncation.' Truncation occurs when the A wave starts to get slightly shorter and flatter. An ideal A

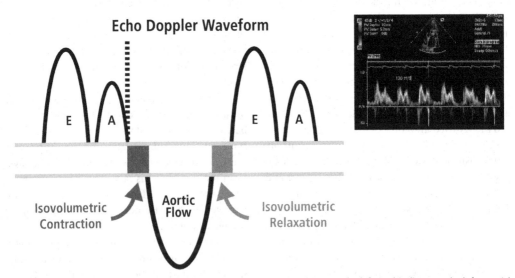

Fig. 15.1 The E and A wave on the Doppler echo can be diagrammed as shown to the left. In this diagram, the left ventricle fills passively with blood (E wave) and completes this process before the left atrial contraction (A wave) commences. The A wave completes before a pause that represents the isovolumetric contraction of the left ventricle. Following the isovolumetric contraction of the left ventricle, blood is pumped out into the body (aortic outflow). *Image used by permission from Dr. Prakash Desai MD, Amarillo Heart Group, Amarillo, Texas, USA.*

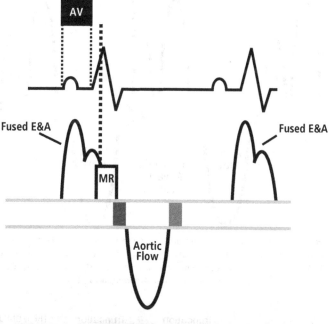

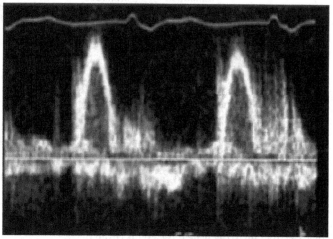

Fig. 15.2 A fused E and A wave on an echo indicates that there is less time for the atrial contribution to ventricular filling and less time for ventricular diastole. Both may reduce the amount of blood that flows into the left ventricle, compromising cardiac output. Furthermore, E and A wave fusion also increases the likelihood of mitral valve regurgitation. *Image used by permission from Dr. Prakash Desai MD, Amarillo Heart Group, Amarillo, Texas, USA.*

wave is symmetrical in that its upslope has the same morphology as its downslope. A truncated A wave will start to show a steeper downslope with some flattening (see Fig. 15.3 and Fig. 15.4).

However, there are some very real limitations to the use of echo as an optimization technique. Firstly, echos are a time-consuming procedure that requires special equipment and trained personnel. Not all device experts are adept at interpreting echo results. Since echos are expensive procedures, it is not practical to use them routinely. For that reason, new algorithms within the

device are helping to meet the challenge of timing optimization.

One timing algorithm (QuickOpt™ algorithm from St. Jude Medical) uses the intracardiac electrogram from the implanted CRT device to optimize timing. A few studies have found that this algorithm correlates closely to the optimization results for AV and VV timing obtained by echocardiography.[2,3]

The QuickOpt™ algorithm was based on the notion that certain mechanical events corresponded to specific portions of the electrogram. While echocardiography can help show the clinician those events

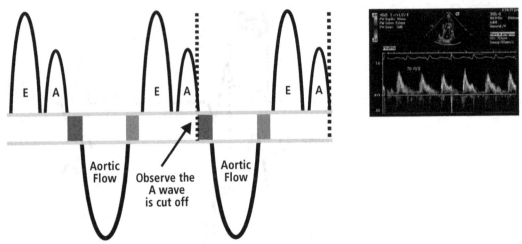

Fig. 15.3 A step-down test from a high AV delay will start with fused E and A waves, then progress to separate E and A waves and finally start to show a separate E and A waves with A wave truncation. Truncation, which shows up as a change in A wave morphology, occurs when the A wave is cut off by isolvolumetric contraction. *Image used by permission from Dr. Prakash Desai MD, Amarillo Heart Group, Amarillo, Texas, USA.*

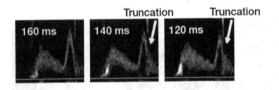

Fig. 15.4 In this echo, the E and A wave are separate at 160 ms, but the A wave undergoes changes in morphology (truncation) at 140 ms which become more pronounced at 120 ms. Specifically, the downslope of the A wave gets steeper and a bit flatter. An ideal A wave is symmetrical, with the upslope and downslope showing the same morphology.

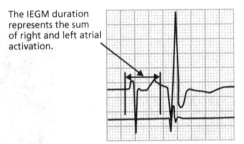

The IEGM duration represents the sum of right and left atrial activation.

Fig. 15.5 AV optimization with QuickOpt™ algorithm. The intracardiac electrogram obtained from the implanted cardiac resynchronization therapy device looks at the local activation of the right atrium and far-field activation of the left atrium. The duration of this P-wave can be used to determine mitral valve closure, which, in turn, is used to calculate the optimal AV delay setting for an individual patient.

with respect to the device's timing cycles, the Quick-Opt™ algorithm uses key landmarks on the intracardiac electrogram to calculate those events (from the P-wave duration and peak of the R-wave) and from there, determine optimal AV timing (see Fig. 15.5).

The algorithm also handles VV timing optimization, that is, setting up ventricular output timing to allow the right and left ventricles to depolarize and contract simultaneously. It uses the intracardiac electrogram to determine interventricular conduction delays by looking at the peak of the R-wave in the right ventricle (RV) versus the peak of the R-wave in the LV. The algorithm then calculates the appropriate offset value so that the CRT device can stimulate the RV and LV in such a way that they contract simultaneously (see Fig. 15.6).

Using this algorithm gives a 97.69% correlation between algorithm results and results obtained by echocardiography (specifically, aortic VTI).[4] The algorithm is accessed by the programmer; the procedure runs semi-automatically. Once the algorithm is initiated, it performs an atrial sensing test, a ventricular sensing test, and an RV pacing test. These tests complete without clinician intervention and take about a minute.

The ease and convenience of this algorithm should allow for timing optimization to become a regular part of any follow-up. Currently, optimiza-

Fig. 15.6 VV Optimization with QuickOpt™ algorithm. The noninvasive test performs paced and sensed tests to obtain the times at which each ventricle depolarizes and contracts. The goal is to have both ventricles contract simultaneously, so the algorithm calculates the appropriate offset value so that the cardiac resynchronization therapy system can stimulate the right and left ventricles in such a way that they contract together.

Delays between right and left ventricular depolarization are measured and offsets are calculated. The goal is to time the right and left ventricular activation so that the paced wavefronts meet near the ventricular septum.

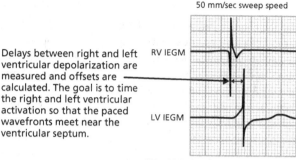

50 mm/sec sweep speed

RV IEGM

LV IEGM

RV to LV Interval = 100 ms (RV followed by LV)

tion by echocardiography is done only in patients who are clearly not responding as expected to CRT and then only about once a year, at the most. However, there is evidence that timing cycles change over time in CRT patients, sometimes in a matter of days. One study found that VV timing delays tend to get progressively shorter, while AV delays tend to do the opposite over time.[5]

References

1 Morris-Thurgood JA, Turner MS, Nightingale AK *et al.* Pacing in heart failure: improved ventricular interac-

tion in diastole rather than systolic re-synchronization. *Europace* 2000; **2:** 271-5.

2 Meine TJ. IEGM based method for estimating optimal VV delay in cardiac resynchronization therapy. *Europace* 2004; **6:** (#149/2).

3 Porterfield *et al.* Device based intracardiac delay optimization versus echo in ICD patients (Acute IEGM AV and PV Study). *Europace* 2006; **8:** (6178).

4 Meine TJ. An intracardiac EGM method for VV optimization during cardiac resynchronization therapy. *Heart Rhythm Journal* 2006; **3:** (AB30-5).

5 O'Donnell D, Nadurata V, Hamer A, *et al.* Long-term variations in optimal programming of cardiac resynchronization therapy devices. *PACE* 2005; **28:** S24-S26.

The nuts and bolts of CRT system optimization

- Optimizing the cardiac resynchronization therapy (CRT) system means adjusting the electrical parameters to impact the mechanical activities (contracting and relaxing) of the heart. This primarily involves setting appropriate values for the timing cycles of atrioventricular (AV) delay and ventricular-ventricular (VV) timing.
- The electrical activation of the heart can be evaluated on a surface ECG, or intracardiac electrogram. However, what is going on electrically may not necessarily match what is going on mechanically. Timing optimization is designed to help align electrical stimulation with the contractions and relaxations of the heart muscle.
- One commonly used method for timing optimization is echocardiography. The most

commonly used types are two-dimensional (2D or 'real time'), motion modality (M-mode), color Doppler echo or spectral Doppler.
- The echo will reveal an E wave and an A wave, which ideally should be distinct (not fused) and complete (not truncated). The E wave represents the diastole (passive filling of the ventricles) while the A wave represents the atrial systole (atrial kick). The AV delay controls the timing of these waves in a CRT patient.
- The optimal AV delay should be as short as possible while allowing for a complete E and A wave. Timing optimization using echo involves a step-down or iterative test from a high AV delay (for instance, 220 ms) down to the lowest AV delay that permits appropriate E and A waveforms.

Continued p. 106.

Continued.

- When the E and A wave are fused, the atria contract before the ventricles have completed their passive filling with blood; this cuts short ventricular diastole.
- When the A wave is truncated, the full atrial contribution to ventricular filling is not received. An ideal A wave has a symmetrical morphology, that is, the upslope and downslope are the same shape. A truncated A wave typically has a sharper, steeper, and possibly flatter downslope.
- A new algorithm uses the intracardiac electrogram obtained from the implanted device to calculate optimal AV delay values and optimal VV timing. This algorithm (QuickOpt™ algorithm, St. Jude Medical) runs a semi-automatic test that takes about a minute to determine optimal timing values. No echo is required.
- The QuickOpt™ algorithm uses the duration of the P-wave (interatrial conduction time) to determine mitral valve closure and thus the optimal sensed and paced AV delay settings. The algorithm uses the peak of the R-wave in the RV and LV to determine the offset between these contractions and thus recommend the optimal VV timing.
- Since QuickOpt™ is not as elaborate, expensive, or involved as echocardiography, it may be used more frequently in CRT patients and on all CRT patients. Currently, echocardiography is typically performed only in so-called 'non-responders' and then only occasionally.
- Timing optimization should be performed frequently, in that timing cycles can vary in patients and tend to change over time. One study suggests that AV delays tend to get longer over time, while VV delays get shorter. This study further discovered that timing cycles change frequently, sometimes in a matter of days or weeks!

Chapter 16

Troubleshooting the Non-Responder

While clinical studies have shown that most patients indicated for cardiac resynchronization therapy (CRT) derive significant clinical benefits from having a CRT device, there is a rather small but important subset of patients that do not seem to improve with a CRT system.[1,2] When a hopeful heart failure (HF) patient receives a CRT system and then fails to improve or even deteriorates further, this can confound clinicians. With a systematic approach to managing non-responders, many of them can be converted to responders (and some minimally responsive patients can be made more responsive). While this systematic approach does not guarantee that all non-responders will improve, it does address several of the key concerns that seem to separate responders from non-responders.

From large randomized clinical studies, we know that patients with New York Heart Association (NYHA) Class III or IV HF, a QRS duration > 120 ms, a left ventricular ejection fraction (LVEF) of ≤ 35% and an LVEDD of ≥ 55 mm are indicated for CRT device therapy. Most of them respond favorably. It is hard to give statistics, since not only did studies vary, but so did the definition of 'response'. In some cases, a CRT responder is a person who showed functional improvement with CRT, typically measured in NYHA Classification score or in distance covered in the hallway walk test. These are 'soft end-points', but still frequently used.

Others have defined responders as those who met certain objective criteria, such as a change of oxygen uptake at the anaerobic threshold during exercise or the reduction of the diameter of the left ventricle (LV). While these are valuable criteria, not all physicians will be able to perform such tests.

Decreased heart size is also used as a marker of CRT response, particularly when it accompanies a change in functional classification or improved tolerance of exercise. To be realistic, in some cases

CRT response might even be defined as stabilization without symptomatic improvement; for example, a patient who remains NYHA Class III and does not progress to NYHA Class IV could be counted as a 'responder'.

For our purposes, we define non-responders as CRT patients who meet one or more of the following criteria:

- Their HF gets worse after they receive a CRT device
- After 6 months of having a CRT device, they have not improved in functional classification and have increased ventricular remodeling
- They initially responded to CRT but now have worsening symptoms.

Patients who could be 'non-responders' by these definitions should be systematically evaluated, since non-response may be due to a number of different factors. The main reasons to which most experts attribute non-response to CRT include: improper patient selection, suboptimal lead placement and inappropriate device programming. In reality, there is much we still have to learn about HF. Despite these limitations, there is a great deal that a systematic approach can do to convert non-responders and even enhance the degree of CRT response in patients who are already responders.

Step 1: patient evaluation

The first step in troubleshooting a non-responder involves a clinical evaluation of the patient's status, particularly with regard to atrial fibrillation (AF), fluid volume and cardiac ischemia. These three conditions can all have a profound effect on not only the patient's overall sense of well-being but also on how well CRT can function.

For some clinicians confronted with a CRT non-responder, the first thought is to correct the device.

While device programming is a key step in troubleshooting the non-responder, it should not be the first step. There are many non-device-related factors that can influence a patient's response to CRT!

Atrial fibrillation

HF patients are at increased risk of developing AF and other forms of atrial tachyarrhythmias. For the sake of optimal hemodynamics and best possible CRT performance, a patient should be in sinus rhythm. This means that methods of rhythm control (drug therapy) rather than pure rate control should be preferred for patients with intermittent runs of high-rate atrial activity. Patients who respond well to drug therapy for AF or cardioversion should be treated to reduce or eliminate AF. This means that one of the ways to help manage a CRT non-responder is to better manage them pharmacologically! Bear in mind, however, that many anti-arrhythmic agents may not work well for HF patients due to potential pro-arrhythmic effects or negative inotropic effects.

Even patients whose atrial arrhythmias can be managed with drug therapy may still experience breakthrough episodes of atrial tachyarrhythmias. HF patients with paroxysmal AF or atrial tachycardia should have a device with a mode switch algorithm to prevent a rapid ventricular response to high-rate atrial activity. When evaluating a non-responder with paroxysmal AF or intermittent atrial tachycardia, make sure that the mode switch algorithm is activated and that the cut-off rate (the atrial rate which initiates the mode switch) is appropriate for the patient. When selecting the cut-off rate, the clinician needs to balance two concerns: the highest ventricular pacing rate the patient can tolerate well and the highest rate the atria might reasonably achieve to keep up with patient activity. For example, a very sedentary patient might do well with a mode switch cut-off rate of about 100 beats/min, while a fitter, more active patient might need a cut-off rate of about 120 beats/min.

Many HF patients have or eventually develop persistent or even permanent AF. For patients likely to experience constant or nearly constant AF, program the CRT system from a dual-chamber mode (typically DDDR) to a single-chamber mode (VVIR). While dual-chamber pacing provides better hemodynamics for the patient, AF counteracts that. A VVIR device uses less battery energy and avoids any possibility of pacing the ventricle at a high rate in response to atrial activity.

All CRT patients should be checked periodically in terms of atrial activity. For those CRT patients in normal sinus rhythm, clinicians need to be wary of the onset of potential atrial tachyarrhythmias. For patients with atrial tachyarrhythmic activity, it is important to monitor AF. AF, like HF, is a progressive condition. Patients who get even short runs of paroxysmal AF do not 'get over them' but tend to get worse over time.

Volume status

Nothing affects the well-being of a HF patient more acutely than their fluid volume and managing volume is a key to all forms of HF therapy, including CRT. Diuretics provide fast relief for congestion, but diuretics need to be carefully monitored; it is very easy for a patient to end up taking too much (pre-renal azotemia or too much nitrogen in the blood) or too few (congestion). A congested or azotemic patient may respond poorly to CRT for reasons of fluid volume rather than device issues. Volume status can be controlled with reasonable efficacy using pharmacological methods (diuretics, particularly loop diuretics).

Cardiac ischemia

The cardiac condition of the CRT patient should be periodically evaluated with respect to ischemic heart disease, i.e. coronary artery disease (CAD). CAD occurs when plaque builds up on the interior of the coronary arteries that supply the heart muscle itself with oxygenated blood. If the coronary arteries become occluded or clogged, the heart gets less oxygen-rich blood than it needs to function. This can cause some of the heart muscle to die and become ischemic. Ischemia can affect the patient's overall condition and increase symptoms of fatigue and dyspnea. Furthermore, worsening ischemia can negate the benefits of CRT to the point that a patient appears to be a 'non-responder' when in reality he may be a CRT responder suffering from CAD.

Physicians should refer ischemic patients to appropriate specialists (if required) and patients may be considered for angiography or revascularization.

Angiography is a catheter-based technique in which a balloon-type catheter is inserted gently into the occluded vein and then inflated to widen the vessel diameter. In some cases, a stent may be inserted, which is a little 'scaffold' that can help physically prop open the artery. Angiography can sometimes be done in a catheterization lab as an out-patient procedure, but may require a hospital stay.

Revascularization involves a surgical approach to 're-route' vessels that serve the myocardium. The most familiar type of revascularization procedure is the coronary artery bypass graft procedure (CABG) or simply bypass. In this procedure, a healthy section of vessel is taken (often from the patient's upper leg or other part of the body) and is then sewn into place around the outside of the heart in such a way that it can 'bypass' the clogged artery. A double bypass involves doing this for two clogged arteries, and so on with triple and quadruple bypass procedures. A bypass is a very invasive but relatively safe and highly effective procedure that typically requires a hospital stay of several days.

Step 2: device interrogation

Once the patient's overall condition is reviewed and addressed, the CRT device should be interrogated and checked. CRT devices, like any sort of cardiac rhythm management devices, require periodic follow-up assessments, which will be covered in greater detail in Chapter 25. However, any time a patient is not responding well to CRT, the next step is to evaluate right-ventricular (RV) and LV capture and atrioventricular (AV) and VV optimization of the system.

RV and LV capture

Although CRT systems should be followed with the same care and diligence as other implantable cardiac rhythm management devices, troubleshooting the non-responder involves some of the same steps as well. The CRT device should be interrogated and programmed settings checked. The status of the device should be checked: has the device been reset to backup or is the battery running down? Assuming the device appears to be in working order, a chest X-ray should be ordered to verify that the leads have not become dislodged. Lead dislodgement, particularly

on the left side of the heart, may occur even in the chronic system. Damage to the lead can also occur and can be checked by looking at the lead impedance values. (Lead impedance is not a programmable value and is read when the device is interrogated. The manufacturer states acceptable lead impedance values for any given lead in a range; the actual lead impedance varies depending on numerous factors. However, any change of $> 200\,\Omega$ in lead impedance value, particularly in a short period of time, strongly suggests damage to the lead or a loosening lead connection to the device.)

When troubleshooting the non-responder, it is particularly important to look at RV and LV capture. Although part of any routine follow-up session, capture assessment is crucial for troubleshooting the non-responder, since when capture is lost, CRT is essentially turned off.

Capture threshold testing may be performed using the semi-automatic capture test on the programmer in order to to assess appropriate capture in both RV and LV. (Atrial capture testing is not crucial to troubleshooting the non-responder, but may be performed if the clinician feels there is reason to suspect atrial capture problems.) New output parameter settings should be programmed if needed to assure proper capture.

It may be worth noting here that capture, although fundamental to device performance, is not always easy to maintain. A patient's capture threshold, i.e. how much energy it takes to capture the heart reliably, varies with many factors. There is some degree of normal daily variation in the capture threshold and thresholds can change somewhat with posture and meal times. Drugs can have a more profound effect on capture thresholds, and certain drugs are known to affect thresholds significantly. Furthermore, cardiac ischemia and disease progression also influence thresholds. A device that captured the heart previously may fail to capture the heart in the future, particularly in patients with serious cardiac disease. For that reason, capture testing becomes an ongoing part of following any CRT patient!

AV and VV optimization

Like capture testing, AV and VV optimization becomes an ongoing part of following any CRT patient, and it is particularly important to troubleshooting the non-responder. The AV delay can have a significant impact on systolic function (see Fig. 16.1).

A good rule of thumb in AV delay optimization is to program the AV delay to about 75% of the patient's native PR interval, i.e. the interval from intrinsic atrial contraction to intrinsic ventricular contraction. The AV delay needs to be this short in order to guarantee continuous ventricular pacing; CRT works only when the patient is paced in the ventricle as close to 100% of the time as possible. On the other hand, the AV delay can be too short. If it is programmed too much out of this proportion (three-quarters of the PR interval), the result may be pacing the LV as the left atrium is contracting.

A recommended method of AV delay optimization testing was described in Chapter 15. Using either echocardiography or the QuickOpt™ algorithm, optimal settings for the sensed and paced AV delays and VV timing can be determined.

While AV optimization regulates how atrial and ventricular contractions synchronize, VV optimization attempts to harmonize the activities of the right and left ventricles. In first-generation CRT devices, the ventricular output pulses for right and left sides of the heart fired simultaneously. However, for some patients, one of the outputs (RV or LV) might better occur slightly in advance of the other. Allowing one side of the heart to pace first (called pre-activation) can improve cardiac output in some individuals, i.e. increase the benefits of CRT in that patient. Unfortunately, there is no simple formula for how this should work. In some patients, LV pre-activation improves cardiac output, while in others, RV pre-activation might have the same effect.

VV optimization (covered in more detail in Chapter 15) is influenced strongly by the etiology of HF and the possible presence of other cardiac disease. For example, ischemic tissue can slow conduction

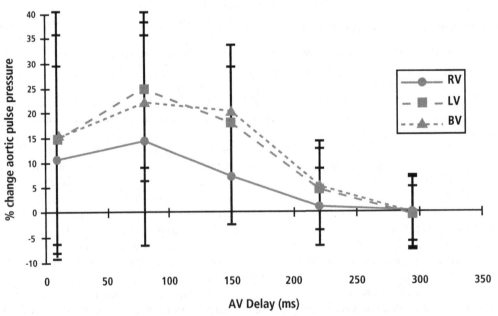

Fig. 16.1 The effect of the atrioventricular (AV) delay setting on systolic function. The length of the AV delay affects the heart's systolic function (defined as aortic pulse pressure) and varies by chamber. When the AV delay is too long, it allows for late left-ventricular (LV) activation, resulting in more opportunity for mitral regurgitation and an elevated LV end diastolic pressure. An AV delay that is too short may allow for pre-systolic mitral regurgitation and result in shortness of breath and malaise. An AV delay that is too short may actually undermine CRT altogether. Source of chart: Auricchio A, Stellbrink C, Block M *et al.* Effect of pacing chamber and atrioventricular delay on acute systolic function of paced patients with congestive heart failure. The Pacing Therapies for Congestive Heart Failure Study Group. *Circulation* 1999; **99**:2993–3001.

time. A patient with ischemic LV tissue may require even longer VV intervals (i.e. more LV pre-excitation) than a patient without ischemia.

Step 3: dyssynchrony evaluation

CRT devices address the mechanical dyssynchrony of the heart, specifically those that prevent the LV from contracting as a unified, coherent whole and other timing factors (such as VV and AV timing) that prevent the heart from beating as an effective pump.

Echocardiographic evaluation of mechanical dyssynchrony is still in its early stages, but already we know that a good variable to look at is 'septal to posterior wall motion delay' of the LV. This defines the time lag between the contraction of the ventricular septum and the contraction of the back wall of the LV. Ideally, the ventricle should contract as a whole unit, so the delay should be minimal. As a rule of thumb, this variable (sometimes abbreviated SPWMD) should be < 130 ms. In fact, SPWMD values < 130 ms are strong predictors of CRT response.

Another variable for echo studies of CRT patients is interventricular mechanical delay (IVMD), which is captured on echo by looking at the ECG, aortic outflow, and possibly pulmonary outflow. IVMD can be thought of as the time it takes from the onset of ventricular electrical activation (output pulse from device or native electrical impulse) until blood starts to pump out of the heart (from LV to aorta or from RV to pulmonary artery). As a rule of thumb, the IVMD value should be < 40 ms.

If these values fall outside these general guidelines, the next step is possible lead revision. Lead revision involves a surgical procedure to move the pacing leads to more optimal locations or to implant a new lead in a better position. If a new lead is implanted, it is often acceptable to leave the old lead in place after unplugging it from the pulse generator and capping it.

Lead revision is a serious step, but one that may ultimately be of great benefit to certain patients. Leads that are damaged or loosen from the pulse generator (generally determined by chest X-ray or lead impedance values during device interrogations) require replacement, while suboptimally placed leads are a matter of clinical judgment. Every surgical revision

carries with it all of the risks of surgery and lead removal is associated with additional risks.

Step 4: evaluate mitral regurgitation

Mitral regurgitation (MR) occurs when blood that should be going out from the LV into the aorta ends up going backward, up toward the left atrium through the mitral valve. MR decreases cardiac output and can severely impact CRT response. In fact, persistent MR can cause non-response.

Sometimes MR can be controlled or at least managed by AV delay optimization, but in other cases, valvular disease or damage makes that impossible. For some patients, mitral valve repair may be required.

Mitral valve repair procedures are major surgical interventions that carry with them all of the associated risks of surgery. As such, careful clinical consideration is necessary. Not all patients with CRT systems and persistent MR may be good candidates for this type of surgery.

Conclusion

Getting good CRT response involves certain steps prior to device implantation. Patient selection is an important factor; not every patient with HF is a candidate for CRT. The primary indication for CRT devices involves the presence of some form of mechanical dyssynchrony. Once a patient undergoes CRT device surgery, it is crucial that the LV lead be implanted in the best possible location. Even the textbook candidate for CRT will not respond well to stimulation therapy if the LV lead is poorly placed.

After the CRT device is implanted, many diseases can impact the effectiveness of CRT and turn patients into non-responders or poor responders. These factors include atrial rhythm disorders, particularly AF, cardiac ischemia, and persistent mitral regurgitation. The patient's volume status can also influence how well they responds to CRT, but this can often be adjusted with changes in the diuretic regimen.

What does the clinician do when a CRT non-responder fails to improve, although they have been thoroughly examined and all possible 'non-response' factors are addressed? In the presence of severe HF or cardiac disease, such patients may be encountered. Once all known factors are addressed, the persistent non-responder may be considered for alternative treatment methods. Such therapies include a left-ventricular assist device (LVAD) or a heart transplant.

These treatment measures are extreme, but should be clinically considered. HF remains a dangerous and complex syndrome that sometimes requires extreme treatment measures.

References

1   Abraham WT, Fisher WG, Smith AL *et al.* MIRACLE Study Group. Multicenter InSync Randomized Clinical Evaluation: Cardiac resynchronization in chronic heart failure. *N Engl J Med* 2002; **346:**1845–53.

2   Auricchio A, Stellbrink C, Sack S *et al.* Long-term clinical effect of hemodynamically optimized cardiac resynchronization therapy in patients with heart failure and ventricular conduction delay. *J Am Coll Cardiol* 2002; **39:**2026–33.

The nuts and bolts of troubleshooting the non-responder

- The non-responder to cardiac resynchronization therapy (CRT) is a the patient who meets at least one of these three criteria:
  Worsening heart failure
  No change in New York Heart Association classification in the presence of ventricular remodeling
  Initial favorable response to CRT with now worsening symptoms.
- Even in properly selected patients (those indicated for CRT, i.e. those with evidence of mechanical dyssynchrony), about a third do not respond to CRT.
- Troubleshooting the non-responder should be done systematically and involves an evaluation of the patient's clinical status, device interrogation, an evaluation of dyssynchrony and a check for mitral regurgitation.
- Three clinical conditions that can impact CRT response are atrial tachyarrhythmias [particularly atrial fibrillation (AF)], the patient's volume status and cardiac ischemia (coronary artery disease).
- If a CRT patient has AF, attempts should be made to maintain sinus rhythm. This involves the approach to AF management known as 'rhythm control' rather than rate control. If AF can be managed in this way, the mode switch algorithm should still be programmed carefully to prevent rapid ventricular pacing in response to runs of high-rate atrial activity. In the presence of persistent or permanent AF, the CRT system should be programmed to VVIR mode (i.e. no atrial sensing at all).

- Non-responders should be checked for device status (good battery status) and lead impedance values. If lead impedance values vary by > 200 Ω in a short time (such as between check-ups), this strongly suggests damage to the lead or a loose lead connection with the pulse generator. A chest X-ray can further confirm proper lead fixation and status. Damaged, poorly connected or dislodged leads must be surgically revised.
- When troubleshooting the non-responder it is important to check capture in all chambers, since many factors can affect proper capture. It is not unusual for a patient to lose capture, even if they had it previously. If capture is lost, device output settings (pulse amplitude and pulse width) must be adjusted. Note that patients are quite likely to have different ventricular capture thresholds in the right ventricle (RV) and left ventricle (LV).
- The atrioventricular (AV) delay should be checked for an optimal setting in the non-responder. As a rule of thumb, a good AV delay for a CRT patient is about 75% of his intrinsic PR interval. This relatively short AV delay helps assure continuous ventricular pacing, which is essential to CRT. However, if the AV delay is too short, it can undermine CRT stimulation and increase symptoms. An AV delay that is too long encourages mitral regurgitation.
- VV optimization defines how the ventricles contract with respect to each other. Sometimes patients benefit when one ventricle is paced slightly in advance of the other. This pre-

Continued.

Continued.

excitation varies by patient and is hard to predict without careful evaluation. Some patients benefit from LV pre-excitation, while others do better with RV pre-excitation.

- Ischemic tissue slows conduction time. Thus, a patient with an ischemic LV (from coronary artery disease or a prior myocardial infarction) may require a longer VV interval with LV pre-excitation than a non-ischemic patient.
- Echocardiographic evaluation of mechanical dyssynchrony shows how well the heart is physically contracting and relaxing. Two guideline parameters are septal to posterior wall motion delay (SPWD) and interventricular mechanical delay (IVMD).
- SPWD could be thought of as the time lag between the contraction of the interventricular septum (the wall between the ventricles) and the contraction of the back wall of the LV. An SPWD value < 130 ms is a predictor of CRT response. Patients with an SPWD value > 130 ms should be considered for a possible lead revision.
- IVMD defines the time it takes from the onset of electrical stimulation of the ventricles (either naturally or artificially by the CRT device) until blood pumps out of the heart into the aorta (measured as aortic outflow) or the pulmonary artery (measured as pulmonary outflow). The IVMD should be < 40 ms, otherwise lead revision should be considered.
- Lead placement plays a major role in how well a CRT device can resolve mechanical dyssynchrony. Many non-responders may be potential candidates for LV lead revision. Lead revision (particularly lead removal) is a surgical procedure with risks and potential benefits that must be carefully considered.
- Mitral regurgitation (MR) should be evaluated as a possible contributing factor (or cause) of CRT non-response. Some CRT non-responders with MR may be potential candidates for mitral valve repair. Again, this surgical intervention carries associated risks, which demand careful clinical consideration.
- It is not possible to troubleshoot all CRT non-responders out of their non-responsive state to a responsive one. For such persistent non-responders, alternative approaches, such as a left-ventricular assist device (LVAD) or cardiac transplant, may be considered.

Chapter 17

Defibrillation Basics

Heart failure (HF) patients are at risk of dangerous ventricular tachyarrhythmias and sudden cardiac death (SCD). There is a popular misconception among clinicians that the risk of SCD is greatest among New York Heart Association (NYHA) Class I and II HF patients, but that the risk decreases with advanced HF. It is true that more NYHA Class III and IV HF patients die of pump failure than of SCD, but the actual risk of SCD increases as NYHA classification goes up. The only reason more NYHA Class III and IV patients die of pump failure is that pump failure deaths increase even more rapidly. To make SCD even more insidious in HF patients, it can occur in HF patients with no previous evidence of arrhythmias.

The SCD-HeFT clinical trial actually found that prophylactic implantable cardioverter-defibrillator (ICD) devices [defibrillators without cardiac resynchronization therapy (CRT) functionality] implanted in certain HF patients reduced mortality.[1] With this landmark study emerged a new patient population: the primary-prevention patient or the HF patient who derived a significant mortality benefit from receiving an ICD even without documented evidence of a potentially life-threatening tachyarrhythmia.

Since CRT offered specific clinical benefits to the subset of HF patients with mechanical dyssynchrony and since ICDs offered mortality benefits to HF patients even without documented tachyarrhythmias, it was logical for engineers to work to create a device that combined the rescue function of an ICD with a CRT system. This CRT plus defibrillator device, sometimes called the CRT-D system, found immediate clinical resonance. In the USA, far more CRT-D systems are implanted than CRT pacemakers (without defibrillation).

For that reason, clinicians who deal with CRT patients need to know the basics of defibrillation therapy. Unlike CRT stimulation, which provides therapeutic benefit by constantly pacing or resynchronizing the heart, a defibrillator offers simply a rescue function. It cannot suppress or act to prevent ventricular tachyarrhythmias, but it does work to rescue a patient once such a potentially lethal rhythm disorder commences.

In order to do this, a defibrillator must be able to sense cardiac signals, diagnose potentially dangerous rhythms and then deliver therapy.

Defibrillator sensing

Probably the greatest engineering challenge in developing a CRT-D system involves reliable sensing for the defibrillator. While the ventricular signals generated by normal CRT stimulation would be fairly large and stable, intrinsic ventricular activity associated with potentially fatal ventricular tachyarrhythmias and ventricular fibrillation (VF) are often notoriously small and erratic. The CRT-D system must be extremely sensitive in order to detect these small, unstable signals. Yet a very sensitive device risks picking up other low-amplitude signals, like T-waves, far-field signals (i.e. paced activity from the other chamber) and even muscle noise. Furthermore, conventional pacemakers and ICDs have taught device specialists that there are dangers to both 'over-sensing', or making the device overly sensitive, and 'undersensing', or making the device insensitive to incoming signals. For defibrillation purposes, oversensing might involve sensing signals that are not really indicative of a ventricular tachyarrhythmia and delivering a painful and unnecessary shock. Undersensing is even worse; a necessary shock therapy might not be delivered at all because the device fails to detect the ventricular tachyarrhythmia!

CRT-D devices rely on automatic, dynamically self-adjusting sensitivity algorithms to meet this formidable challenge. Every major CRT-D device manufacturer offers some form of this special algorithm; this book will look at the algorithm used in St Jude Medical CRT-D devices. When dealing with a new or unfamiliar CRT-D system, it is always a good idea to refer to the product manual, which contains the specifics on that particular device model. Note that not only do manufacturers' algorithms vary, but sometimes devices by a single manufacturer will vary by model also. This is not due to whimsy on the part of the manufacturers; all device manufacturers work continuously to improve and refine the sensitivity algorithm and other device algorithms. Changes in algorithm reflect the manufacturers' commitment to keep improving products.

When the device picks up a ventricular signal, it launches a timing cycle known as the sensed refractory period. During that time, the device measures the peak of the maximum amplitude that occurs. Note that device signals are digitally rectified and filtered in such a way that they are positive (no negative deflections from the baseline). This peak value is stored as Threshold Start (see Fig. 17.1). When the sensed refractory period expires, the Threshold Start defines, in terms of a percentage, how sensitivity is set for the next cardiac cycle. While Threshold Start is programmable, let us assume a generally acceptable value of 50%. This means sensitivity for the next cardiac cycle is 50% of the peak value of the last cycle (Threshold Start). If the peak value or Threshold Start was 8 mV, then the sensitivity for the next cardiac cycle is 4 mV (50% of 8 mV). There is a linear decline from the Threshold Start down to the programmed maximum sensitivity value which describes what ventricular signals would be sensed (see Fig. 17.2).

A programmable function called Decay Delay may be further programmed, which causes the Threshold Start value to plateau for a short period before beginning its decline to baseline (see Fig. 17.3).

The sensitivity function of a CRT-D system is largely automatic and governed by a few relatively straightforward parameter settings (such as the percentage value of Threshold Start and the optional programmability of Decay Delay). It is possible to undertake more fundamental reprogramming of the sensitivity function, but such steps should always involve consultation with the manufacturer's representative or technical services department.

Diagnosing arrhythmias

Once the CRT-D system detects incoming ventricular signals, it needs a reliable method of sorting out the activity in order to determine if any represent a potentially life-threatening ventricular tachyarrhythmia. Diagnostic methods have to be rapid and accurate. The two main errors to avoid are diagnosing dangerous arrhythmias when none is occurring (resulting in a distressing, battery-draining and inappropriate shock) or the potentially catastrophic error of failing to rescue a fibrillating heart.

Fig. 17.1 Threshold Start in implantable cardioverter-defibrillator sensing. The Threshold Start value is determined by the highest peak or maximum amplitude measured during the sensed refractory period. A programmable percentage of the peak value sets the Threshold Start value. In this case, the maximum amplitude was 4 mV and the Threshold Start was programmed to 50% or 2 mV. The Threshold Start declines in linear fashion and is used to sense the next cardiac cycle. In order to be sensed, a ventricular signal has to be large enough to be seen outside the shaded area.

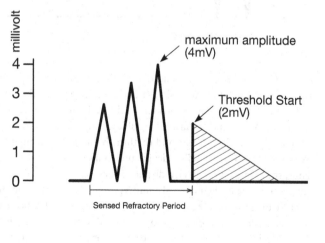

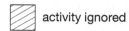

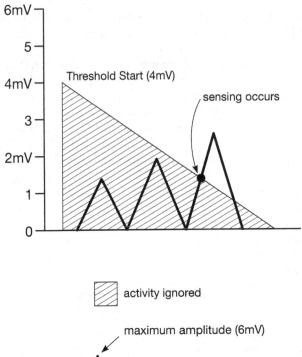

Fig. 17.2 Threshold Start in implantable cardioverter-defibrillator sensing. Ventricular signals that occur in the shaded area are ignored. However, a signal that can break through the shaded area is large enough to be sensed and counted by device. Note that a signal may be sensed on the upward or downward slope, depending on which is the first to break out of the shaded zone.

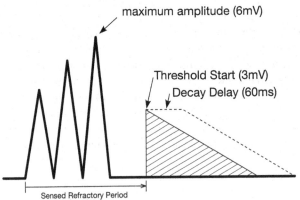

Fig. 17.3 Extending the Threshold Start value. In this example, a 60-ms Decay Delay value is programmed which causes the Threshold Start to hold steady for 60 ms before declining in linear fashion.

The CRT-D device has broad diagnostic categories: normal sinus rhythm (NSR), VF and ventricular tachycardia (VT), which are further subdivided into VT1 ('slow' VT) and VT2 ('fast' VT). Unlike clinicians, who rely on a variety of rate and rhythm characteristics for diagnosis, a CRT-D device uses only rate. Thus, sometimes these device diagnostic categories are not the same as their clinical counterparts.

Each diagnostic category (NSR, VT, VF) is associated with a therapeutic response. For NSR, the device decides that there is no need for any electrical therapy. For VF, the device delivers maximum-energy shock therapy. For dangerous arrhythmias in the ventricle that are not VF, the clinician may opt to have less-than-maximal shocks delivered (so-called 'cardioversion') or even antitachycardia pacing (ATP).

The rates that define these categories can be programmed by the clinician in terms of cut-off values. For example, NSR might be anything from 60 to 100 beats/min, VT might be 100–200 beats/min and VF might be any rate above 200 beats/min. The VT category might be further subdivided so that VT1 was 100–180 beats/min and VT2 was 180–200 beats/

min. However, not all patients require so many subdivisions.

When determining the rate cut-offs and categories for a particular patient, it is useful to consider the patient's history of arrhythmias and how likely they are to respond to cardioversion or ATP. For example, a patient known to have more than one type of rhythm disorder, including well-tolerated VT as well as more dangerous faster forms of VT or VF, could benefit from programming separate therapeutic responses for slow VT, fast VT and VF. A primary-prevention patient not known to have any history of arrhythmias probably should be programmed only for NSR and VF. Patients with a history of VT may be known to respond well to ATP. If a patient can tolerate VT reasonably well and responds favorably to ATP, this is a good initial therapeutic strategy, since ATP is painless therapy and does not drain the battery as much as shock therapy. The drawbacks to ATP are that it can be ineffective or, even worse, accelerate a VT into a faster and more dangerous arrhythmia (see Table 17.1).

While zones are defined by rates stated in beats/min, the CRT-D device measures the corresponding intervals. Since patients with known or potential rhythm disorders are prone to erratic heart beats, the CRT-D device does not count intervals in isolation, but uses a system of interval averaging. Interval averaging avoids the possible miscounting of intervals that could occur with a premature ventricular contraction (PVC) or occasional unusual event.

Interval averaging involves looking at the current interval (CI) and then comparing it with the average interval (AI), which is defined as the average of the last four intervals immediately preceding the CI (see Fig. 17.4).

Binning involves counting intervals by zone until the prescribed number of intervals in a particular zone is reached. Binning is easy to understand when the CI and AI fall in the same zone. However, sometimes the AI and CI will be in different zones. When that occurs, the device must decide how to count the interval. In St Jude Medical devices, when either the AI or CI is NSR, then the interval is discarded, i.e. not binned. Otherwise, when the AI and CI differ, the interval is counted in the faster zone because the device errs on the side of patient safety (see Table 17.2).

Once the programmed number of required intervals in a particular zone is achieved, the device diagnoses the rhythm based on that zone and proceeds to therapy. NSR is a zone and although the device will 'bin' intervals into NSR, NSR never results in therapy delivery of any kind. It is possible not only to program the number of intervals necessary for a bin to be full, but to program different numbers for different zones. For example, a clinician might program 20 intervals for VT1, 12 intervals for VT2 and eight intervals for VF. In general, the faster and more dangerous the arrhythmia, the fewer intervals should be required to reach diagnosis.

Table 17.1 CRT-D configurations

Configuration	Categories	Patient profile
	(rate ranges are programmable; ranges below are examples only)	
1 Zone	NSR (< 200 beats/min) VF (> 200 beats/min)	Primary-prevention patients and those known to be unlikely to respond to ATP or cardioversion
2 Zones	NSR (< 120 beats/min) VT (120–200 beats/min) VF (> 200 beats/min)	Patients known to experience reasonably well-tolerated VT that responds to ATP or cardioversion
3 Zones	NSR (< 120 beats/min) VT1 (120–160 beats/min) VT2 (161–200 beats/min) VF (> 200 beats/min)	Patients known to have multiple VTs that are stable, reasonably well tolerated and respond to ATP or cardioversion

NSR, Normal sinus rhythm; VT, ventricular tachycardia; VF, ventricular fibrillation; ATP, antitachycardia pacing therapy.

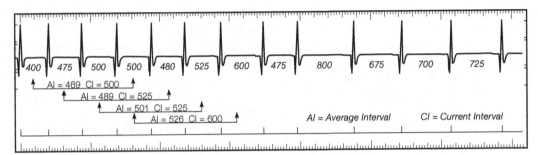

Fig. 17.4 How intervals are counted. Interval averaging works by averaging four intervals and then comparing that value (average interval or AI) to the next current interval (CI). In this case the four intervals to be averaged were 400, 475, 500 and 500 ms, resulting in an average interval value of 468.75 ms, which the device would round up to 469 ms. The next interval or CI would be compared with 469 ms.

Table 17.2 Binning in the two-zone configuration

Current interval	Average interval	Bin
NSR	NSR	NSR
VT	VT	VT
VF	VF	VF
VT	NSR	Discarded
VF	NSR	Discarded
VF	VT	VF
VT	VF	VF

While intervals do not have to be consecutive to count toward diagnosis, they must occur within a prescribed range. Again, the range is programmable within a range of settings. A typical value might be a VT diagnosis when 12 out of 16 consecutive intervals are VT. Once a diagnosis is made in any zone other than NSR, the device proceeds to therapy.

Therapy

An ICD has three basic types of therapy: shock, cardioversion and ATP. While many CRT-D patients will not require all three types of therapy to be programmed, it is important to understand the differences between them.

Shock therapy is sometimes called high-voltage therapy or maximum therapy. It consists of a large bolus of electrical energy delivered to the heart all at once at the highest settings programmed by the clinician. Shock therapy may be described in terms of volts (700–800 V is typical) or joules (30–36 J). When this large amount of energy is delivered to the

heart, it 'jolts' the heart out of the tachyarrhythmia and restores normal sinus rhythm.

In device therapy, cardioversion is defined as a low-energy shock, i.e. a shock, but at a value (volts or joules) below the maximum setting. (Note that cardioversion has other clinical definitions as well; this is specific to implantable defibrillators.) For example, cardioversion might be a shock at 500 V (see Fig. 17.5).

Determining the appropriate size of the shock involves three issues:
- What is the patient's defibrillation threshold (DFT), if known?
- Is the shock intended to terminate a non-lethal VT or a potentially deadly VT?
- Is the patient known to respond well to lower-energy shocks?

The DFT is defined as the minimum amount of energy required to defibrillate the heart reliably. DFT testing may be done at device implant by inducing VF and then allowing the device to terminate the arrhythmia. Depending on the patient and clinical circumstances, several inductions and terminations may be done in a step-down protocol or one or two inductions and terminations are used to simply determine safe DFT values. In some cases, the implanting physician may forego DFT testing at implant. Since DFT testing requires inducing, observing and then trying to convert a potentially deadly rhythm disorder, it requires that the patient be deeply sedated or under general anesthesia. It can be a nerve-wracking procedure for the implant team and may require a crash cart or outside intervention.

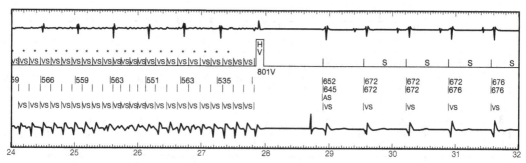

Fig. 17.5 Shock therapy. In this printout, ventricular fibrillation is detected and a high-voltage shock (HV) is delivered, restoring the patient to normal sinus rhythm.

For some primary-prevention patients or in cases where a CRT-D device will only be used to terminate potentially life-threatening episodes of VT or VF, the physician may not do DFT testing at implant and simply program therapy to maximum value.

However, if a patient is known to have a fairly low DFT, it can be wise to program cardioversion to save potential battery energy for the device. CRT-D devices allow clinicians to program multiple therapies so that cardioversion can be attempted first and, if that fails to convert a dangerous rhythm disorder, followed immediately by high-energy therapy at maximum settings. While cardioversion spares device energy and may be less stressful for the patient (although it is doubtful a patient can truly detect the nuances of 500 V versus 750 V), the potential danger in cardioversion is that it may prolong the time a patient has to spend in VT before life-saving therapy is delivered. Therefore, careful clinical consideration is required. In general, patients who are not expected to need shock therapy often or who are not known to have slower VTs that respond to lower-energy shocks, can probably be well served by programming only high-energy shocks.

What happens when an arrhythmic episode diagnosed by the device terminates spontaneously? This might occur when a very short run of VT or even VF occurs and then resolves on its own. The CRT-D system is designed to charge up to capacity and deliver therapy quickly, but even so, the rhythm disorder may self-terminate before that. If the device is 'committed', it commits to deliver therapy even if it appears that the rhythm is back to NSR. Committed devices are mainly older systems. Today, most devices are 'non-committed,' which means that if

NSR is detected after a rhythm disorder has been diagnosed but before therapy is delivered, the CRT-D device will abort therapy. The energy charged up in the capacitors of the device is gradually and painlessly bled off and the patient receives no shock (see Fig. 17.6).

Some patients with known VTs respond well to programmed stimulation designed to terminate their arrhythmia or ATP. ATP is not painful; in fact, some patients are not even aware that they receive therapy. It can reduce the number of painful shocks to the patient, and it does not present much drain to the device battery. While ATP from the EP lab has the somewhat deserved reputation of being complicated, most CRT-D devices allow for fairly straightforward and even intuitive programmability of ATP parameters.

The best candidates for ATP are patients with re-entrant monomorphic VT who are hemodynamically stable and tolerate the VT well. Conversely, ATP is unsuitable for patients with unstable arrhythmias and those who are symptomatic or could be hemodynamically compromised by their rhythm disorder. Thus, the majority of CRT-D patients are not likely to be candidates for ATP.

Every zone (except NSR) can have its own therapy programmed. For example, in a 1 zone configuration, VF will be treated with a high-voltage shock. In a 2 zone configuration, a clinician could program the device so that VT is treated with cardioversion and VF is treated with a high-voltage shock. It is also possible to program multiple therapy attempts in a particular zone; for example, VT might be treated first with cardioversion and then with high-voltage therapy.

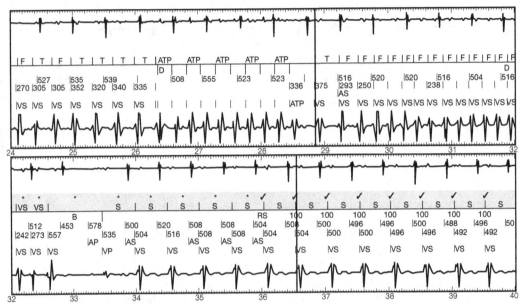

Fig. 17.6 Record of an arrhythmia. In this tracing, a non-committed device diagnoses ventricular tachycardia (VT) and delivers antitachycardia pacing therapy (ATP), which accelerates the VT into ventricular fibrillation (VF). The device starts to charge to deliver high-voltage therapy (top strip), but in the lower, continuous strip, the VF self-terminates and normal sinus rhythm (shown here as S) resumes. The device aborts the shock and the patient receives no therapy. Had the device been a committed system, the patient would have received therapy and it would have appeared in the lower strip.

Once therapy is delivered, the device 'redetects' or checks the rhythm to be sure that NSR is restored. The period immediately following delivery of any shock therapy can cause the heart to be somewhat vulnerable. Post-shock pacing parameters (PSP) are special parameter settings that go into effect immediately after therapy delivery (shock, cardioversion or ATP). These parameters include a pause, PSP rate, PSP output settings, PSP mode and PSP duration.

The PSP pause defines how many seconds should elapse after therapy and before onset of PSP; a typical value might be 5 s. Pacing immediately after shock might be pro-arrhythmic. A special lower-than-normal PSP base rate is recommended, again to counteract possible pro-arrhythmic effects of faster pacing settings. Cardiac tissue stressed by

therapy may have a temporarily elevated capture threshold, so pulse amplitude and pulse width are usually set to much higher values, even maximum settings for PSP. The PSP mode should be the same as the regularly programmed mode with the exception of rate response; if a patient was previously programmed to DDDR, then the PSP mode should be DDD. Finally, PSP duration defines how long PSP parameters are in effect. The programmable range is from 30 s to 10 min.

Reference

1   Bardy GH, Lee KL, Mark DB *et al*. Amiodarone or an ICD for congestive heart failure. *N Engl J Med* 2005; **352**:225–37.

The nuts and bolts of defibrillation basics

- Heart failure (HF) patients are at risk of sudden cardiac death (SCD) and that risk increases with SCD, although in New York Heart Association Class III and IV the risk of dying of pump failure increases even more significantly.
- SCD-HeFT best defines the primary-prevention HF patient: a patient with no prior evidence of arrhythmias. Conventional implantable cardioverter-defibrillators decreased mortality significantly in this group.
- Most cardiac resynchronization therapy (CRT) systems implanted in the USA are CRT-D devices which combine CRT stimulation with defibrillation for rescue from potentially life-threatening ventricular tachyarrhythmias.
- Defibrillators must sense ventricular activity, diagnose potential rhythm disorders and deliver therapy.
- Defibrillators sense ventricular activity with an automatic, self-adjusting, dynamic sensitivity algorithm. This means that sensitivity is automatically adjusted for each cycle.
- Automatic sensitivity algorithms are necessary for defibrillation because ventricular fibrillation (VF) signals are often low amplitude and erratic signals that can be hard to detect; however, if a defibrillator were adjusted to look always for very small signals, it could easily but inappropriately sense T-waves, muscle noise, or atrial pacing outputs and count them as ventricular events.
- The CRT-D device categorizes ventricular activity by zones, which are defined by rates. Rates are programmable within certain ranges. Thus, to the device normal sinus rhythm (NSR) is a rate category and has nothing to do with actual rhythm characteristics.
- The most elaborate device configuration programmable is three zones, which allows for NSR (normal sinus rhythm), VT1 (slow VT), VT2 (fast VT), and VF. Programming configurations of 1 and 2 zones are available and may be more common for HF patients.
- The device diagnoses rhythm disorders by counting intervals at varying rate ranges and binning them. Intervals do not have to be consecutive but they must fall within a certain range of consecutive intervals (such as 12 out of 16 intervals). The number of intervals required to fill a bin is programmable and may differ by zone. For example, VT might be diagnosed when 12 out of 16 consecutive intervals are VT, but VF is diagnosed when eight out of 16 intervals are VF.
- In order to avoid being fooled by an occasional premature ventricular contraction (PVC), the device counts intervals by comparing the current interval (CI) against the average value of the last preceding four intervals (average interval or AI). When both intervals are in the same zone, that zone is binned. When either the AI or CI is NSR, the interval is trashed and not binned at all. When the AI and CI fall in different zones (but neither is NSR), the interval gets binned in the faster zone.
- When any bin (except NSR) is filled to capacity, the device proceeds to therapy. Therapy may be a high-voltage shock, cardioversion (lower-than-maximum voltage shock), or antitachycardia pacing (ATP). It is possible to program different therapies for each zone and, within a zone, several therapies can be programmed. Thus, VT may be treated first with ATP, then with cardioversion, and then with high-voltage therapy.
- To determine the type of therapy the patient needs, it may be useful to know the patient's defibrillation threshold (DFT). The DFT is the lowest amount of energy required (in volts or joules) to defibrillate the heart reliably. DFT testing can be done at implant, but it is a challenging procedure that is sometimes skipped, particularly in primary-prevention patients.
- In primary-prevention patients or in patients who do not receive DFT testing, it is typical to program only high-voltage therapy. For patients known to have multiple rhythm disorders (VT and VF) or those with known and fairly low DFTs, it can be useful to program cardioversion and then high-voltage therapy.
- Patients with multiple rhythm disorders and re-entrant monomorphic VT that is well tolerated

Continued p. 124.

Continued.

may benefit from ATP. ATP is also useful for patients known to have VT that responds well to programmed stimulation (this may be established in EP testing). ATP offers some benefits and drawbacks for such patients. On the one hand, it is painless therapy which does not take much battery energy and which can safely and effectively treat some rhythm disorders. On the other hand, when ATP does not work well, it can prolong the time a patient spends in a potentially dangerous VT and may even accelerate a VT.

• When a non-committed device diagnoses a rhythm disorder and prepares to deliver therapy, it will abort that therapy if NSR is detected before therapy delivery. On the other hand, a committed device will deliver the therapy no matter what. Most modern defibrillators are non-committed.

• After therapy, the cardiac tissue is traumatized and may require a short period of pacing at special parameter settings. This is called post-shock pacing (PSP) and usually involves pacing at higher outputs, a lower base rate, and a non-rate-responsive mode. PSP usually starts a few seconds after therapy delivery (this is programmable) and lasts for only a matter of minutes (also programmable).

Chapter 18

Advanced Defibrillation Functions

Today's CRT-D devices could be thought of as full-featured implantable cardioverter-defibrillators (ICDs) with cardiac resynchronization therapy (CRT) pacing capabilities. While the basic rescue function of a defibrillator is fairly easy to understand, the implantable ICD has to be on constant standby in the body, ready to charge up and deliver high-voltage therapy in a matter of moments. While the basics of how a CRT-D system senses intrinsic cardiac activity and arrives at a diagnosis might seem straightforward, most clinicians know that real life is rarely as clear-cut at those textbook examples. That is why CRT-D devices offer some advanced defibrillation features aimed at helping clinicians better manage their patients.

SVT discrimination

Defibrillators were designed to treat life-threatening ventricular tachyarrhythmias, which can be defined as rapid ventricular activity of ventricular origin. Another common rhythm disorder—which on the surface looks very much like a ventricular tachyarrhythmia—is the supraventricular tachycardia (SVT), named because it originates above the ventricles (supra-ventricular). An SVT is often characterized by rapid ventricular activity, but in this case it is the rapid ventricular response to high-rate intrinsic atrial activity, in other words, atrial tachycardia or atrial fibrillation.

While high-voltage therapy is necessary and absolutely appropriate to treat ventricular tachycardia (VT), it is inappropriate for SVT. But how can a CRT-D device tell them apart, particularly since devices make their diagnoses based on rate? The answer is a suite of features known collectively as SVT discriminators.

The actual amount of so-called 'inappropriate therapy' is unknown. One study reported a 14% incidence of inappropriate therapy in ICD patients,[1] but earlier studies (using older technology) reported even higher rates.[2] Clearly, the presence of known atrial tachyarrhythmias, in particular atrial fibrillation (AF), is a risk factor for inappropriate therapy, but inappropriate therapy can potentially affect any device patient.[3]

Inappropriate therapy sounds more benign than it really is. When a patient gets an inappropriate shock, he is exposed to the full energy of a high-voltage shock. While patients vary in terms of how they experience therapy delivery, most patients find the shock delivery upsetting, stressful and painful. Furthermore, therapy delivery can distress the whole family, who may be concerned about the patient's well-being or take time off from work to rush the patient to the emergency room. Patients who have trouble adjusting to life as a 'device patient' may find therapy psychologically unsettling. In addition, shocks place a burden on the device's battery. Receiving shock therapy may limit a patient's ability to drive (many physicians preclude patients from driving for a time period after they get shocked) as well as their willingness to get out of the house.

For those reasons, SVT discriminators can make device therapy more specific [specifically targeting true VT and ventricular fibrillation (VF)] without compromising sensitivity (making sure no VT or VF episode is missed). The theory behind SVT discrimination is based on the same clinical judgments made every day by doctors and nurses who look at a patient's ECG or intracardiac electrogram to evaluate a rhythm disorder. For example, a doctor looking at an ECG of a patient with a high ventricular rate would be likely to use the rhythm tracing to answer several questions:

- What is the patient's atrial rate? Is the patient experiencing some sort of atrial tachyarrhythmia? (The presence of an atrial tachyarrhythmia strongly suggests SVT rather than VT.)

- Did the rapid ventricular rate start gradually or did it begin abruptly? (SVT tends to 'warm up' gradually, while VT has a sudden onset.)
- Is the ventricular rate stable? (SVT tends to produce an erratic ventricular rhythm, while VT is more stable.)
- Do the ventricular complexes on the tracing look 'normal' or is there some distortion? (A ventricular beat conducted from the atria should have a 'normal' look, even if the rhythm is faster. Thus, normal QRS complexes indicate SVT. Ventricular beats originating in the ventricles for a true VT will have a distorted morphology.)

These normal clinical questions are the very questions that the CRT-D system will ask in its attempts to discriminate an SVT from a VT. While all currently available CRT-D systems offer SVT discriminators, there can be differences by devices, even from a single manufacturer. This book will discuss the features of St Jude Medical CRT-D systems; the product manual is the best resource for the specifics for any given CRT-D model. Note that most CRT-D devices offer several types of SVT discriminator algorithms. It is a matter of clinical judgment as to which of these algorithms should be activated. While it is sometimes appropriate to turn on all of the available SVT discriminators, the more discrimination algorithms are active in a given patient, the more difficult it becomes for any rhythm disorder to rise to the level of treatable VT. Many patients are well served with one or two algorithms only. While it is possible to deactivate all SVT discriminators in a patient, that would mean that any rapid ventricular rate could provoke high-voltage therapy. Thus, it is important to match the available SVT discriminators to the patient. There are four main SVT discriminators: Rate Branch, Interval Stability, Sudden Onset and Morphology Discrimination.

Rate Branch

Rate Branch is the most fundamental SVT discriminator, in that it compares the atrial rate activity to the ventricular rate activity, much as a clinician might examine a rhythm strip to see if a patient with a fast ventricular rate is experiencing any type of atrial tachyarrhythmia. Rate Branch requires an atrial lead to sense in the atrium (most CRT-D patients will have an atrial lead in place). When a rapid ventricular rate is diagnosed by the CRT-D device, the device checks the simultaneous level of atrial activity and arrives at one of three determinations: either the atrial rate is faster than the ventricular rate (this suggests an atrial tachyarrhythmia or SVT), the atrial rate is slower than the ventricular rate (this suggests VT), or the atrial rate and the ventricular rate are the same (this suggests sinus tachycardia, which is a form of SVT) (see Fig 18.1).

Rate Branch can inhibit therapy or allow the device to advance toward therapy delivery (see Fig. 18.2), but most of us in clinical practice know that rhythm disorders can be deceptive. For example, what if the patient has chronic AF and also simultaneously develops a true VT? For that reason, it may be useful to employ another SVT discriminator that helps sort out rapid ventricular rates in the presence of AF.

Interval Stability

AF is a rapid, erratic rhythm which conducts inconsistently through the atrioventricular (AV) node,

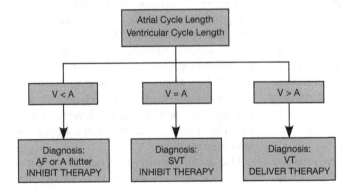

Fig. 18.1 Rate Branch. Rate Branch compares the atrial and ventricular rates to reach its conclusion about the rhythm in question. Rate Branch is one of the most fundamental supraventricular tachycardia discriminators and may be the basis for other discrimination algorithms.

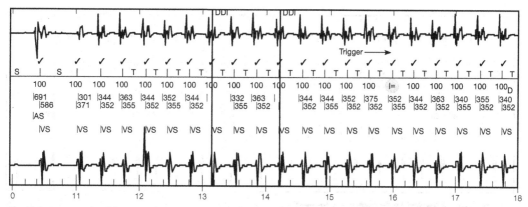

Fig. 18.2 An example of therapy inhibition. Rate Branch inhibits therapy after a series to tachycardia intervals are diagnosed (the row of Ts in the upper half of the tracing). Rate Branch found a one-to-one correspondence of atrial activity to ventricular activity (A = V) and decided that the rhythm was a supraventricular tachycardia. Thus, the device inhibited rather than delivered therapy. This is shown by the highlighted I= on the strip below the row of Ts. (I means inhibited and = refers to the A = V rate branch.)

provoking an irregular ventricular rhythm. Interval Stability is a special algorithm which examines interval stability, under the theory that a VT will have stable intervals, while an SVT will cause unstable ventricular intervals.

To accomplish this, the CRT-D device looks at a number of VS–VS intervals during an episode. The number of intervals the algorithm checks is programmable (for example, 12). It compares the changes between intervals during this run of 12 intervals by a programmable value known as the interval stability delta (or just delta). Using a typical delta value of 80 ms, the algorithm would check 12 VS–VS intervals during an episode of high-rate ventricular activity. If the VS–VS interval changed by more than 80 ms in those 12 intervals, the algorithm would decide that the interval stability was 'irregular', allowing it to diagnose AF with rapid ventricular response and inhibiting therapy.

On the other hand, if no VS–VS intervals changed by more than 80 ms in those 12 intervals, the CRT-D system would decide that the VS–VS intervals were stable, allowing it to diagnose a VT, which would cause the device to advance to therapy delivery.

Interval Stability can be used alone or together with Rate Branch. The combination may be particularly appropriate for CRT-D patients with known or suspected AF. Note that Rate Branch requires an atrial lead to sense the atrium, but Interval Stability does not. Thus, for the CRT-D patient with known

or suspected AF and a device system without atrial sensing (either no atrial lead or one that does not sense properly), Interval Stability can still work to discriminate SVTs from VT (see Fig. 18.3).

Sudden Onset

Sinus tachycardia occurs in patients who have both an atrial tachycardia and an intact conduction system. Sometimes sinus tachycardia is perfectly appropriate, for example, when a person is exercising or under stress. At other times, sinus tachycardia may be the 'normal' response to a relatively slow atrial tachycardia (not AF). CRT-D patients susceptible to sinus tachycardia (i.e. patients who have intact conduction and are either active or may experience atrial tachycardia) present a special challenge to the device, particularly if their 'normal' sinus tachycardia may occur at rates that overlap with rates of a VT. For example, what about a CRT-D patient who experiences 'slow VT' at around 120 beats/min but also experiences sinus tachycardia rates of 100–130 beats/min? How can the device reliably discriminate an SVT from a VT at 120 beats/min?

It has been observed in such patients that a sinus tachycardia typically starts out gradually and builds up to faster and faster rates, often as physiological demand increases. On the other hand, VT tends to start abruptly. Just as a doctor might scan an ECG to see if a rapid ventricular rate commenced gradually or all at once, the Sudden Onset algorithm looks at

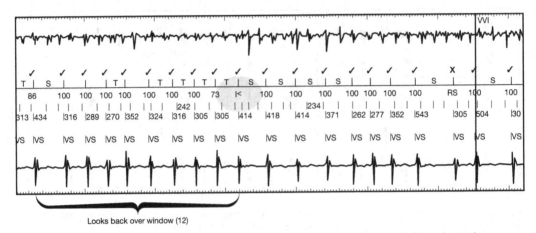

Fig. 18.3 Another example of therapy inhibition. In this example, a run of tachycardia intervals (Ts on the strip) occurs, but the Interval Stability algorithm is active. In this case, the algorithm determined that the atrial rate was faster than the ventricular rate (A < V) and decided the rhythm disorder was a supraventricular tachycardia. This caused therapy to be inhibited. This is indicated in the annotations as I<, where I means inhibition and < refers to the A < V Rate Branch.

the change or delta in interval measurement from a non-tachycardia interval to a tachycardia interval. As an example, let us assume a Sudden Onset delta at a typical value of 100 ms (the delta value is programmable). The Sudden Onset algorithm looks to see if the transition from non-tachycardia to tachycardia interval was less than or greater than 100 ms. If the change is > 100 ms, then VT is diagnosed. If the change is < 100 ms, then SVT is diagnosed and therapy is inhibited (see Fig. 18.4).

Morphology Discrimination

The QRS complex on the ECG is the visual record of the ventricular contraction, and its morphology or shape varies with the origin of the depolarization. For example, most clinicians have observed that a

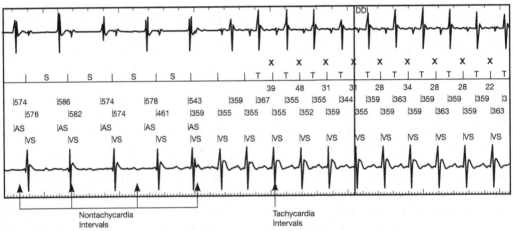

Fig. 18.4 More therapy inhibition. The Sudden Onset Discriminator compares non-tachycardia intervals with tachycardia intervals and looks at the change or delta. A programmable Sudden Onset delta determines the cut-off value. If the change from non-tachycardia interval to tachycardia interval exceeds the delta, the device considers this to be sudden onset, diagnoses ventricular tachycardia and proceeds to deliver therapy. If the change from non-tachycardia interval to tachycardia interval is less than the delta value, the device considers this not to be sudden onset, diagnoses supraventricular tachycardia and inhibits therapy.

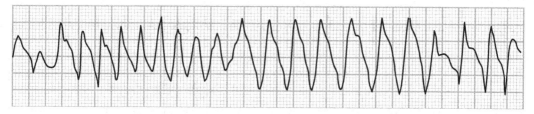

Fig. 18.5 Polymorphic ventricular tachycardia (VT). A polymorphic VT is a rhythm disorder involving multiple sites of origin of the ventricular arrhythmia. Note that each origin provokes a differently shaped QRS complex.

paced QRS looks different (wider and sometimes with a little notch) than an intrinsic QRS (narrower, sharper, no notch). A patient with a polymorphic VT has a rhythm disorder with multiple (poly) origins and thus QRS complexes of varying shapes (see Fig. 18.5).

A patient experiencing an SVT with a rapid ventricular response will have relatively 'normal-looking' QRS complexes since they are naturally conducted from the atria to the ventricles. A patient with VT will have a different QRS morphology, since the rhythm disorder arises in the ventricles. While there can be considerable variation in QRS morphology in SVT versus VT between patients, the morphology distinctions are relatively consistent and clear-cut within a single patient (see Fig. 18.6).

Morphology Discrimination first captures a template of the patient's QRS morphology in normal sinus rhythm. This step is typically done at implant or in an early follow-up session. It can be set up to update automatically, in that the CRT-D system may be programmed to get new templates at periodic intervals. Furthermore, the template can be manually updated in any programming session. Updated templates can be important, since QRS morphology may change over time, in particular in patients with such serious conditions as heart failure.

When the device detects a possible rhythm disorder, the Morphology Discrimination algorithm initiates a scoring algorithm in which it compares the 'normal' template against the QRS of the suspicious rhythm. The match is reported as a percentage, with 100% an exact match. The percentage match that counts as a true match is a programmable value; a typical programmed percentage value might be 60% match counts as a match. Also programmable is the number of intervals that the device must find

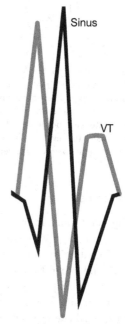

Fig. 18.6 QRS during sinus rhythm versus during ventricular tachycardia. QRS morphology varies by the origin of the rhythm. A QRS that originates from the sinus node tends to be taller, narrower and sharper than a QRS of ventricular origin.

this degree or more of match. If the CRT-D system can count the programmed number of complexes that match the template 60% or more (or whatever the programmed percentage), then the device determines that the arrhythmia is an SVT. The logic is that if the complex looks like a sinus complex, the rhythm is likely to be an SVT.

If, after the programmed number of intervals, the device cannot match the sinus template to the QRS complex, a non-match is determined. The device decides that the rhythm in question is a VT and will advance toward therapy (see Fig. 18.7).

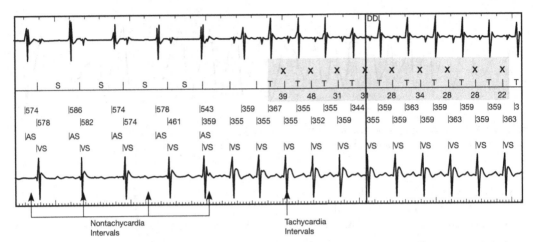

Fig. 18.7 Morphology Discrimination leading to therapy. Morphology Discrimination goes into effect as soon as a rhythm disorder was detected (shaded area). The row of Ts indicates ventricular tachycardia (VT) intervals. Below the Ts is a series of numbers starting with 39. These are the percentage figures for the match (39% match, 48% match, 31% match and so on). Above the row of Ts, the symbol X appears. Each X indicates a tachycardia interval for which no match was made. In this example, the system was programmed to seek out a 60% match in five out of eight tachycardia intervals. The device could not make a match (not even in a single interval), which means the device determines the rhythm disorder is a VT. The CRT-D system would begin to prepare to deliver therapy.

Special features

The most important function of a CRT-D system in the presence of a VT or VF is deliver high-voltage therapy. While discrimination algorithms and antitachycardia and other features exist to help minimize exposure to inappropriate shocks, it can be crucial that the device does not waste too much time with ineffective therapies or attempting unsuccessful therapies if the patient is truly experiencing a life-threatening ventricular arrhythmia. Thus, when SVT discriminators are used, it is important to activate some timing features that prevent prolonged exposure to unsuccessful therapies. These are VT Therapy Timeout and SVT Discrimination Timeout.

VT Therapy Timeout

The purpose behind VT Timeout is that high-voltage therapy gets delivered quickly to a patient in a potentially lethal ventricular tachyarrhythmia. This timer can be set to a number of different programmable settings (from 10 s to 5 min) and a good typical value is 20 s. When programmed in this manner, the timer will allow the device to wait only a maximum of 20 s before high-voltage therapy is delivered.

The approach is designed to ensure that the patient receives adequate therapy quickly. When programmed effectively, the VT Timeout feature allows clinicians to program lower-voltage cardioversion shocks or even antitachycardia pacing therapy with confidence, knowing that if they do not convert a VT quickly, high-voltage therapy will be delivered promptly.

VT Timeout is a timer that begins as soon as the first tachycardia interval in the rhythm disorder is binned. When it times out, it overrides any other programmed therapy and goes immediately to high-voltage shock.

SVT Discrimination Timeout

Most CRT-D devices can be set up with efficient SVT discriminators to help prevent inappropriate shocks when the patient experiences rapid ventricular response to an SVT. However, SVTs can sometimes last for a very long time and the patient needs relief from the rapid ventricular response. SVT Timeout sets a time limit in terms of how long a CRT-D system can withhold therapy in the presence of a rhythm the device recognizes as an SVT. Programmable from 20 s to 60 min, a good typical setting might be 30 s. (For patients who experience frequent, long-lasting spells of SVTs that they tolerate well, longer timeouts, even 10 or 20 min, might be appropriate.)

When the SVT Timeout expires, therapy is delivered.

Both VT Timeout and SVT Timeout are available to treat only VT. VF should be treated with immediate high-voltage therapy.

Putting it all together

For the primary-prevention patient with no known rhythm disorders or patients with only VF, programming therapy is often quite straightforward, but many patients have multiple rhythm disorders and may tolerate some quite well, at least for a short period. The decision as to which advanced features to program becomes highly individualized! Although it may seem complicated at first, these advanced features give the clinician incredible flexibility in fitting therapy to meet the specific requirements for virtually any type of CRT-D patient.

First of all, for patients with only VF or primary-prevention patients, the device configuration offers only one zone (VF) and one therapy (high-voltage shocks). As the configuration expands to two or three zones (VT and VF or VT1, VT2 and VF), it may be useful to impose some algorithms to help sort out potential SVTs from VTs. Note that the more

SVT discriminators are used, the more discriminating the device becomes. This means a device with all discrimination algorithms in use will scrutinize every rhythm disorder much more critically than a device with just a single discrimination algorithm activated. For that reason, most clinicians will program one or two discriminators (typically Rate Branch as the basis, and then possibly Morphology Discrimination) as a good start. If the patient is known to have sinus tachycardias that 'confuse' the CRT-D device, Sudden Onset can be added to the mix. If the patient is known to have AF with rapid ventricular response, Interval Stability might be added instead (see Table 18.1).

References

1 Rinaldi CA, Simon RD, Baszko A *et al*. A 17-year experience of inappropriate shock therapy in patients with implantable cardioverter-defibrillators: are we getting any better? *Heart* 2004; **90**:330–1.

2 Nunain SO, Roelke M, Trouton T *et al*. Limitations and late complications of third generation implantable cardioverter defibrillators. *Circulation* 1995; **91**:2204–13.

3 Brugada J. Is inappropriate therapy a resolved issue with current implantable cardioverter defibrillators? *Am J Cardiol* 1999; **83**:40D–44D.

Table 18.1 Special defibrillation features. Care must be taken by the clinician when programming special defibrillation features; not every feature is appropriate for every patient. In fact, programming too many highly specific features can make the device overly selective in terms of identifying dangerous tachyarrhythmias; likewise, not programming any such features can set the stage for the device to deliver inappropriate therapy. The judicious use of these features can improve defibrillation specificity and sensitivity.

Advanced defib features	What it does	Why you would program it	Why you would not program it
Rate Branch	Compares atrial rates with ventricular rates	Suitable for most patients; however, if patient is known to have both AF and VT, it is probably useful to add Interval Stability	Not available unless there is a properly sensing atrial lead; if the atrial lead is damaged, fails to function, or is compromised, this algorithm will no longer work
Interval Stability	Compares VS–VS intervals to see if ventricular activity is stable (stable VS–VS indicates VT, while unstable VS–VS indicates SVT)	Useful for patients with known AF and VT. If there is no atrial lead, this can be programmed instead of Rate Branch. When used with Rate Branch provides 'safety net' that no AF and VT are occurring simultaneously	If the patient is known to have VT with some degree of interval instability, do not program this or program the delta value carefully. Probably not necessary for patients without known AF who are using Rate Branch
Sudden Onset	Compares non-tachycardia intervals with tachycardia intervals and compares against a delta to see if onset was gradual or abrupt	Useful for patients who may be susceptible to sinus tachycardia (i.e. with intact conduction and atrial tachycardia) particularly if a sinus tachycardia might occur at or around the same rate as a true VT	Not useful for patients with AF or those with poor or non-existent AV conduction
Morphology Discrimination	Compares sinus QRS with QRS in suspicious rhythm and matches based on percentage for a certain number of intervals (such as 60% match in 5 out of 8 intervals)	Useful for most patients with SVTs. Note that an atrial lead is not required	Not useful if the patient does not have SVTs
VT Timeout	Limits time that less-than-maximum therapy is delivered to treat a VT	Useful when cardioversion or ATP might break a VT, but where the patient's exposure to a VT should be limited as much as possible	Cannot be programmed for VF and is not useful when the patient does not tolerate VT well or becomes hemodynamically compromised quickly
SVT Timeout	Limits time that SVT discriminators can inhibit therapy and launches therapy, even if the rhythm disorder might truly be an SVT	Ideal for patients with known SVTs, particularly those susceptible to longer spells of SVTs or patients who do not tolerate SVTs well (or both)	Not available without SVT discriminators. There is a lot of flexibility in programming this timer. Patients who require quick relief from SVTs should be programmed to short durations, while those who tolerate SVTs well can be programmed to longer timer periods

AF, Atrial fibrillation; VT, ventricular tachycardia; SVT, supraventricular tachycardia; AV, atrioventricular; ATP, antitachycardia pacing; VF, ventricular fibrillation.

The nuts and bolts of advanced defibrillation functions

- Supraventricular tachycardias (SVT) originate above the ventricles and ventricular tachycardias (VT) originate within the ventricles. While both can be characterized by rapid ventricular activity, defibrillation is most appropriately directed at VT.
- Therapy delivery to an SVT is called 'inappropriate' and can cause the patient to experience a distressing, painful shock that drains battery life from the device.
- SVT discriminators are algorithms in the CRT-D device designed to help distinguish SVT from VT. They include: Sudden Onset, Interval Stability, Rate Branch and Morphology Discrimination. All of them look for basically the same things that a clinician would look for on an ECG or electrogram when trying to determine the nature of a particular rhythm disorder.
- Rate Branch is an algorithm which compares the atrial rate with the ventricular rate. If A > V, the device categorizes the rhythm as AF or atrial flutter. If A = V, the device decides that it is a sinus tachycardia (SVT). In both cases, therapy delivery is inhibited. If A < V, the device sees this as VT and advances to therapy delivery.
- Interval Stability is an algorithm which examines a series of consecutive VS–VS intervals to see if the intervals are stable or erratic. To do this, it uses an X out of Y pattern (e.g. any 8 intervals out of 12 consecutive intervals) and compares them with a programmable delta value. If the programmed number of intervals (8) varies by more than the programmed delta, the rhythm is categorized as unstable. An unstable rhythm is likely to be a rapid ventricular response to AF rather than a true VT. If the rhythm is unstable, therapy delivery is inhibited.
- Rate Branch plus Interval Stability is a good combination for patients with known AF and the likelihood of having simultaneous episodes of both VT and AF. In such cases, Rate Branch alone might fail to discriminate SVT from VT (A > V), but the addition of Interval Stability could help 'uncover' a VT in the presence of AF.

- Sudden Onset determines if an arrhythmia started abruptly (likely to be VT) or gradually (more likely to be an SVT). To do this, it looks at a number of intervals within a consecutive range (the X out of Y pattern) and compares the change in intervals with a programmable delta. If the change is greater than the delta, the onset was sudden (VT, therapy is delivered), but if the change is less than the delta, the onset was gradual (SVT, therapy is inhibited).
- Sudden Onset is particularly valuable for patients who are susceptible to appropriate sinus tachycardias that could occur at rate ranges of actual episodes of VT. For example, a patient who might get a sinus tachycardia of 120 beats/min during exertion could also be experiencing a genuine VT at 120 beats/min.
- Morphology Discrimination compares a template of the patient's intrinsic QRS complex in sinus rhythm with the QRS complexes during a suspicious episode. This is based on the fact that an intrinsic QRS conducted from the atria will have a different appearance on an ECG from a QRS of ventricular origin. The 'normal' QRS tends to be sharper, taller and narrower than the QRS of a VT, which is often wider and may have a notch.
- Morphology Discrimination compares the patient's sinus template with complexes during a suspected tachycardia and rates each complex based on a percentage match. For example, a clinician may program that a match of ≥60% counts as a match and six out of 10 consecutive complexes must match. If Morphology Discrimination matches a sufficient number of complexes, the rhythm disorder is viewed as an SVT and therapy is inhibited. On the other hand, if Morphology Discrimination cannot make the programmed number of matches, the rhythm disorder is counted as VT and the device proceeds to therapy delivery.
- VT Therapy Timeout (or VT Timeout) is a timing cycle that prevents less-than-maximum therapy delivery to a VT after a certain period of time. For instance, if VT is diagnosed and the

Continued p. 134.

Continued.

device delivers antitachycardia pacin1g therapy (ATP) or low-voltage shocks, VT Timeout can be programmed so that after a programmable length of time (e.g. 20s), the CRT-D automatically advances to high-voltage therapy. The purpose of VT Therapy Timeout is to avoid exposing the patient to prolonged periods of ineffective therapy.

• SVT Discrimination Timeout (SVT Timeout) is a timing cycle that prevents SVT discriminators from inhibiting therapy for a prolonged period of time during which the patient is in SVT. For example, SVT Timeout can be programmed to 5 min. This would allow SVT discriminators to inhibit therapy delivery in the presence of an SVT, but, after 5 min, the device would automatically deliver therapy. The purpose of SVT Discrimination Timeout is to avoid exposing the patient to prolonged periods of high-rate ventricular activity, even if they are of atrial origin.

• Care must be taken when programming SVT discriminators and special features like VT Timeout and SVT Discrimination Timeout. Every SVT discriminator makes the device more 'specific', i.e. it makes the device just a bit more unlikely to see a rhythm disorder as a true VT and deliver therapy. On the other hand, the proper use of SVT discriminators and special features can reduce inappropriate shocks and make device therapy much more tolerable for the patient.

• SVT discrimination algorithms work only when the device is configured to two or three zones; SVT discriminators are never used when the CRT-D system diagnoses VF. When VF is diagnosed, the device delivers maximum therapy immediately.

• Primary-prevention patients probably do not need SVT discriminators, in that their devices are likely to be more simply configured (one zone: VF).

• Very few patients actually need all SVT discriminators. The most fundamental discriminator is Rate Branch, followed by Morphology Discrimination. Sudden Onset should be used when patients are known to have sinus tachycardias that could overlap in terms of rate ranges with true VT. Interval Stability should be used for patients with known AF and rapid ventricular response.

Chapter 19

Advanced CRT ECG Analysis

ECG analysis of the cardiac resynchronization therapy (CRT) system focuses on three primary questions:

- Is the device capturing both ventricles?
- Is the left-ventricular (LV) lead in its proper place, i.e. is there any evidence of micro- or macrodislodgement?
- Is there any remarkable device or rhythm behavior that may need to be addressed?

The clinician must first be able to discern readily on a surface ECG what right-ventricular (RV) pacing looks like compared with LV pacing and both compared with true biventricular (BV) pacing. For example, when doing a capture test, if the device starts out pacing BV and then LV capture is lost, the ECG will show a transition from BV to RV pacing. When LV capture is restored, the ECG will shift from RV pacing to BV.

The surface ECG will vary in morphology depending on where and how the device is pacing. On Lead I, the QRS morphology will show up positive (upward deflection from baseline) for RV pacing and more or completely negative (downward from baseline) for BV pacing. In fact, on Lead I a BV QRS complex may look almost identical to an inverted RV complex! (see Fig 19.1). On Lead III, the LV complex will show up as more positive than the BV, again, sometimes looking like an upside-down version of the same complex (see Fig. 19.2). To visualize better why these complexes look the way they do, it is important to review how the electrical energy captured on the ECG is traveling through the heart (see Fig. 19.3). BV energy tends to create a more negative morphology on the tracing than either RV pacing alone or LV pacing alone. Because of the way the electrodes are placed, Lead I transmits a graphic depiction of what is going on in the right side of the heart, while Lead III shows the same image of the left side.

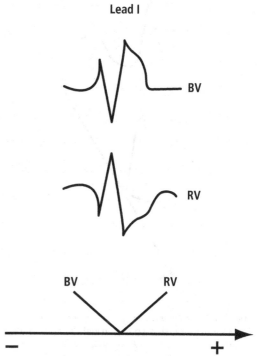

Fig. 19.1 QRS complexes on Lead I. A biventricular (BV) complex shows up as more negative on Lead I than a corresponding right-ventricular (RV) complex. In fact, the BV complex may look like an inverted RV complex! Lead I shows mostly right-sided cardiac activity.

When the heart is paced from the RV or LV alone, the resulting QRS complex on the surface ECG is characteristically longer than the QRS complex in BV pacing. Should the ventricular contraction be initiated by a paced output from either the RV or LV, the electrical energy takes longer to radiate out across both ventricles and cause depolarization than it does when both sides are paced at or close to the same time. Thus, a tighter, taller QRS complex is more indicative of BV pacing than a wider, more rounded QRS complex.

Lead III

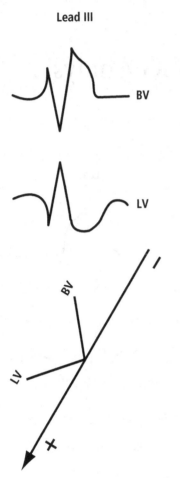

Fig. 19.2 QRS complexes on Lead III. On Lead III, the waveform depicts what is going on in the left side of the heart. The biventricular (BV) paced QRS complex is more negative than the left-ventricular paced QRS complex. Again, sometimes the BV complex will look like the right-ventricular complex upside down.

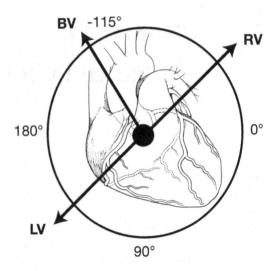

Fig. 19.3 Right-ventricular (RV), left-ventricular (LV), biventricular (BV) waveforms. The ECG is a visual depiction of cardiac activity. In any paced ECG, the morphology or shape of the QRS complex varies depending on the direction the electrical energy is traveling through the heart. BV pacing creates a more negative waveform on the ECG compared with RV pacing alone or LV pacing alone.

The morphology of the QRS complex will vary by pacing type (RV only, LV only, BV), by lead (Lead I, II, and III are of the most interest to device specialists) and by patient (see Fig. 19.4). It is recommended that clinicians following CRT patients preserve RV, LV and BV Lead I and Lead III morphologies on record, since changes in paced complexes (in particular the BV and LV complexes) can indicate possible LV lead dislodgment.

When evaluating the paced ECG from a CRT patient, it can also be useful to examine the relative morphologies of QRS complexes. When the QRS morphology changes on a particular lead, the chances are good that there has been a change in how the device is pacing the heart (see Fig. 19.5).

A sudden change in QRS morphology can indicate a loss of capture, which may be anticipated (such as during a capture threshold test) or spontaneous. Sometimes, loss of capture is intermittent (see Figs 19.6 and 19.7).

Fusion and pseudofusion are the cause of much confusion in any paced ECG, and these phenomena can occur in CRT pacing as well as conventional pacing. A fused beat occurs when an electrical stimulus 'collides' with an intrinsic event in such a way that the stimulus contributes to the beat but does not entirely cause it. A fusion beat has a distinct 'hybrid' morphology, in that it is neither entirely paced nor entirely sensed. When fusion occurs, the electrical stimulus contributes to the paced beat but it is 'wasted energy' in that the heart was starting to beat on its own anyway (see Fig. 19.8).

Pseudofusion occurs when an electrical stimulus falls exactly on top of a sensed event. The result is

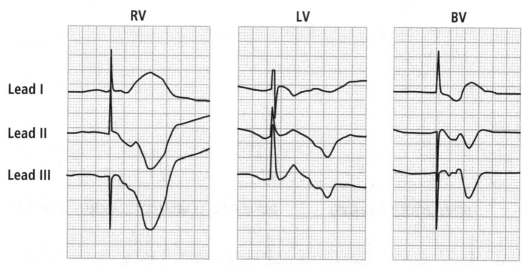

Fig. 19.4 QRS morphology by lead and chambers. Each of these nine tracings shows a ventricular depolarization (QRS complex). The QRS morphology varies by lead and by type of pacing (right-ventricular differs from left-ventricular and both differ from biventricular pacing).

Fig. 19.5 Transitions from biventricular (BV) to left-ventricular (LV) or right-ventricular (RV) pacing in an older tied-output device. The first two QRS complexes in all tracings show BV pacing, while the last two show RV only (right side) or LV only (left side). Should LV capture be lost, the device would change from BV pacing to RV only pacing. On Lead I, this will show up as a QRS complex that becomes more positive, even dramatically more positive, but there will be little or no evidence of the change on Lead III. Should RV capture be lost, the device would shift from BV pacing to LV pacing only. On Lead I, there is little evidence of the transition, but on Lead III, the QRS complexes become more positive.

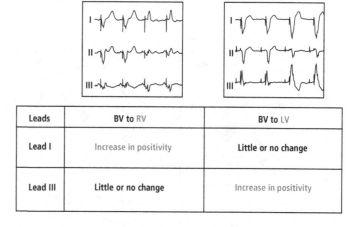

Leads	BV to RV	BV to LV
Lead I	Increase in positivity	Little or no change
Lead III	Little or no change	Increase in positivity

that the output pulse is delivered once the heart was already beating; the output spike appears on top of the paced beat. The morphology of the pseudofusion beat is similar to the morphology of a true sensed event; the pacemaker spike is gratuitous. The spike contributes nothing to the beat and also represents a waste of energy.

The confusion about fusion and pseudofusion concerns what they are (and are not) and what they mean. First, fusion and pseudofusion are not uncommon, so clinicians need to recognize that such beats will occur. Second, fusion actually confirms capture, because the hybrid fused morphology shows that the electrical energy is depolarizing the heart, even though the heart was trying to beat on its own anyway. Pseudofusion neither confirms nor disproves capture. Last, but most important, fusion and pseudofusion are primarily timing problems

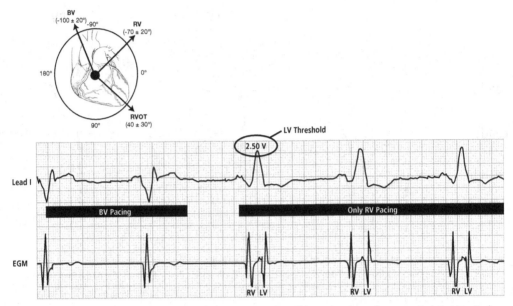

Fig. 19.6 Threshold test in which left-ventricular (LV) capture was lost. This tracing comes from a capture test in a tied-output device. The first complexes show biventricular pacing. The deflection of the QRS suddenly turns positive, indicating here that LV capture is lost and the patient is receiving only right-ventricular (RV) pacing. This is evident from Lead I. Confirming evidence can be seen on the surface ECG, where, during RV pacing, there is evidence of a sensed LV beat. The RV pacing output paces the RV (causing the main depolarization), which then travels to the LV and causes a slightly delayed sensed event.

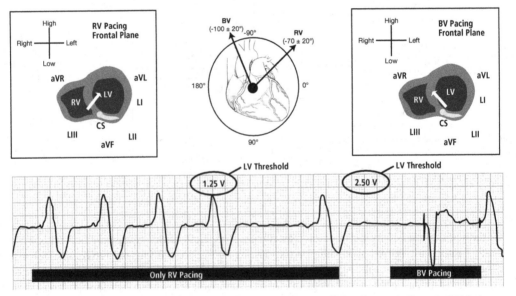

Fig. 19.7 Cardiac resynchronization therapy (CRT) capture test in a tied-output device. Capture testing on a CRT device may be done semi-automatically or manually. The right ventricle (RV) and left ventricle (LV) often have different capture thresholds and may require different output settings (pulse amplitude and pulse width). In this case, RV pacing is tested until the point where capture is lost. Note that during RV pacing, the QRS is wide and somewhat rounded. In this particular strip, the RV pacing threshold was 1.0 V at 0.4 ms pulse duration. The device tries to resume biventricular (BV) pacing but the LV threshold is 2.5 V; this means the initial settings result in another RV-only paced beat. When the LV output increases about 2.5 V, BV pacing resumes. The BV-paced QRS complex is more negative (downward deflection), narrower and sharper.

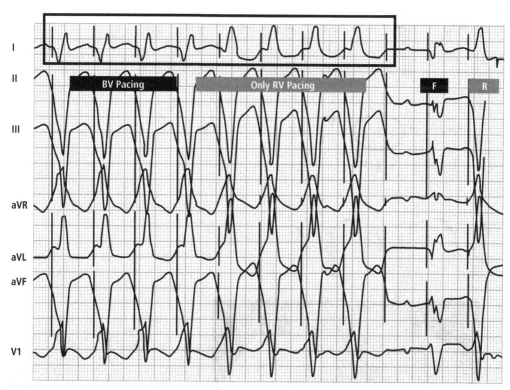

Fig. 19.8 Capture test in an older, tied-output CRT device. The beat marked F has a unique morphology, unlike the paced RV beat but also unlike a sensed beat. This is an example of fusion, which is actually evidence of capture. Fusion is a timing issue. Its occasional appearance on rhythm strips is not uncommon and may not require troubleshooting.

rather than output issues. When fusion or pseudofusion occur occasionally, there is probably no troubleshooting action required. However, should fusion or pseudofusion persist, it is important to recognize that the heart is beating intrinsically at a rate close to the pacing rate. For CRT patients, one approach is to increase the pacing rate (for example, if fusion occurs frequently at 60 pulses/min, a good troubleshooting technique would be to increase the pacing rate to 70 pulses/min). Another troubleshooting technique for CRT might be to decrease the atrioventricular (AV) delay, that is, to allow for less time to elapse between atrial stimulation and ventricular stimulation. Since AV timing optimization is such an important factor in CRT success, this technique should be undertaken only if the AV can be shortened in such a way that it does not otherwise compromise therapy.

Sometimes the location of the LV lead allows it to pick up intrinsic or paced atrial activity and to sense it mistakenly as ventricular activity. Conventional dual-chamber pacemakers and implantable cardioverter-defibrillators have grappled with the issue of 'far-field R-wave sensing', which occurs when the atrial channel of the conventional device picks up the large ventricular signals and inappropriately counts them as sensed atrial events. This phenomenon is similar—it involves one channel inappropriately sensing signals from the other channel, but it works the other way around. In this case, the LV lead senses atrial activity and counts it as intrinsic ventricular events (see Fig. 19.9).

Far-field P-wave sensing would not happen in a conventional dual-chamber device, because such systems have only one lead in the RV and the RV is simply not close enough to the atria to pick up the smaller-amplitude signals generated by atrial activity, even paced atrial activity. The reason far-field P-wave sensing occurs in CRT devices is specific to the nature of the LV lead: placed in one of the coronary veins that wrap around the outside of the heart, it may well be located near or even on

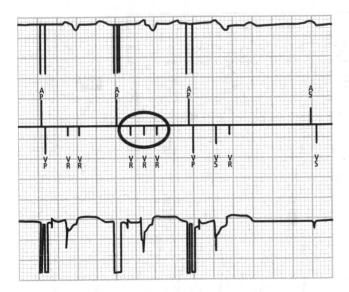

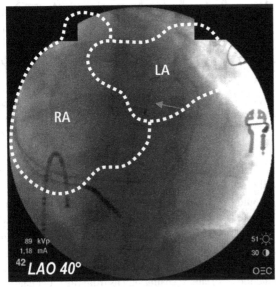

Fig. 19.9 Far-field P-wave sensing. The circled events on the tracing are examples of double-counting caused by far-field P-wave sensing from the left-ventricular (LV) lead. The best way to determine far-field P-wave sensing is to look for markers or annotations showing a sensed ventricular event which does not have a corresponding QRS complex on the tracing. (Note that in this example, the second of those sensed ventricular events is a true sensed ventricular event, but the first one is a far-field P-wave.) Far-field P-wave sensing occurs when the LV lead can sense paced events from the right atrium; this occurs in certain patients because of where the LV lead is placed with respect to the right atrium (see heart diagram).

top of the lower portion of the atria. This problem is precluded in many CRT-D systems by not allowing LV sensing.

There are two dangers of far-field P-wave sensing. First, counting P-waves as sensed ventricular events will inhibit CRT pacing. The goal of any CRT system should be as close to 100% CRT pacing as possible. For that reason, anything that inhibits CRT pacing counteracts the benefits of CRT.

For patients with a CRT-D device, far-field P-wave sensing can result in something known as 'double-counting'. Double-counting is not actually poor counting; it refers to the fact that the device is falsely counting ventricular events that never occurred. As a result, a CRT-D device may determine that the patient is experiencing a sudden spell of rapid ventricular activity and deliver inappropriate therapy.

Far-field P-wave sensing is primarily a problem of LV lead sensitivity. Atrial activity, even paced, has relatively small signals compared with ventricular signals, so it should be possible to set sensitivity in such a way that the device is insensitive to smaller atrial signals while remaining appropriately sensitive to true ventricular activity.

In summary, looking at a CRT tracing can be a challenge, but it always comes back down to the basics. It is important to look at the morphologies of the QRS complexes and to recognize that changes in the QRS complex (shape or how positive or negative the waveform is) generally indicate that something has changed in the CRT function. For that reason, it is a good idea to not only be familiar with CRT

rhythm strips in general, but to keep on record specific examples of that patient's morphologies from previous follow-up visits. A change in morphology of paced activity from one visit to the next strongly suggests that something has changed, which can indicate a potential problem.

CRT rhythm strips usually involve multiple leads, although, for most practical purposes, Leads I, II, and III provide the clinician with the needed information along with the electrograms.

Remember that the normal 'ECG stuff' can also occur in CRT tracings. That means that fusion and pseudofusion can occur, and the occasional premature ventricular contraction may also make an appearance (see Fig. 9.10).

RV = Rv Pacing Only
LV = LV Pacing Only
I = Intrinsic Activity (Normal Sinus Rhythm)

PF = Pseudofusion
PVC = Premature Ventricular Contraction

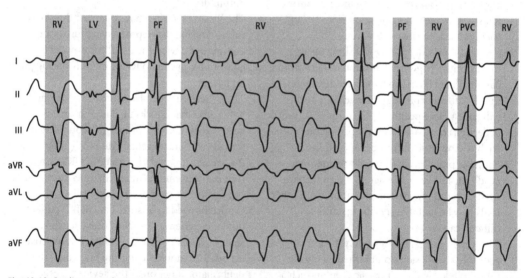

Fig. 19.10 Cardiac resynchronization therapy (CRT) tracings. This CRT tracing may look complex, but it actually covers all of the basics! There are five different morphologies on the strip. Events marked RV are right-ventricular (RV) pacing only. The second complex, marked LV, is the only example on the strip of left-ventricular (LV) pacing only. The two events labeled I are normal sinus rhythm, i.e. an intrinsic beat. The two events marked PF are pseudofusion; notice that they look like intrinsic beats but there is a pacing spike. The event marked PVC is a premature ventricular contraction.

The nuts and bolts of advanced CRT ECG analysis

- ECG analysis of any cardiac resynchronization therapy (CRT) system should check that the device is capturing both ventricles and that the left-ventricular (LV) lead is functioning properly. Furthermore, rhythm strip evaluation of the CRT system should look for any unusual cardiac behavior.
- The QRS complex will have a different morphology (shape) when the ventricles are paced biventricular (BV) versus right-ventricular (RV) only or LV only. Although there is considerable variation among patients, BV complexes tend to have shorter QRS durations and to be more negative than RV only or LV only complexes.
- When the ECG of a tied-output device reveals a transition from BV to RV pacing, LV capture is lost. Conversely, the transition from BV to LV pacing reveals the loss of RV capture.
- On Lead I, RV only pacing will show up as more positive (upward deflection of QRS from baseline) than BV pacing. On Lead III, there may be little morphology change. LV pacing will have a more positive QRS complex (upward deflection) compared with BV pacing on Lead III, but show little difference on Lead I.
- For most practical rhythm strip evaluations, Lead I, II, and Lead III tracings are all that are needed. Naturally, extra information from other leads may be useful in specific instances or difficult cases.
- CRT rhythm strips may also show fusion or pseudofusion. Fusion occurs when an output pulse 'collides' with an intrinsic event in such a way that the output pulse contributes to but does not entirely cause the depolarization. A fused beat has a distinct and unique morphology; it does not look like a true paced or sensed beat. Pseudofusion occurs when the output pulse falls right on top of the intrinsic contraction. Pseudofused beats look like intrinsic beats but with a pacemaker spike on top.
- Fusion is proof of capture (the spike influences the QRS morphology, indicating capture), but

pseudofusion neither proves nor disproves capture. Both fusion and pseudofusion waste battery energy but occasional occurrences of fusion or pseudofusion may not be harmful or worth addressing. Fusion and pseudofusion are both timing problems; increasing the pacing rate or shortening the atrioventricular (AV) delay can help. (However, the AV delay should only be changed with care, since AV timing optimization is crucial to CRT success.)
- Capture testing for any CRT system should be done in a step-down test starting with a high output and decreasing gradually.
- Modern devices offer independent outputs and semi-automatic capture tests. However, in clinical practice, you may run into older, tied-output devices.
- The RV and LV often have different threshold values. During the step-down capture test in a tied-output device, the usual pattern will be to go from BV pacing to RV or LV only pacing, to no pacing.
- The LV lead may be placed in such proximity to the atria that it picks up paced or intrinsic atrial signals and inappropriately counts them as sensed ventricular events. This is called 'far-field P-wave sensing' and may occur in CRT systems (but not conventional dual-chamber pacemakers or implantable cardioverter-defibrillators).
- Clinicians need to be sure that CRT-D patients do not experience far-field P-wave sensing, since it causes 'double-counting' of ventricular events. Such double-counting may cause the defibrillator function of the device to suspect a ventricular tachyarrhythmia, resulting in the delivery of inappropriate therapy.
- The best approach to manage far-field P-wave sensing is to adjust the sensitivity setting of the LV channel in such a way that it is insensitive to P-waves but still sensitive to the much larger ventricular signals.
- The goal of CRT is as close to 100% pacing as possible, but it is still not uncommon to see intrinsic events, including an occasional

Continued.

Continued.

premature ventricular contraction, on a CRT tracing.

- It is good practice to keep examples of rhythm strips from previous follow-up visits in the patient's records. A change in QRS morphology can be indicative of a lead problem, device problem, or other device setting that may require clinical attention. Furthermore, there is considerable variation in QRS morphology among patients and it is a good idea to have templates of a particular patient's ventricular morphologies on hand.

Chapter 20

DFT Management in CRT-D Patients

The defibrillation threshold (DFT) is the minimum amount of energy required to reliably defibrillate the heart. A cardiac resynchronization therapy (CRT)-D device offers patients not only the benefits of CRT stimulation, it also offers the life-saving safety net of defibrillation in the event of sudden cardiac death (SCD) or other potentially life-threatening ventricular tachyarrhythmias. However, this rescue therapy works only when the amount of energy delivered to the heart is adequate to defibrillate the quivering heart. For a variety of reasons, DFTs deserve very special consideration by clinicians, particularly since defibrillation will work only if the amount of energy delivered meets or exceeds the patient's DFT.

DFT testing may be done at implant, but it requires that a life-threatening ventricular tachyarrhythmia be induced and a shock delivered from the device. A capture threshold can be tested with a step-down protocol (decreasing the output by small increments until capture is lost and then stepping up to restore capture to home in on the actual threshold value); however, DFT testing is far more arduous for the patient, nerve-wracking for the implant team and expensive in terms of battery energy. For those reasons, DFT testing at implant may be abbreviated and a DFT established when a particular, relatively low amount of energy suffices to defibrillate the heart. For example, if a patient can be defibrillated during implant at 10 J, that setting may then serve as the official DFT, although it is quite possible the true DFT may be somewhat lower.

There are three main problems with DFTs:
- Some patients have high DFTs at implant
- Some patients with normal DFTs at implant will experience an increase in DFTs at some point in their lives
- These two conditions are impossible to predict.

Defibrillation works by sending a large amount of energy all at once to the myocardium in an effort to depolarize all of the cells at one time. This wave of energy might be thought to 'reset' the electrical timing of every single cell in the heart. After defibrillating energy is delivered, there is usually a brief moment of time when the heart rests and then the heart's normal electrical conduction activity resumes. Although this initial 'normal activity' may be a bit wobbly at first, the heart soon regains its normal rhythm. After all, a life-threatening ventricular tachyarrhythmia is an electrical malfunction; resetting the electrical activity may be all that is required to stop the re-entry circuits.

There are many things that can potentially affect DFTs. First, it is clear from clinical experience that DFTs are not static values. It is also clear that we do not even appreciate all of the factors that can influence a DFT. However, we know of a few:
- DFTs can change with disease progression, myocardial lesions, advancing ischemia, and systolic dysfunction
- Advancing age can increase DFTs[1]
- Greater body size increases DFTs
- Wider QRS, higher New York Heart Association (NYHA) class and lower ejection fraction are all associated with increased DFTs
- As left-ventricular (LV) dilatation worsens, there is evidence that the DFTs increase
- Some drugs can affect DFTs, the most famous of which is amiodarone.[2]

While there are no specific clinical studies that prove that CRT-D patients are at greater risk of high DFTs than conventional implantable cardioverter-defibrillator (ICD) patients, it does appear at first glance that many of the factors associated with high DFTs are common among CRT-D patients. Thus, there is really no reason to assume that CRT-D patients are at any less risk of high or rising DFTs than other defibrillation patients; they may even be at heightened risk.

While there are known risk factors for rising DFTs, these DFT changes may be otherwise clinically silent. One retrospective study of 122 conventional ICD patients found 24 so-called 'critical findings' in 18 patients, including DFT rises of 25 J or more! Thus, even if a patient has a normal DFT at implant, there is no guarantee that the DFT will remain normal over the patient's lifetime!

The best way to manage DFTs is to know the tools that are available and how to use them. One of the first things to evaluate when selecting an appropriate CRT-D system for a patient is the amount of energy that the device can deliver to the heart. Product labeling and other descriptive materials will typically state energy in terms of two very different things: stored energy and delivered energy. Stored energy refers to how much energy the capacitors can store when charging to deliver high-energy therapy. While stored energy may be of theoretical interest to engineers, it really does not have much significance clinically. Of clinical importance is the delivered energy, which reports how much energy the device is capable of actually sending to the myocardium. Stored energy is always higher than delivered energy, which may be why some manufacturers like to report it so prominently. However, what is important is how much energy your patients can actually count on receiving, and that is expressed only in delivered energy. Most CRT-D devices can deliver upward of 30 J. As a general rule, it is wise to implant higher-energy CRT-D systems for the simple reason that it is impossible to predict which patients will need these higher-level settings.

However, most experienced clinicians have been in the situation where even the highest outputs on a high-output device are inadequate. Fortunately, there may be some other techniques that can help clinicians to manage high DFTs.

Programmable pulse width/tilt

Today, we know that pacing and defibrillation are more similar than we once thought. When a pacemaker output is delivered to the myocardium, it captures and causes a depolarization if the energy of the stimulus (the so-called 'output parameters') is sufficient to control the heart electrically. In pacing,

output parameters are called pulse amplitude (voltage) and pulse width or pulse duration (milliseconds) and both together define how much energy the output pulse sends to myocardial tissue.

A defibrillation waveform is similar to a pacemaker output—on a much larger scale! While clinicians typically program the pacing output by setting voltage and millisecond values, defibrillation waveforms are typically programmed by the amount of energy (joules) that they deliver. Calculating joules may require more mathematics than most clinicians are comfortable with: it is a function of voltage (pulse amplitude), duration (pulse width), as well as impedance and other factors. However, what can be confusing to clinicians is that pulse amplitude (voltage) and pulse duration (pulse width) are not programmable in the same way for defibrillation as for pacing.

Recent advances in the science of defibrillation have demonstrated that defibrillation is most effective at certain voltage levels and at certain pulse durations. In other words, it is not always the 'total energy package' that matters, it is the relationship of voltage and duration that is involved in the energy equation. The duration of the waveform is particularly important. Since a defibrillating wavefront needs to electrically 'reset' the myocardial cells, it must be long enough to accomplish that, but not too long.

The first defibrillators used a monophasic waveform, i.e. a waveform that was pretty similar in shape to a pacing output pulse, just on a much larger scale. However, today we know that a biphasic waveform works much better at defibrillating the heart. A biphasic waveform consists of two phases in reversed polarity (see Fig. 20.1). The prevailing theory as to why a biphasic waveform works more efficiently at defibrillating the heart than a monophasic waveform is that the first phase of the waveform does not quite 'get' all of the myocardial cells. Some that are very close to the waveform may get a bit too much energy and others, more distant from the waveform, may not get enough energy to depolarize completely. The second phase then sweeps up these overly or undercharged cells to assure that everything depolarizes. This very simplistic explanation is what scientists sometimes call the 'burping' response of the biphasic waveform.[3]

Not all devices allow clinicians to program the pulse width of a defibrillation waveform. The dura-

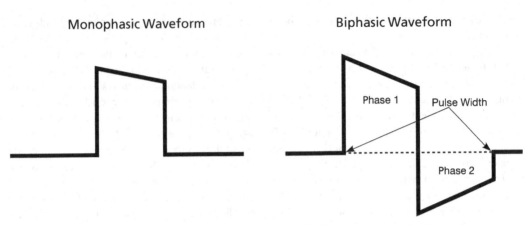

Fig. 20.1 Monophasic vs. biphasic waveforms. The first implantable defibrillators used a monophasic or single-phase waveform. Today we know that biphasic waveforms are more effective at defibrillating the heart. A biphasic waveform consists of an initial positive phase, immediately after which polarity is reversed and a negative phase follows.

tion of the waveform is controlled by a parameter known as tilt, which can be a bit counter-intuitive. Tilt defines how rapidly the energy delivered at the initiation of the output declines over time. A setting of 65% tilt (fairly common and even a default setting on some defibrillators) allows for the first phase of a biphasic waveform to decrease to 65% of its initial energy. A 50% tilt setting (which one manufacturer is now using as a default setting in shipped devices) allows the first phase of the biphasic waveform to decrease to 50% of its initial energy. In a roundabout way, these tilt settings define the pulse duration. A 50% tilt allows for a shorter pulse width than a 65% tilt (see Fig. 20.2).

Defibrillation waveforms can be optimized so that the maximum efficiency is delivered at the smallest possible amount of energy. Studies have shown that an initial phase of about 4 ms duration is actually more efficient than an initial phase of, say, 8 ms duration, and that the second phase of a biphasic waveform ought to be even shorter than the first phase.[4] By optimizing a waveform in this way, less total energy may be able to defibrillate the heart.

The importance of pulse width of the defibrillation waveform extends to special situations. One study found that patients taking amiodarone—which is associated with elevated DFTs—could be defibrillated with less energy if the second phase of the biphasic waveform was programmed to a 2-ms pulse duration compared with a 5-ms duration. Ac-

tually, reducing the duration of the second phase of the biphasic waveform lowered the DFT for all patients, even those in the control group.[5]

Many devices offer programmable tilt settings and adjusting the tilt, in particular making the tilt correspond as well as possible to a pulse width setting of 4 ms in the first phase, can optimize the waveform. Some devices (St Jude Medical) offer the clinician the option of directly programming the pulse width. This provides even greater control of this key optimization strategy. In such cases, the pulse width is programmed (4 ms is a good starting value) and the tilt is correspondingly adjusted. In many instances, a defibrillation waveform insufficient at one pulse width may be effective at a different pulse width even at the same voltage! This technique is so valuable in terms of optimizing defibrillation energy that it should be the first line of defense.

Leads and polarity

Defibrillating energy is delivered through the right-ventricular (RV) lead into the heart. Lead location is crucial to defibrillation success. For that reason, when troubleshooting a chronic rise in DFT, it may be worth checking the RV defibrillating lead. Some devices allow the lead to be checked using a not-quite-high-voltage shock and checking impedance values (this is called the high-voltage lead integrity check in St Jude Medical devices). While this feature is very useful in ascertaining lead efficiency, it does

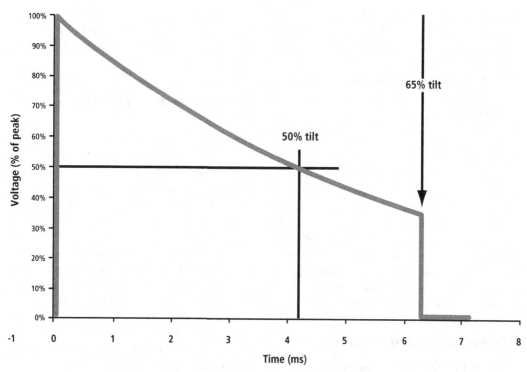

Fig. 20.2 Tilt. Tilt was originally an engineering way to help define pulse duration by describing the percentage decrease of energy from the initiation of the output over time. Although clinicians can control the pulse width of the defibrillation waveform by programming tilt, the tilt value may not allow for much fine-tuning!

deliver a shock which patients will probably experience as uncomfortable or even painful.

An RV lead fixated in a distal location typically has the best defibrillation results. However, in a CRT-D system, the RV lead also has a pacing function that means it should be attached to the interventricular septum. If the lead is positioned too proximally, it may impact defibrillation efficacy.

Other ways to check lead integrity are to look at impedance values over the past several follow-ups. Most lead manufacturers today state the acceptable impedance values for their leads in broad ranges of values. Many factors can impact lead impedance, so it is not unusual to have several hundred ohms variation between the high and low end of acceptable impedance values. However, once implanted, lead impedance values should remain fairly stable. While slight variation in impedance values is perfectly normal over the life of an implanted system, any sudden change of $\geq 200\,\Omega$ strongly suggests damage to the lead. Leads can become dislodged (either slightly in a microdislodgement or grossly in a macrodislodge-

ment) or fractured in the body. Sometimes leads can loosen within the generator ports or their insulation can get nicked or compromised. An X-ray is the next step when lead damage is suspected.

The shocking energy that travels through the lead can be delivered with the RV serving as either the anode (positive pole) or cathode (negative pole). This is programmable in some CRT-D systems, and many clinicians are inclined to adjust this in the face of high DFTs. However, pooled findings from a variety of studies suggest that programming the RV as the anode (which is the shipped setting for St Jude Medical CRT-D systems) is the better choice in terms of defibrillation efficacy 88% of the time.[6] This means that for most patients, making sure that the RV is the defibrillation anode is the right choice.

Defibrillation energy to the heart, like any electrical energy, must travel in a circuit. That circuit can be formed by the defibrillation electrode on the proximal end of the RV lead and the pulse generator itself (sometimes nicknamed 'hot can') in a unipolar configuration or the circuit can be made between the electrode at the proximal end of the RV lead and the superior vena cava (SVC) coil, a more proximal electrode on the RV lead named SVC coil because it ends up being located in or near the superior vena cava. When the defibrillating energy travels from RV tip to SVC coil, this is similar to a bipolar circuit (smaller antenna). Changing the SVC coil (either to ON or OFF) may have an effect on the DFT. In some devices, this change must be made at implant, but other CRT-D systems allow the SVC coil to be programmed using the programmer, even post-implant (St Jude Medical). There have been studies that report early evidence to support the notion that a change in SVC programming can increase defibrillation efficacy.[7] It is unclear why this works and may, in fact, go back to the notion of optimized waveforms. It is possible that changing the vector or pathway the defibrillating energy travels may actually shift the waveform to a more optimized morphology.

Troubleshooting high DFTs

A high DFT usually shows up unexpectedly, either at implant or in follow-up testing or as a result of failed therapy. When DFT testing at implant reveals a high DFT, the implant team may be able to compensate for it by:

- Using a high-output device and programming the output to high or maximum values
- Relocating the RV lead; in many cases, lead position impacts defibrillation efficacy
- Optimizing the waveform, ideally by programming the pulse width of the first phase of the biphasic waveform to about 4 or 5 ms and the second phase to 3 ms
- Changing the SVC by programming on or off.

Just because a patient has normal DFTs at implant (or even over time) does not mean that a DFT cannot suddenly (and silently) become dangerously elevated. For such chronically implanted systems, the strategy should include:

- Adjusting the pulse width of the defibrillating waveform (biphasic, first phase 4 or 5 ms pulse width, second phase 3 ms pulse width)
- Increasing the energy output of the defibrillating waveform, if possible
- Changing the SVC (from on to off or vice versa).

Obviously, surgical revision to reposition the leads, implant a higher-energy device, or change the

SVC coil situation (in non-St Jude Medical devices) may be required, but these should be undertaken only once these non-invasive tactics have been exhausted.

What effect does CRT-D have on DFTs?

This intriguing question is one that we have only just begun to thoroughly investigate. Medical literature has reported on the phenomenon of high and rising DFTs and their possible management for about a decade, but will CRT-D patients experience a different clinical course with respect to DFT management?

From the known risk factors for high DFTS, it appears that the kind of patient who would be likely to receive a CRT-D system is also the kind of patient who would be likely to have a high DFT. In particular, systolic dysfunction, higher NYHA class, and amiodarone are known to elevate DFTs and are frequently seen in CRT-D patients. However, there are no actual clinical data to support this; it is just an inference.

The established benefits of CRT could possibly counteract high DFTs. For example, higher NYHA class is associated with higher DFTs. We know that CRT systems can improve functional characteristics in patients, including lowering NYHA class. Could that possibly help stabilize DFTs? CRT is also associated with higher ejection fractions and improved systolic function. Again, these might possibly stabilize DFTs. There is no hard evidence for these things, but they do offer us some intriguing possibilities.

Managing high and rising DFTs is crucial to the success of any implanted defibrillation system, whether conventional ICD or advanced CRT-D system. Fortunately, today's devices give the clinician many tools to help troubleshoot the defibrillation waveform and manage high DFTs in a broad spectrum of patients.

References

1   Tokano T, Pelosi F, Flemming M *et al.* Long-term evaluation of the ventricular defibrillation energy requirement. *J Cardiovasc Electrophysiol* 1998; **9:**916–20.
2   Pelosi F Jr, Oral H, Kim MH *et al.* Effect of chronic amiodarone therapy on defibrillation energy requirements

in human. *J Cardiovasc Electrophysiol* 2000; **11**:736–40.

3 Kroll MW. A minimal model of the single capacitor biphasic defibrillation waveform. *Pacing Clin Electrophysiol* 1994; **17**:1782–92.

4 Swerdlow CD, Brewer JE, Kass RM, Kroll MW. Application of models of defibrillation to human defibrillation data: implications for optimizing implantable defibrillator capacitance. *Circulation* 1997; **96**:2813–22.

5 Merkely B, Lubinski A, Kiss O *et al.* Shortening of the second phase duration of biphasic shocks: effects of class III antiarrhythmic drugs on defibrillation efficacy in humans. *J Cardiovasc Electrophysiol* 2001; **12**:824–7.

6 Kroll MW, Tchou PJ. Testing of Implantable Defibrillator Functions at Implantation in Clinical Cardiac Pacing and Defibrillation. Philadelphia: WB Saunders 2000.

7 Gold MR, Olsovsky MR, DeGroot PJ *et al.* Optimization of transvenous coil position for active can defibrillation thresholds. *J Cardiovasc Electrophysiol* 2001; **11**:25–9.

The nuts and bolts of DFT management in CRT-D patients

- The DFT (defibrillation threshold) is the minimum amount of energy required to defibrillate the heart consistently and reliably. Unfortunately, DFTs are not static values and may change with disease progression, age, drug interactions and other factors.

- While cardiac resynchronization therapy (CRT)-D patients are likely to have some of the risk factors for high or rising DFTs (including compromised systolic function, lower ejection fractions, higher New York Heart Association Class), there is an intriguing (but unproven) possibility that the benefits of CRT-D might help ameliorate these risks (improving systolic function, stabilizing ejection fractions, improving functional capacity).

- Drugs can affect DFTs. Amiodarone, in particular, is associated with increased DFTs.

- Defibrillating energy is defined in joules (units of energy), but the actual defibrillating waveform is defined by voltage (pulse amplitude) and time (pulse duration).

- Defibrillating waveforms can be monophasic (one phase) or biphasic (two phases). Biphasic waveforms have been clinically established to be more effective at defibrillating the heart.

- CRT-D device labeling often states both stored energy and delivered energy for the system; these are two different things. Stored energy refers to how many joules can be stored in the device's capacitors. Delivered energy refers to how many joules can be sent to the heart to defibrillate it. Delivered energy is the value that matters to clinicians.

- The defibrillation waveform can be optimized by adjusting its pulse width. Optimal values for most patients are a 4–5-ms pulse width in phase one and a 3-ms pulse width in phase 2.

- Not all CRT-D systems allow pulse width to be programmed directly. In some cases, pulse width has to be determined by adjusting the tilt value. Tilt refers to how much the voltage declines over time. Programming 65% tilt means that the waveform will have whatever pulse width it takes to go from the initial energy to a 65% decay. Thus, 50% tilt defines a shorter pulse duration than 65%.

- Defibrillating energy is delivered in an electrical circuit. This circuit may consist of the right-ventricular (RV) distal electrode and the pulse generator can ('hot can' or 'active can' configuration) or it may be formed by the RV distal electrode to a superior vena cava coil. Changing the defibrillating circuit alters the shocking vector or the route the defibrillating waveform travels through the heart. A change in the shocking vector may make defibrillating energy more effective.

- For the vast majority (88%) of patients, the shock should be delivered with the RV electrode serving as the anode (positive pole). Allowing the RV electrode to act as the cathode is not advantageous in most patients.

- Lead integrity should always be checked when confronting high DFTs, since lead problems may manifest as suddenly elevated DFTs.

- Since DFTs can and do change over time and with many other factors (probably several of which we do not even know at the moment), it is wise to check DFTs periodically.

Chapter 21

Atrial Fibrillation

If you have worked in some area of cardiology for any length of time, you have no doubt encountered patients with atrial fibrillation (AF). As a rhythm disorder, AF is more common than ventricular tachyarrhythmias. While there is still some debate about the exact statistics, about 10–30% of all heart failure (HF) patients today also have AF, and AF occurs most often in those with severe heart failure.[1,2] AF represents a therapeutic challenge, even in otherwise robust patients, and managing AF in patients with HF is a double challenge.

Despite the fact that AF is a common arrhythmia, there remains much we do not understand about this rhythm disorder and there are a few myths in the clinical community and general population about the disorder. AF is characterized by very rapid, seemingly chaotic and disorganized atrial activity, which typically causes a rapid and equally irregular ventricular response (see Fig. 21.1). The ventricular response to AF varies by patient and depends largely on the state of the patient's intrinsic conduction pathways. AF has been roughly grouped into three main categories defined by the characteristics of the rhythm disorder: paroxysmal, persistent, and permanent. Paroxysmal AF, as the name implies, starts suddenly, resolves spontaneously, and may be asymptomatic. Runs of paroxysmal AF may be of very short duration, but if they last longer or provoke symptoms, they may be managed successfully with medication. Persistent AF lasts longer and requires medical intervention (chemical or electrical cardioversion) to convert. Persistent AF is more troublesome and rarely occurs without symptoms. Permanent or chronic AF is refractory to medical intervention and, as the name states, does not go away.

One of the first 'myths' about AF is that these three states are specific and distinct. They are actually more like guidelines with blurred divisions.

They are best interpreted as describing the progressive nature of AF. Although AF may start out as a short-duration, asymptomatic and 'manageable' rhythm disorder, it eventually progresses to a drug-refractory permanent disorder.

Another 'myth' about AF is that it is one thing. Current thinking—and the debate is far from over—is that there may be more than one type of AF. The first major and enduring theory of AF involves the multiple wavelet hypothesis. This theory, first proposed in 1962 by G. K. Moe, held that AF started when several places in the atria started spontaneously to generate electricity. The resulting waveforms radiated outward and bumped into each other, creating more electrical energy. Meanwhile, the atria were trying to depolarize in response to these many outputs and the resulting little waves, with the ventricles struggling to keep up.[3]

It was our understanding of the multiple wavelet theory that led to one very effective but highly invasive surgical approach to AF, namely the maze procedure. In the maze procedure, a surgeon ablates a pattern or 'maze' of atrial tissue to disrupt the propagation of these multiple wavelets. A more sophisticated, less invasive approach is the so-called 'catheter maze', radio-frequency catheter ablation which creates the maze of disrupted cardiac tissue (see Fig. 21.2).

More recently, cardiologists in France have made an astonishing discovery, namely that some AF appears to be caused by impulses generated from a single focal point rather than multiple foci.[4] They were successful in treating some AF patients with catheter ablation of tissue only at the focal point.[5] Interestingly, the single focus of such AF cases tends to be in the pulmonary vein rather than the atrium.

Whether AF is caused by multiple wavelets or a single focal point is not readily discerned on a surface ECG. Both the multiple-focus AF and single-

Atrial Tachycardia

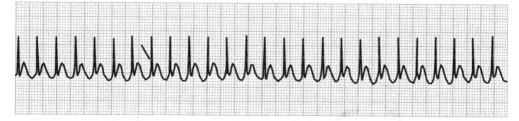

Atrial Flutter

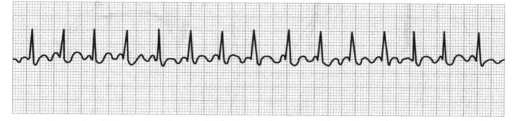

Atrial Fibrillation

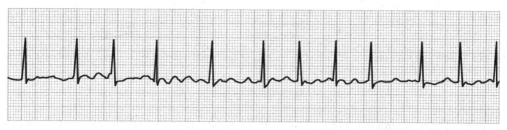

Fig. 21.1 Atrial tachycardia versus atrial flutter and fibrillation. Atrial tachycardia is slower than atrial fibrillation, which is characterized by very rapid, irregular atrial activity and an irregular but often rapid ventricular response.

focus AF create similar ECG patterns and provoke similar symptoms, while exposing patients to similar risks. While the mechanism that initiates AF is not clearly understood yet, it is believed that AF is maintained by multiple wavelets of re-entry.[6]

The last 'myth' about AF that needs to be dispelled is that AF is a relatively harmless rhythm disorder. One study found that the mortality rate among HF patients with AF was 34% higher than among HF patients without AF.[1] Another study of HF patients found during 1 year of follow-up that there was a greater mortality risk if the patient had AF.[7] While AF clearly worsens the outlook for HF, it is unclear at this time whether AF causes more deaths or whether AF is a marker for worsened HF.

AF may occur in HF patients because the disease process affects the atrial myocardial tissue or because the atria become flabby and extended out of shape as a result of pressure or volume overload in the ventricles. The atria may remodel over time. A vicious cycle develops: the AF makes the HF worse, and the HF aggravates the AF. The rapid ventricular response provoked by the AF can induce cardiomyopathy.

It is such a commonly observed comorbidity with HF that it is important for clinicians to develop a management strategy. When dealing with AF, there are two main schools of thought in terms of treatment. Clinicians can try to restore sinus rhythm (i.e. get the atria out of fibrillation) or they can slow the ventricles (i.e. not worry about the AF and just control the ventricular response). These two approaches are often nicknamed 'rhythm control' (for those who want to restore sinus rhythm) and 'rate control' (for those who try to manage only the ventricular response). While most clinicians have the intuitive sense that rhythm control is the preferable method, the jury is still out in terms of clinical evidence. Fur-

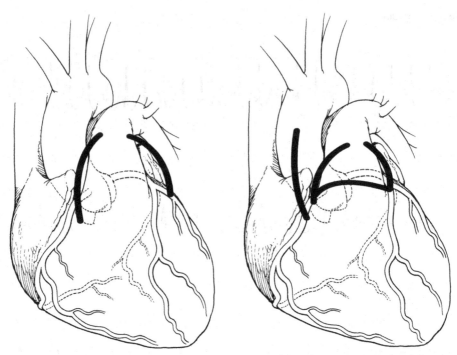

Fig. 21.2 The catheter maze procedure. The black lines on these two hearts (anterior and posterior views) show potential areas of scar formation after a catheter maze procedure.

thermore, rhythm control may not be possible in some cases. So just how do you manage AF in the HF patients?

Drugs have always been a frontline approach in terms of dealing with AF, but HF complicates the picture in terms of what drugs will work. Quinidine is the only antiarrhythmic agent approved for treating AF in HF patients, but other Class I antiarrhythmics (procainamide, disopyramide, flecainide, propafenone) and Class III drugs (sotalol and amiodarone) have been used off-label. The biggest consideration in using any of these antiarrhythmics is their paradoxical side-effect of creating new arrhythmias. Some antiarrhythmic drugs also have negative inotropic effects (decreasing the vigorousness of the cardiac contraction) as well as pro-arrhythmic effects. It should not be surprising that many antiarrhythmic drugs are actually associated with an increased death rate in HF patients with AF.[8] Amiodarone stands alone as an antiarrhythmic not associated with an increased mortality rate in patients with HF, and it has demonstrated efficacy in managing rhythm disorders. Although not ap-

proved in the USA for the treatment of AF, amiodarone is sometimes used off-label in HF patients with AF. The problem with amiodarone is that is has toxic effects and some patients do not tolerate it well. In randomized trials, amiodarone is often (41% of the time) discontinued even when it appears to be effective.[9] Dofetilide has been proposed as an alternative to amiodarone.

Another approach to managing AF with drugs involves slowing the ventricular rate. This could be accomplished with digoxin, which is often used in HF patients. Digoxin will not convert AF, but it can slow the ventricular rate, which may alleviate symptoms.

Patients with persistent or permanent AF also need anticoagulation therapy (typically warfarin), since AF carries with it the increased risk of stroke. The association of strokes and AF has long been established and is present even in AF patients without HF. The idea is that AF causes blood to pool in the atria rather than be pumped through the cardiac system. Over time, this stagnant blood can clot. If a clot forms and stays in one place, it is called a thrombus (plural thrombi); if the clot forms and breaks free and starts to travel out into the circulatory system, it is called an embolism (plural emboli). Both thrombi and emboli can cause strokes by blocking the flow of oxygen-rich blood to the brain. The thrombus does this by clogging an artery like a plug. The embolism causes a stroke by traveling upstream until it gets lodged in or near the brain and then plugs up blood flow. Warfarin and other anticoagulants help prevent blood clots from forming.

However, strokes are not the only reason that AF poses big problems for HF patients. AF essentially takes the atria out of their proper role in terms of providing an atrial kick to enhance ventricular filling. This diminishes cardiac output. The rapid atrial rate and ensuing rapid ventricular response increase demand, decrease ventricular filling time and end up decreasing coronary perfusion. The rapid ventricular response may not allow for optimal pumping action, both by shortening the systole and the diastole; this further exacerbates HF. Rapid ventricular activity can aggravate or even cause dilated cardiomyopathy. In fact, in HF patients with dilated cardiomyopathy, it is far more important to manage the rapid ventricular response than the atrial rhythm.

In some patients with permanent AF, it may be prudent to perform an ablation to disrupt the conduction pathway between atria and ventricles. This does nothing to address the AF, which will continue unabated, but it stops the rapid ventricular response which is associated with symptoms and worsening cardiomyopathy. (This approach will be covered in detail in Chapter 22.)

The frustrating aspect to managing AF in the HF patient is that every effective approach carries with it risks that may be worse than the AF itself! For decades now, clinicians have known that pacing the atrium can help contain atrial tachyarrhythmias.

In fact, it has been observed that dual-chamber pacing (i.e. pacing the atrium as well as the ventricle) reduces the occurrence of atrial tachyarrhythmias when compared with single-chamber pacing (pacing the ventricles only). While it is far from proven, it is believed that the mechanisms of atrial pacing that reduce atrial tachyarrhythmias are the fact that atrial pacing eliminates atrial pauses (which can throw off the rhythm) and works to counteract the 'dispersion of refractoriness'. During the cardiac cycle, the atria

depolarize, then repolarize. Following depolarization, the atrial tissue is briefly refractory. However, with multiple, rapid-fire atrial impulses, the atria are not uniformly refractory. Instead, refractoriness occurs unevenly in pockets, interfering with the atria's natural ability to conduct electricity. This uneven refractoriness is described as the 'dispersion of refractoriness' and contributes significantly to atrial arrhythmias. Pacing the atrium helps to restore normal timing cycles and normal refractoriness of the atrial myocardium as a whole.

While conventional dual-chamber pacing might manage some high-rate atrial activity, it was then observed that frequent atrial pacing 'overdrives' or take controls of the atria, whenever the atrium was paced at a rate higher than the intrinsic rate. In other words, pacing the atrium keeps the atrium beating at the paced rate providing the pacing occurs at a rate sufficiently fast to keep any native activity from breaking through. Some conventional pacemakers and implantable cardioverter-defibrillators (ICDs) were equipped with so-called 'overdrive algorithms' which paced the atria at relatively high rates. The idea behind this overdrive pacing was that pacing the atria—even if it was slightly faster than the normal rate—would discourage AF from starting. Furthermore, the pacing could be done in a way that harmonized with ventricular activity, at least to some extent. The biggest drawback to these overdrive algorithms was that the atrial pacing rate had to be programmed to a set value and left at that value. For patients with intermittent atrial tachyarrhythmias, a permanently high atrial rate could be uncomfortable and it certainly put an unnecessary drain on the device battery.

Fortunately, some cardiac resynchronization therapy (CRT)-D devices today have algorithms to help manage high atrial rates. One of the most intriguing is an algorithm called the AF Suppression™ algorithm (St Jude Medical), which was designed to suppress AF before it could start.

The AF Suppression™ algorithm is a dynamic atrial overdrive algorithm, meaning it adjusts itself automatically to a rate that is slightly higher than the patient's intrinsic atrial rate. If the patient's natural atrial rate is slow or normal, then the algorithm may not be activated at all. As the patient's atrial rate starts to ramp up, the algorithm is activated, but only to pace the atria at a rate slightly higher than the patient's base rate. If the patient's intrinsic atrial rate goes back down, the algorithm ramps down or may go off. With this sort of automatic algorithm, the atrial paced rate is never far off from what the patient's own rhythm demands (see Fig. 21.3).

The AF Suppression™ algorithm is programmed on or off, with other settings that allow the clinician to fine-tune the algorithm for individual patients. It looks for two intrinsic atrial events (or P-waves) out of a 16-cycle window. If it finds those two P-waves in any 16 consecutive cycles, it assumes an overdrive rate. The overdrive rate is based on the intrinsic atrial rate and is typically 5–10 beats/min faster. The algorithm remains in effect for a programmable number of overdrive cycles. At that point, the algorithm enters the rate recovery phase and extends the pacing interval back down to the original overdrive rate. As it recovers the rate, intrinsic atrial activity (if

it continues to break through) will reset the clock on the number of overdrive cycles (see Fig. 21.4).

In the clinical trial ADOPT-A, the programmable number of overdrive cycles for the algorithm (which was called Dynamic Atrial Overdrive at the time of the study) was set to 15 cycles. This appears to be a good default setting for most patients. The ADOPT-A study found that the AF Suppression™ algorithm reduced AF burden in patients. This is the only clinically proven AF suppression algorithm available in a CRT-D device.

When programming AF Suppression™ on, there are a few important things to remember:
- The Maximum Sensor Rate (MSR) of the CRT-D device is still the device's 'speed limit'. The atrium cannot be overdriven faster than the MSR.
- The ventricular pacing rate is tied to the atrial rate; you cannot program a separate atrial and

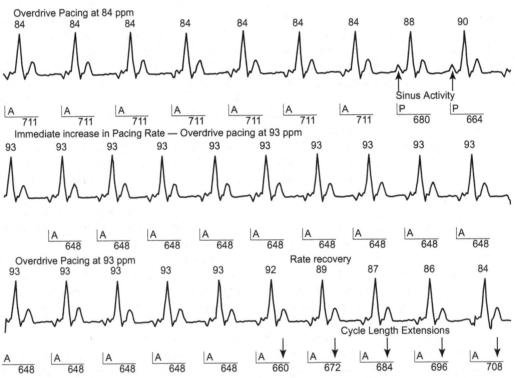

Fig. 21.3 The AF Suppression™ algorithm. In this example using a conventional pacemaker, the atrium is paced at 84 pulses/min to start (note the A markers on the strip, indicating atrial paced events). For the first several complexes that is sufficient to 'overdrive' the atrium. When a couple of intrinsic atrial events break through (end of upper strip, annotated P), the algorithm automatically and immediately increases the atrial overdrive rate to 93 pulses/min, again overdriving the atrium. When the programmed number of overdrive cycles expires, the algorithm enters the rate recovery phase (bottom strip). If the intrinsic atrial rate permits, the algorithm gradually extends the timing cycles to return to the original paced atrial rate of 84 pulses/min.

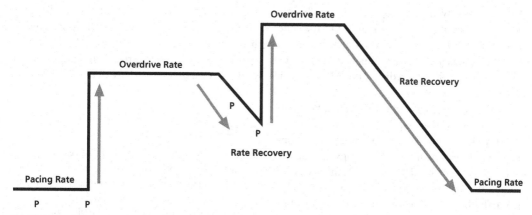

Fig. 21.4 The AF Suppression™ algorithm. When a P-wave is sensed, it initiates a 16-event window. If another P-wave is sensed in that window, the algorithm launches overdrive pacing based at a rate slightly above the patient's base rate. The overdrive rate continues for a programmed number of cycles (typically 15) and then slows during the rate recovery phase. However, if atrial activity breaks through during the recovery phase (two P-waves in 16 consecutive events) then overdrive pacing restarts.

ventricular rate. As a result, you should be sure that the patient can tolerate the ventricular pacing rates you program.

• One intrinsic atrial event breaking through starts the 16-event window. If another P-wave occurs in that window, the overdrive algorithm starts.

AF Suppression™ is not compatible with hysteresis, a function found in conventional pacemakers and ICDs but not CRT or CRT-D systems. Hysteresis is an algorithm designed to encourage as much intrinsic activity as possible. CRT systems try to pace 100% of the time, and the AF Suppression™ algorithm seeks to pace the atrium as much as possible.

Besides suppressing AF before it starts, the AF Suppression™ algorithm offers another powerful advantage to the CRT-D patient: it plays a major role in reducing inappropriate shocks. Shocks are delivered when the CRT-D system 'thinks' that the patient is experiencing a dangerous ventricular tachycardia (VT). However, sometimes that VT is actually the rapid ventricular response to a supraventricular tachycardia (SVT). While SVT discriminators work well, the AF Suppression™ algorithm goes a step farther. With its design to suppress SVTs, it clearly will reduce the SVTs that 'fool' the CRT-D device into delivering a shock.

CRT-D patients who experience frequent shocks, have multiple arrhythmias, or who have received known inappropriate therapy deliveries are excellent candidates for the AF Suppression™ algorithm, even if they have no documented history of AF. While many device patients have AF at the time of implant, AF can develop suddenly in people with no previous history of it. The occurrence of inappropriate therapy indicates the presence of SVTs with rapid ventricular response. While this may not be classic AF, the AF Suppression™ algorithm can still be useful.

For such patients, the AF Suppression™ algorithm should work in concert with other SVT discriminators, such as Rate Branch, Morphology Discrimination and Interval Stability. When the device is overdriving the atrium, therapy will not be delivered. However, the AF Suppression™ algorithm can pace the atrium only up to the maximum sensor rate and should be set at a rate the patient can tolerate ventricular pacing. For that reason, it is possible for atrial activity to 'break through' the algorithm at rates above the overdrive possibilities. In such instances, the SVT discriminators would be the next line of defense to prevent inappropriate shocks.

While it is possible for the atrial rate of an HF/AF patient to break through at rates higher than anything the algorithm can overdrive, this occurrence is not frequent. The idea behind the AF Suppression™ algorithm is that it watches every single atrial beat and overdrives the atrium to the point that AF cannot ever get started. This does not guarantee there will never be any breakthrough AF; that is when the SVT discriminators come in handy. On the other hand, the ADOPT-A study showed that in conventional pacemaker patients with paroxysmal AF, the algorithm significantly reduced the AF burden in patients who used it.

Managing the HF patient with AF can be an ongoing challenge that requires monitoring, adjustment and a strong patient commitment to compliance. Drugs remain a first therapy, but adding another drug to the HF patient's pill box is not something that should be undertaken lightly. While antiarrhythmics may work at helping to control AF, they should be used with extreme caution in HF patients.

Surgical approaches to AF can be curative, but not all AF patients are candidates for surgery. Focal ablation is a promising new technique that remains elusively on the horizon for us today. Surgical ablations or catheter maze procedures may work for some HF patients; however, patients with severe HF may not be good candidates for any type of elective cardiac surgery.

The HF/AF patient with a CRT or CRT-D device actually may have some advantages over the non-device patient, in that the device may offer powerful algorithms to control high atrial rates. First, forced atrial pacing appears to benefit some patients with atrial tachyarrhythmias, so normal CRT-type stimulation may reduce high-rate atrial activity in and of itself. Second, automatic mode switching can 'disconnect' atrial tracking so that the patient does not experience rapid ventricular response to AF. Fast ventricular response is actually responsible for many of the characteristic symptoms of AF (palpitations, dizziness, weakness, lightheadedness) and can contribute to dilated cardiomyopathy. In that respect, automatic mode switching is a 'rate control' approach to the management of AF. Finally, atrial overdrive algorithms, in particular the AF Suppression™ algorithm, were designed to help suppress AF before it can start.

These device features are encouraging additions to the arsenal of tools we have in fighting AF in HF patients.

References

1 Dries DL, Exner DV, Gersh BJ *et al*. Atrial fibrillation is associated with an increased risk for mortality and heart failure progressions in patients with asymptomatic and symptomatic left ventricular systolic dysfunction: a retrospective analysis of the SOLVD trials. *J Am Coll Cardiol* 1998; **32**:695–703.

2 Stevenson WG, Stevenson LW, Middlekauff HR *et al*. Improving survival for patients with atrial fibrillation and advanced heart failure. *J Am Coll Cardiol* 1996; **28**:1458–63.

3 Alessie A. Experimental evaluation of Moe's multiple wavelet hypothesis of atrial fibrillation. In: Cardiac Electrophysiology and Arrhythmias. Zipes DP, *et al*., eds. Orlando, FL: Grune and Stratton 1985:265–75.

4 Haissaguerre M, Marcus FI, Fischer B, Clementy J. Radiofrequency catheter ablation in unusual mechanisms of atrial fibrillation: report of three cases. *J Cardiovasc Electrophysiol* 1994; **5**:743–51.

5 Jais P, Haissaguerre M, Shah DC *et al*. A focal source of atrial fibrillation treated by discrete radiofrequency ablation. *Circulation* 1997; **95**:572–6.

6 Zipes DP. Atrial fibrillation: a tachycardia-induced atrial cardiomyopathy. *Circulation* 1997; **95**:562–4.

7 Middlekauf HR, Stevenson WG, Stevenson LW. Prognostic significance of atrial fibrillation in advanced heart failure: a study of 390 patients. *Circulation* 1991; **84**:40–8.

8 Stevenson WG, Stevenson LW. Atrial fibrillation and heart failure. *N Engl J Med* 1999; **341**:910–11.

9 Amiodarone trials meta-analysis investigators. Effect of prophylactic amiodarone on mortality after acute myocardial infarction and in congestive heart failure: meta-analysis of individual data from 6500 patients in randomised trials. *Lancet* 1997; **350**:1417–24.

The nuts and bolts of AF

- Atrial fibrillation (AF) is one of the most common rhythm disorders [its incidence exceeds that of ventricular tachycardia (VT)] and is frequently seen in the clinical setting.
- AF is a comorbidity of heart failure (HF); together they form a vicious circle with each one aggravating the other. Anywhere from 10% to 30% of all HF patients have AF, and the worse the HF gets, the more likely a patient is to develop AF.
- There are three gradations of AF: paroxysmal (resolves spontaneously), persistent (requires medical intervention), and permanent (chronic).
- AF is progressive, which means that it keeps getting worse. Patients with paroxysmal AF will progress over time to persistent and eventually permanent AF.
- Permanent AF is drug refractory, but paroxysmal and persistent AF respond to medical treatment.
- The two main theories about AF today are Moe's multiple wavelet hypothesis (AF starts when many areas of the atrium fire all at once) and the focal theory (AF starts from a single rapidly firing source, often in the pulmonary vein).
- AF is typically treated with antiarrhythmic drugs but the negative inotropic properties of these agents (particularly Class I antiarrhythmics such as procainamide, disopyramide, and so on) and their proarrhythmic properties make them potentially dangerous for HF patients.
- Some AF patients may be candidates for surgical interventions such as the maze procedure (invasive, requiring a sternotomy) or a catheter maze procedure (less invasive). These procedures ablate many areas of the atrium (in a pattern or maze formation) to prevent conduction of atrial arrhythmias from multiple sources.
- Other surgical approaches for AF include atrioventricular nodal ablation and focal ablation (the latter is not approved in the USA to date but appears promising).
- The two main approaches to AF management involve rhythm control (trying to restore sinus rhythm to the atria) and rate control (not worrying about the AF but slowing the ventricle's rapid response). Drugs such as digoxin can work to slow rapid ventricular response.
- Amiodarone is not approved in the USA for treating AF but is sometimes used off-label to help suppress ambient arrhythmias, including VT and AF. Amiodarone does not appear to increase mortality in HF patients, unlike other antiarrhythmic agents.
- Patients with persistent or permanent AF should receive anticoagulation therapy, since they are at increased risk of stroke.
- Device therapy may offer some benefits to AF patients. Conventional pacemaker patients who are paced in a dual-chamber mode (atrial plus ventricular pacing) have fewer problems with atrial tachyarrhythmias than single-chamber (ventricular pacing only) patients. Forced atrial pacing can help control the atrial rate.
- Overdrive pacing has been available for years in conventional pacemakers; it allows the pacemaker to control or overdrive the atrium by pacing faster than the intrinsic atrial rate.
- Many cardiac resynchronization therapy (CRT) and CRT-D systems offer atrial overdrive algorithms. The only clinically proven one of these is the AF Suppression™ algorithm, which is dynamic and adjusts automatically to overdrive the atrium at a rate slightly above the intrinsic rate.
- Forced atrial or overdrive pacing probably helps control AF and other forms of atrial tachyarrhythmias by eliminating pauses and reducing the dispersion of refractoriness in the atria.
- The ADOPT-A clinical study found that the AF Suppression™ algorithm (St Jude Medical) reduced AF burden in pacemaker patients. The algorithm was designed to suppress AF before it can start.
- The AF Suppression™ and other overdrive algorithms are of particular benefit for the CRT-D patient in that the suppression of AF (the most common supraventricular tachycardia) may help reduce inappropriate therapy delivery.

Chapter 22

CRT in Post-AV Nodal Ablation Patients

An entirely new indication for cardiac resynchronization therapy (CRT) device therapy opened up recently when results of the Post-AV-Nodal Ablation Evaluation (PAVE) study were published in late 2005. PAVE patients were not necessarily heart failure (HF) patients (although some were) and the devices they received had no defibrillation function. Instead, PAVE patients had undergone an elective atrioventricular (AV)-nodal ablation procedure to help manage chronic atrial fibrillation (AF). This procedure surgically ablates tissue in the AV node that electrically connects the fibrillating atria from the ventricles. Without an intact conduction pathway, the ventricles are left to beat on their own. For that reason, most AV-nodal ablation patients receive a permanent pacemaker for iatrogenic (physician-induced) heart block.

Nicknamed 'ablate-and-pace' procedures, AV nodal ablation with subsequent permanent pacemaker implantation is a safe, effective procedure associated with significant symptomatic relief.[1,2] In terms of AF management, ablate-and-pace is a technique for rate control (slowing the rapid ventricular response to AF) rather than a rhythm control approach (ablation does nothing to stop AF). Since the rapid ventricular rate is what causes symptoms in most patients, ablate-and-pace patients generally do well with this surgery. In fact, the long-term efficacy of AV nodal ablation and permanent pacemaker implantation is around 98–100%.[3]

AV nodal ablation is not appropriate therapy for every AF patient. The typical candidate for this type of surgery is a patient with drug-refractory permanent AF who is troubled by the rapid ventricular response provoked by the atrial rhythm disorder. It requires the patient to undergo ablation (typically done by radiofrequency catheter in the catheterization laboratory) and receive a permanent pacemaker. It is estimated that in 2003, only about 2% of all AF patients in the USA opted for this procedure.[4] These low numbers may have to do with access to care, the number of trained clinicians to handle such cases, and the overall condition of the patient (debilitated patients might not want to undergo catheterization and device implant).

Up until PAVE, the ablate-and-pace patient typically received a basic single-chamber (VVI) pacemaker with a single pacing lead placed at or near the apex of the right ventricle. While dual-chamber pacemakers (with atrial pacing) seem redundant, there actually are some clinicians who advocate dual-chamber devices in AV nodal ablation patients, since some post-AV-nodal ablation patients do eventually revert to sinus rhythm.[4]

There are a few things to consider about ablate-and-pace therapy. Despite advocates of dual-chamber pacing, most of these patients remain in AF and must maintain lifelong anticoagulation therapy. Ablation is a surgical procedure that carries with it the usual risks of any surgery, plus all ablation procedures carry with them an increased risk of polymorphic ventricular tachycardia (VT).[2] Post-AV-nodal ablation patients should be paced at higher-than-normal rates, typically around 80 or 90 pulses/min, for the first month or two after ablation in order to help prevent such rhythms. Furthermore, it appears that AV nodal ablation encourages pacemaker dependency, i.e. patients become asystolic without pacing.

PAVE was the first clinical trial to explore the use of CRT-P systems in this small but important patient population. After all, PAVE patients all had chronic, medically refractory AF. Chronic AF tends to promote tachycardia-induced cardiomyopathy. Many AF patients have some degree of left-ventricular dysfunction, if not full-blown HF. Recent evidence from the DAVID clinical trial[5] and other sources[6] were strongly suggesting that pacing the heart from

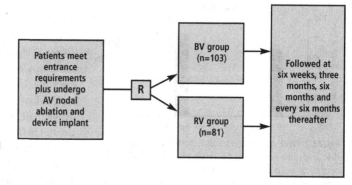

Fig. 22.1 PAVE study design. The PAVE study included patients undergoing atrioventricular nodal ablation for atrial fibrillation and subsequent device implantation. Patients were randomized (R) into two groups and followed at 6 weeks, 3 months and 6 months.

the apex of the right ventricle could aggravate HF in patients with systolic dysfunction. [Although MADIT II was not a HF study, substudy analysis suggested that while devices decreased mortality in patients with left-ventricular (LV) dysfunction, they increased HF hospitalizations. This caused much discussion in the cardiac rhythm management world. However, it must be emphasized that MADIT II was not a study about the role of right-ventricular (RV) pacing in worsening HF and trying to read meaning into any sort of substudy data is controversial by definition.]

PAVE patients did not have to have impaired LV function or heart failure to enroll. In fact, New York Heart Association (NYHA) Class IV HF was an exclusion criterion for the PAVE trial. There were no requirements for patients to have a specific left-ventricular ejection fraction (LVEF) value. At baseline, that is, the point of enrolment into the study, the mean LVEF value in PAVE patients was 46%, which most clinicians would consider normal.

CRT was explored in these patients to see if pacing both right and left ventricles (not necessarily the atrium) might be more beneficial than pacing from the RV apex alone. The PAVE study set functional end-points, i.e. the study tested how patients could perform in the standard 6-min hallway walking test as well as scores on a standard quality of life (QOL) questionnaire. PAVE also looked at LVEF scores.

Patients in PAVE were elective AV nodal ablation patients randomized into two groups: those who received a conventional single-chamber pacemaker and those who received a CRT device. In the study, the devices were called biventricular (BV) pacemakers, which is another term for CRT-P devices.

PAVE was not a study about morbidity or mortality, merely how well patients did after ablate-and-pace compared by devices. The study design was simple and straightforward (see Fig. 22.1).

PAVE followed patients for 6 months. All PAVE patients received a cardiac rhythm management device (single-chamber conventional or biventricular, i.e. CRT-P device) with rate response. All patients were programmed to rate response ON with the rate response sensor optimized at 4 weeks post implant. The pacing base rate was programmed to 80 pulses/min in all patients.

At the end of 6 months, all of the BV patients had a significantly greater improvement in how much distance they could cover in the 6-min walk test compared with the RV (conventional) patients. The BV patients could cover 31% more ground 6 months post implant than they did at implant. The important thing to remember when looking at the PAVE study data is that both RV and BV patients improved. Ablate-and-pace with a VVI pacemaker was already a safe, effective therapy. The PAVE findings are that BV patients improved significantly more than RV patients in terms of how far they could walk in that test (see Fig. 22.2).

In QOL scores, both BV and RV patients improved at 6 months, but in this case the difference was not significant. QOL scores are subjective by nature (they simply measure how patients report they feel) and since all patients felt better after the procedure, perhaps the distinction in terms of 'how much better' they felt was hard to quantify with this particular test vehicle.

As a secondary end-point of the study, LVEF scores were measured at baseline, at 6 weeks and

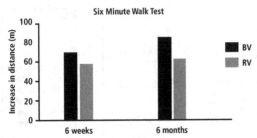

Fig. 22.2 PAVE primary end-point. Both biventricular (BV) and right-ventricular (RV) patients in the PAVE study improved in how far they could walk in 6 min at 6 months versus 6 weeks. However, BV patients showed a significantly greater improvement than RV patients.

again at 6 months. Baseline LVEF scores were taken from the patient's medical records at enrolment and were not captured; thus, it is possible that some baseline LVEF scores were not current. However, LVEF scores at 6 weeks and 6 months were obtained for all PAVE patients. At 6 weeks and 6 months, the differences in LVEF scores between BV and RV patients were significant (see Fig. 22.3). Of great interest for CRT in general is the fact that BV patients did not improve significantly over time; their LVEF scores remained stable. By contrast, RV patients had LVEF scores that decreased over time. In fact, in the RV group, the LVEF decreased a mean 3.1% at 6 weeks and a mean total of 3.7% at 6 months. The PAVE results confirm what other studies sug-

gest: RV patients make systolic function worse over time.

When PAVE results were stratified by LVEF scores, it showed that the lower the patient's LVEF score was, the more they improved with CRT. For example, in PAVE patients in the BV group with an LVEF of ≤ 45%, there was a significant 73% improvement in the 6-min walk test versus RV patients. On the other hand, BV patients with an LVEF of > 45% showed no significant improvement over RV patients. When patients were stratified by NYHA Class, it was found that Class II and III patients in the BV group showed a significant 53% improvement in the 6-min walk test compared with the RV group. There was no significant difference between BV and RV patients in the PAVE patients in Class I. Thus, it could be summarized that patients with impaired systolic function (as evidenced by a low LVEF score or a high NYHA classification) derive greater benefit from BV pacing compared with RV pacing than patients with more normal systolic function.

CRT-P devices should be considered for all patients undergoing an elective AV nodal ablation to manage AF, particularly those who have an LVEF ≤ 45% or who have NYHA Class II or III HF. Clinical judgment suggests that PAVE findings might well be extended to patients of similar pathophysiology, even if they do not submit to an AV nodal ablation. Such patients would be those with a standard bradycardia pacing indication plus severe AV nodal conduction disorder (i.e. patients with complete heart block in which the atria are electrically dissociated from the ventricles).

In reviewing PAVE data, an important conclusion to reach is that RV pacing made patients worse and patients with compromised systolic function derived more benefit from BV than those with more normal systolic function. This suggests that patients with relatively normal LV function are better able to compensate for RV pacing than those who are already weakened by LV dysfunction.

PAVE has advanced our knowledge of CRT-P systems by expanding its potential to a small but extremely interesting patient population. The benefits of CRT clearly are far greater than initially examined, and it is likely that future studies will show other populations in which CRT pacing is clinically preferable to pacing from the RV apex.

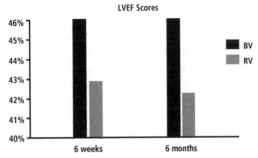

Fig. 22.3 Left-ventricular ejection fraction (LVEF) scores in PAVE. Biventricular (BV) patients had mean LVEF scores of 46%, which remained constant over the 6 months of the study, while right-ventricular (RV) patients showed deterioration of LVEF function over 6 months. Thus, BV patients did not improve in terms of LVEF scores, but RV patients got worse. The difference was significant at 6 months.

References

1 Kay GN, Ellenbogen KA, Giudici M *et al.* The Ablate and Pace Trial: a prospective study of catheter ablation of the AV conduction system and permanent pacemaker implantation for treatment of atrial fibrillation. APT Investigators. *J Interv Card Electrophysiol* 1998; **2**:121–35.

2 Morady F. Radio-frequency ablation as treatment for cardiac arrhythmias. *N Engl J Med* 1999; **340**:534–44.

3 Queiroga A, Marshall JH, Clune M *et al.* Ablate and pace revisited: long term survival and predictors of permanent atrial fibrillation. *Heart* 2000; **101**:1138–44.

4 Queiroga A, Marshall JH, Clune M *et al.* Ablate and pace revisited: long term survival and predictors of permanent atrial fibrillation. *Heart* 2003; **89**:1035–8.

5 Wilkoff BL, Cook JR, Epstein AE *et al.* Dual-chamber pacing or ventricular backup pacing in patients with an implantable defibrillator: the Dual Chamber and VVI Implantable Defibrillator (DAVID) trial. *JAMA* 2002; **288**:3115–23.

6 Karpawich PP, Rabah R, Haas JE. Altered cardiac histology following apical right ventricular pacing in patients with congenital atrioventricular block. *PACE* 1999; **22**:1372–7.

The nuts and bolts of CRT in post-AV nodal ablation patients

- The PAVE study expanded cardiac resynchronization therapy (CRT)-P device indications to include patients who have undergone an elective atrioventricular (AV) nodal ablation for chronic atrial fibrillation (AF) and receive a subsequent cardiac rhythm management device to handle the resulting heart block. This procedure is nicknamed 'ablate-and-pace'.

- Ablate-and-pace patients were previously indicated for a conventional single-chamber pacemaker with a single lead placed in the apex of the right ventricle.

- AV nodal ablation for chronic AF is usually done with radiofrequency (RF) catheter ablation techniques in a cardiac catheterization laboratory. The procedure is not common; it is done in about 2% of all AF patients. Not all AF patients are candidates for AV nodal ablation.

- AV nodal ablation has been done successfully for many years and has a strong positive record for safety and efficacy.

- AV nodal ablation electrically dissociates the atria from the ventricles; the atria keep fibrillating, but without an electrical connection to the ventricles, there is no rapid ventricular response. Patients receive a pacemaker to help keep the ventricle beating appropriately.

- The PAVE study enrolled patients who were undergoing AV nodal ablation for chronic (i.e. medically refractory) AF and randomized them into two groups: one group received a single-chamber conventional pacemaker and the other a biventricular stimulation device or CRT-P system.

- PAVE had no inclusion criteria for left-ventricular function [such as left-ventricular ejection fraction (LVEF) score] or heart failure [New York Heart Association (NYHA) Classification], although NYHA Class IV was an exclusion criterion.

- Although PAVE patients did not necessarily have heart failure (HF) and might have had normal LVEF scores, chronic AF is associated with tachycardia-induced dilated cardiomyopathy and systolic compromise. Thus, many PAVE patients had lower-than-average LVEF scores and had HF.

- The primary end-point of the PAVE study was how far patients could walk in the 6-min hallway walk test; secondary end-points included scores on a quality of life (QOL) questionnaire and LVEF values. These were functional characteristics; PAVE did not present morbidity or mortality data.

- Biventricular (BV) (i.e. patients with a CRT-P system) patients in PAVE could walk significantly farther in the 6-min walk test than right-ventricular (RV) patients, although both BV and RV patients improved.

- QOL scores improved for both BV and RV patients in PAVE with no significant differences.

- At 6 months, BV patients had significantly better LVEF scores than RV patients. Actually, the

Continued p. 162.

Continued.

LVEF values of BV patients remained stable at 6 months post device implant, while RV patients got worse.

- Stratified PAVE results found that BV patients with LVEF scores ≤ 45% derived greater benefit than BV patients with LVEF scores of > 45%. Likewise, BV patients who could be categorized as NYHA Class II or III derived greater benefit from their BV devices than other BV patients in NYHA Class I (or without HF).

- The PAVE trial has ramifications beyond the ablate-and-pace population, in that it shows CRT systems should be considered for patients with a standard pacing indication and a high degree of AV block (such as complete heart block).

Chapter 23

Special CRT Device Features

The evolution of cardiac rhythm management devices is always a progression from basic functionality to sophisticated features aimed at making therapy more effective or quicker and easier for the clinician to oversee or, ideally, both. Cardiac resynchronization therapy (CRT) devices have already had the incredible benefit of being able to incorporate numerous advanced features from pacemakers and implantable cardioverter-defibrillators (ICDs). Their downsized footprint, physiologic shape and sophisticated batteries they owe to earlier devices. Such special features and algorithms as atrial fibrillation overdrive, mode switching, stored electrograms, diagnostic counters and semi-automatic tests were pioneered in earlier cardiac rhythm management devices and incorporated into CRT systems.

Remote patient monitoring systems

As more new features and algorithms are unveiled in other cardiac rhythm management devices, clinicians can expect those functions appropriate to CRT to be integrated into future generations of CRT devices. One of the most exciting developments in terms of new features involves telemedicine or remote patient monitoring. The concept of remote patient monitoring is that a patient need not be physically present in the clinic in order for clinicians to communicate with the implanted device.

Actually, pacemaker technicians 'invented' telemedicine before the term telemedicine was even coined. As far back as the 1980s, pacemaker companies had perfected systems that allowed pacemaker patients to transmit device data over ordinary telephone lines. Known as transtelephonic monitoring (TTM), this 'new technology' allowed patients to have their devices checked without the burden of having to go to the clinic.

The original TTM systems relied on the fact that pacemakers very early on had bidirectional telemetry, a communications system which allowed the device and an external unit called a programmer to talk to each other. Bidirectional telemetry was actually a spin-off of space technology, in that it relied on the same science that allows satellites orbiting the earth to communicate back and forth with stations on the ground. TTM is still in widespread use today for pacemakers. Patients use wrist electrodes or stick-on patch electrodes and an ordinary landline telephone to let the pacemaker download information to a receiving station. TTM does not allow devices to be adjusted or reprogrammed, which is only possible in face-to-face situations, but it can allow a clinic to see how the device is functioning, check on battery status and, if necessary, advise the patient to come into the office.

Allowing remote patient monitoring for ICD patients was more challenging. In the early 1990s, the Housecall™ system, and its current iteration, the Housecall Plus™ system, allowed defibrillation patients to take home a special transmitter unit and let their implanted devices communicate with a receiver at a clinic or monitoring station. The Housecall Plus™ system uses ordinary phone lines for the transmission and, like TTM, does not allow for device reprogramming (see Fig. 23.1). CRT-D devices can also utilize this type of monitoring.

While there are many potential applications for remote patient monitoring technology, probably the most acute need for CRT-D patients is post-therapy monitoring. While there is anecdotal evidence of some defibrillation patients not even being aware of high-voltage therapy delivery, most patients experience shocks as upsetting, sometimes painful, and stressful. The anxiety provoked by a shock (which generally arrives unexpectedly) is often shared by the patient's family. Patients who get therapy deliv-

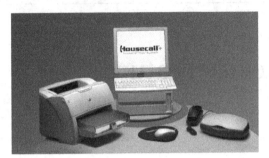

Fig. 23.1 Remote patient monitoring. The Housecall Plus™ remote patient monitoring system is the latest iteration of the first remote patient monitoring system for a cardiac rhythm management device capable of defibrillation. Today, Housecall Plus™ is used to monitor both implantable cardioverter-defibrillators and CRT-D systems.

ery may arrive at emergency rooms or rush to the doctor, even if everything appears to be otherwise in order. Seeking medical consultation immediately after therapy delivery is actually a sensible strategy, but not necessarily one that many already overburdened clinics can tolerate.

Remote patient monitoring can allow a patient to 'check in' with clinical experts following therapy delivery to ensure that everything is all right. Using a remote patient monitoring system like the Housecall Plus™ system, clinicians can review the events leading to therapy and confirm the appropriateness of therapy as well as verify the stability of the patient's current rhythm. Problems can be detected early and patients who might have received inappropriate therapy or whose devices should be adjusted can be counseled to see their physicians for a face-to-face follow-up.

While the technology exists to expand remote patient monitoring, there have been ethical, legal and social considerations which are still being sorted out. A patient who experiences an event and uses a remote monitoring system to check in with his physician never actually speaks to a real clinician. What happens if the patient needs immediate medical attention but his remote transmission gets lost, garbled, or is not reviewed immediately? From early on, remote patient monitoring systems could have tapped into the incredible power of the internet, but there were concerns about privacy. Should people who were wary about typing in their credit card numbers online be sending out their personal med-

ical records into cyberspace? Manufacturers who could build elaborate remote monitoring systems knew that, in the end, they were going to be used by people who were sick and possibly frightened. Would this population, which is largely over the age of 60, be willing to use remote monitoring equipment? Busy clinics faced the organizational issues of how to manage this new inflow of information into their offices. Administrators and government officials had to grapple with reimbursement for this new way of 'doing medicine'.

While much progress will no doubt occur in the coming years, many of the issues surrounding remote monitoring of device patients have been resolved. Improved security on the internet has made it a viable solution for transferring information. Reimbursement and coverage is being clarified, and increasing numbers of patients not only seem to have accepted remote monitoring but actually, in some cases, prefer it to visiting the clinic. The latest advance in remote monitoring is wireless connectivity. The same technology that allows laptop users to go online in certain 'hot spots' can also be used in remote patient monitoring.

The ramifications of wireless remote monitoring are enormous, but not entirely without risk. At the very least, remote patient monitoring from a wireless station is less complicated for patients, some of whom are not particularly comfortable with hooking up to an in-home transmitter. Wireless technology could make automatic follow-up possible. For example, the 'hot spot' might be the patient's bedroom. Follow-up could be programmed to take place automatically at certain intervals during nighttime hours when the patient would probably be asleep. The receiving station could literally initiate and conduct a complete remote monitoring session without the patient's interaction at all.

While automatic follow-up may be possible, it also exposes patients to the potential risk that they may be monitored at times when they do not wish to be and that the receiving station can simply 'take' medical data from their devices at will. While these concerns may seem farfetched, they are already keeping some lawyers busy!

A much more immediate concern with wireless technology is the already overcrowded air. With the popularity of cell phones, wireless laptops and any number of other technologies using the airwaves, there exists the potential for massive interference. The Food and Drug Administration and manufacturers are already trying to work out how to reserve some of the crowded signal space in the air for medical devices. Device monitors are subject to the same interference that can incapacitate cell phones. If every device patient suddenly were to join the wireless network, could we reliably find and monitor them? Or would some of the remote monitoring get 'dropped' like cell phone calls?

At present, there is no technology underway that will allow for long-distance adjustments to device settings. Patients who need their devices reprogrammed for more optimal performance still have to appear at the clinic. While technology might allow for remote programming of devices, there are always potential risks to the patient when changing device parameter settings. For that reason, it is best that the patient be in the presence of medical professionals during device adjustments.

While new device features in cardiac rhythm management systems will no doubt find their way into CRT systems, there are some unique new features designed expressly for CRT.

Integral monitoring systems

Since devices are permanently implanted, it had long been thought that a CRT system could be used to monitor patients as well as deliver therapy. One new feature (OptiVol; Medtronic) continually tracks the patient's fluid status using intrathoracic impedance measurements. The monitor works by measuring fluid build-up in the chest and delivers diagnostic data in the form of trends to clinicians. All currently available CRT systems offer a variety of long-term trend data, including data on high-rate atrial activity and percentage of pacing. These data do not automatically adjust therapy, but can be downloaded and checked to help clinicians make programming decisions.

The QuickOpt™ algorithm

An exciting new algorithm (QuickOpt™ algorithm; St Jude Medical) can help optimize atrioventricular (AV) and VV timing for CRT patients. The number of patients who appear suitable for CRT devices but who end up not responding to therapy remains rela-

tively high. Until recently, the most effective way of managing these so-called non-responders has been to optimize both AV timing (the time from atrial output pulse to ventricular output pulse) and VV timing [the time difference, if any, between right-ventricular (RV) and left-ventricular (LV) outputs]. However, timing optimization typically required echocardiography, a costly and time-consuming procedure. Since optimization relied on obtaining and interpreting an echocardiogram, which could take an hour or more to obtain, timing optimization was reserved for CRT device patients who were clearly deemed non-responders.

Nevertheless, the line between 'responder' and 'non-responder' to CRT is not as clear as some would like to imagine. Many patients with an acceptable level of response to CRT might derive more benefit from therapy if timing could be optimized; however, echo studies were just too elaborate for such patients. Recent evidence now suggests that optimal timing for a patient is not a static thing, but changes quite frequently.[1] In that particular study, 18 out of 18 total patients needed timing cycle adjustments at every follow-up visit. The need for an echocardiogram with each follow-up, not to mention the subsequent timing cycle calculations, seems an overwhelming burden.

The QuickOpt algorithm is an automatic way of calculating AV and VV timing cycles using an intracardiac electrogram (IEGM) and automatic device tests performed with a programmer. The concept behind QuickOpt is that the IEGM contains data, which, when properly analyzed, parallels the findings of a traditional echocardiogram in terms of CRT timing optimization. In fact, one study presented at the Cardiostim meeting in Nice, France, in 2004, found that the QuickOpt algorithm correlated to echocardiography over 97% of the time.[2] Since QuickOpt is an easy, efficient way to optimize timing, it is of potential benefit to all CRT patients, not just the classic non-responder. In fact, several studies on CRT timing optimization show that the majority of CRT patients demonstrate significant improvement from sequential biventricular pacing (i.e. with a timing lag between ventricles) compared with simultaneous ventricular pacing (pacing both right and left ventricles together).[3–6]

The algorithm works by conducting automatic pacing and sensing tests, guided by a clinician at the programmer. For AV timing optimization, the theory is that the total P-wave duration is a good value to use to calculate interatrial conduction time (the time it takes a pacing output in the right atrium to travel throughout both atria). The algorithm accomplishes this by running an 'A Sense Test' (atrial sensing test) and then an 'A Pace Test' (atrial pacing test), during each of which eight IEGM events are measured and then averaged. Using a proprietary algorithm, the optimal values for both sensed and paced AV delays are calculated (see Fig. 23.2).

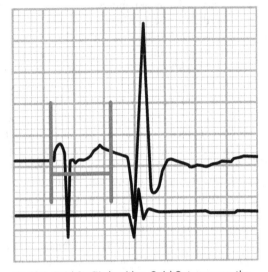

Fig. 23.2 QuickOpt™ algorithm. QuickOpt measures the average duration of the total P-wave in order to calculate interatrial conduction time. Optimal timing is achieved by adding a dynamic interval (delta) to the measured P-wave.

The goal of AV timing optimization is to help maximize preload on the heart and to allow sufficient time for the mitral valve to close properly (before the ventricular contraction commences). While AV timing optimization is crucial for CRT success, it can also be used in dual-chamber ICDs and, in fact, this algorithm is available in the latest generation of products from that manufacturer.

Unique to CRT devices is VV timing optimization. The earliest CRT systems paced both RV and LV simultaneously. While that achieved good results for some patients, it was soon clear that sequential ventricular pacing (pacing one ventricle before the other) was of considerable benefit to the majority of patients. Interestingly enough, there is no set 'formula' for which ventricle is to be paced first or how long the time lag between ventricles should be. There is considerable variation not only among patients but even in a single patient over the course of time! Once again, the QuickOpt™ algorithm measures eight IEGM events to find an average, in this case conducting these tests:

- Ventricular sense test to measure the intrinsic delay between RV and LV (interventricular conduction delay)
- RV pace test to measure the conduction time from the RV to the LV
- LV pace test to measure the conduction time from the LV to the RV.

Based on these average values, the algorithm calculates the appropriate VV timing sequence (see Fig. 23.3). No doubt future generations of CRT systems will include more and more algorithms to

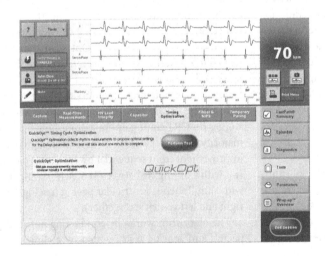

Fig. 23.3 Programming the QuickOpt™ algorithm. After the five QuickOpt automatic test runs and values are calculated, atrioventricular and VV timing can be optimized with a simple programming step.

accomplish timing cycle optimization and other necessary adjustments to make CRT of maximum effectiveness to most patients. (See also Chapter 15.)

References

1 O'Donnell D, Nadurata V, Hamer A, Kertes P, Mohammed W. Long-term variations in optimal programming of cardiac resynchronization therapy devices. *PACE* 2005; **28** (Suppl. 1):S24–6.

2 Meine TJ. IEGM based method for estimating optimal VV delay in cardiac resynchronization therapy. *Europace Supplements* 2006; **6:**14912.

3 Jarcho JA. Resynchronizing ventricular contraction in heart failure. *N Engl J Med* 2005; **352:**1594–7.

4 Cazeau S, Leclercq C, Lavergne T *et al.* Effects of multisite biventricular pacing in patients with heart failure and intraventricular conduction delay. *N Engl J Med* 2001; **344:**873–80.

5 Bristow MR, Saxon LA, Boehmer J *et al.* Cardiac-resynchronization therapy with or without an implantable defibrillator in advanced chronic heart failure. *N Engl J Med* 2005; **350:**2140–50.

6 Abraham WT, Fisher WG, Smith AL *et al.* Cardiac resynchronization in chronic heart failure. *N Engl J Med* 2002; **346:**1845–53.

The nuts and bolts of special CRT device features

- Remote patient monitoring has been around for years with implantable cardiac rhythm management devices in the form of transtelephonic monitoring (TTM) and today's remote patient monitoring systems.
- Remote patient monitoring systems may use ordinary telephone lines (landlines) or the internet or a combination to transmit data from an implanted device to a receiving station. This receiving station may be in a clinic or hospital or a specialized service.
- Cardiac resynchronization therapy (CRT)-D patients may use remote patient monitoring to check on their condition immediately following therapy delivery. This may reduce visits to the local emergency room or to the doctor's office, particularly when an appropriate shock was administered and no further action is required.
- Issues surrounding remote patient monitoring include privacy concerns, wireless transmissions, legal liabilities and reimbursement.
- Remote patient monitoring allows for remote downloading of device and patient data, but does not permit remote adjustment of device parameter settings.
- Some CRT-D systems allow the device to measure congestion in the body through transthoracic impedance measurements. Data from the device can be downloaded via a

programmer and trends from that data can be used to help guide programming.
- The QuickOpt™ algorithm allows for automatic tests which use intracardiac electrogram measurements to help clinicians optimize atrioventricular (AV) and VV timing. The AV timing optimization can be used on a CRT or dual-chamber implantable cardioverter-defibrillator, while the VV timing optimization is for CRT devices. Once the proprietary algorithm calculates the optimal device timing settings, they can be programmed using the programmer.
- The conventional method of timing optimization involves echocardiography, which is an expensive and time-consuming process. Typically, echocardiograms are used only on CRT non-responders to help optimize timing.
- The QuickOpt™ algorithm is easy and effective and can be used on responders as well as non-responders. Medical literature reports that timing optimization for CRT patients should be checked and revised as often as every follow-up session.
- Most CRT patients benefit from timing optimization, even if they might otherwise have been classified as a responder to CRT.
- Interatrial timing values (from atrial output to complete atrial depolarization) help optimize AV delay settings. Knowing interatrial timing

Continued p. 168.

Continued.

allows for maximum preload on the heart and helps assure that the mitral valve closes completely before ventricular depolarization.

- Interventricular timing values (time lag between RV and LV depolarizations or vice versa) help optimize VV timing. In some patients, the RV depolarizes first, in others the LV depolarizes first. The delay between ventricular contractions varies not only among patients but in individual patients over time.

- Medical literature suggests that VV timing optimization confers significant benefits on CRT patients, even those who already have some degree of successful response to CRT.

Chapter 24

Diagnostics

Diagnostics in implantable devices preserve in memory specific information, such as event counts or waveforms, and allow clinicians to download this information later on in any number of user-friendly formats (typically bar charts, graphs or tracings) for subsequent evaluation. While diagnostics provide a vast amount of highly detailed information about how the patient and device have interacted in the follow-up period, only a portion of the total diagnostic information available may be clinically relevant. Even if the patient is doing well, diagnostic data may either confirm that finding or indicate clinically silent problems. When the patient has complaints, diagnostics are the first step to successful troubleshooting.

Cardiac resynchronization therapy (CRT) and CRT-D devices actually do not offer any diagnostic counters or data that are significantly different from the diagnostics available in conventional bradycardia systems (pacemakers) or tachycardia devices [implantable cardioverter-defibrillators (ICDs)]. While the diagnostics may be familiar to clinicians used to dealing with these conventional devices, how they are used can vary for CRT patients. For example, CRT devices should pace the ventricles as much as possible. This means that a histogram showing 50% ventricular pacing could be good news for a conventional ICD patient, but bad news for a CRT-D patient.

Using diagnostics efficiently

Any implanted device has a limited storage capacity in the form of its electronic memory. While manufacturers are constantly upgrading memory function in these devices, just about every device will eventually 'max out' its counters. Most devices simply overwrite the oldest data according to the FIFO

principle (first in, first out). Some counters can be programmed to 'freeze' upon reaching maximum capacity, which preserves the original data but does not record the newest information.

Any time you program new parameter values into a device, you will automatically erase the diagnostic counters (this does not apply to stored electrograms or certain 'lifetime' data). For that reason, review and print out all diagnostic data before you program any CRT device! Diagnostic evaluation should be one of the first steps in any follow-up session, not the last. This is good practice, in any case, since you will need the information from diagnostic counters to help make the best programming choices.

Even if you do not reprogram any parameter settings during a follow-up visit, you should still manually clear the diagnostics when you are done. This ensures that at the next follow-up you will have only the latest and thus most relevant diagnostic information.

Many modern programmers will alert the clinician when new or potentially important diagnostic information has been stored in memory. While clinicians should always evaluate all diagnostic counters in any follow-up session, this system of alerts helps to ensure that nothing significant is inadvertently overlooked.

Every CRT and CRT-D device on the market today offers good diagnostic data. However, manufacturers may vary in how they present diagnostic information and the names they assign to various diagnostic functions, as well as the way data are presented. Furthermore, not all devices will have the most sophisticated level of diagnostic information available and diagnostic functions will vary by device capability (for instance, CRT-P devices will not offer tachycardia diagnostics). What follows is a good general overview. For more specific information on any given device, consult with the appropriate manual or manufacturer. Manufacturers offer excellent training programs on the specifics of their products.

Pacing diagnostics

Although CRT is quite different from conventional bradycardia pacing, the diagnostic functions are similar. For clinicians used to working with pacemakers, CRT diagnostics will seem very familiar! However, the fundamental objective of CRT stimulation is to get as close to 100% pacing as possible, while the objective of most conventional pacemakers is to offer pacing support only when absolutely necessary. Therefore, these similar-looking diagnostic reports must be viewed from a different perspective for the CRT patient compared with the pacemaker patient.

One of the most useful pacing reports is the Event Histogram, a counter which tabulates every beat of the heart and categorizes it by type or pacing state (see Fig. 24.1). The Event Histogram then offers data in the form of a bar chart (histogram), as well as counts in absolute numbers (total number of events), and the highly useful percentage (how much of the time, stated as a percentage of total time, spent in each state).

The pacing states in CRT are described by initials, whereby AS is a sensed atrial event, AP is a paced atrial event, VS is a sensed ventricular event, VP is a paced ventricular event and PVC is a premature ventricular contraction (see Table 24.1).

Using an Event Histogram, pacing states should be assessed with an eye to promoting as close to 100% ventricular pacing as possible. The Event Histogram and other diagnostic tools just provide the information; in the following chapters on follow-up and troubleshooting, we will discuss ways of making appropriate device adjustments.

Another useful diagnostic tool is the Heart Rate Histogram (see Fig. 24.2), which displays cardiac activity by rate ranges rather than pacing states. The Heart Rate Histogram also shows paced versus sensed activity in the form of color-coding on the bar chart. The Heart Rate Histogram shows only ventricular activity (even when there is an atrial lead in place), which eliminates any potential confusion that might be caused by possible atrial tachyarrhythmias. When reviewing a Heart Rate Histogram, clinicians should look for:

- The percentage of paced activity versus sensed activity
- Rates that match the patient's activity level; a sedentary patient with lots of high-rate activity could indicate disease progression, rapid ventricular response to atrial tachyarrhythmias or possible certain forms of so-called 'slow VT'
- If the patient has a rate-responsive system, inappropriately programmed sensor parameter set-

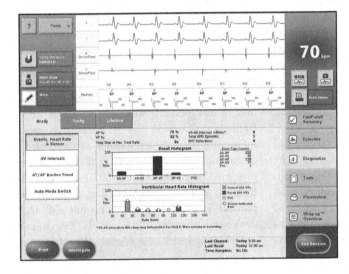

Fig. 24.1 Event Histogram from cardiac resynchronization therapy (CRT)-D system. The Event Histogram records every heartbeat since the last follow-up session and categorizes them by pacing states. The results can be reviewed as bar charts or absolute numbers. This diagnostic report can be crucial to successful CRT because the goal of CRT is to achieve as close to 100% pacing as possible.

Table 24.1 Pacing states and their role in cardiac resynchronization therapy (CRT)

Pacing state	What is going on	Role in CRT
AP–VP	The device delivers an atrial output pulse which captures the atrium; it then delivers a ventricular output pulse to capture the ventricle	This is an optimal pacing state for the CRT patient; it should be as close to 100% as possible
AP–VS	The device delivers an atrial output pulse which captures the atrium, but before it conducts to the ventricles an intrinsic ventricular depolarization occurs	The ventricles are beating on their own, so there is no CRT. This state should be as close to 0% as possible
AS–VP	The atria contract on their own; the device delivers ventricular output pulses to pace the ventricles	This state occurs when the patient's own atrial rate is faster than the base rate. While not ideal, a patient in AS–VP pacing is still receiving the benefits of CRT
AS–VS	The atria contract on their own and the ventricles contract on their own; there is no pacing at all.	The patient is not receiving any CRT. This state should be as close to 0% as possible
PVC	The ventricles contract spontaneously without an intervening atrial contraction or paced atrial event. Sometimes known as a PVE or premature ventricular event	PVCs do happen, so a small amount of them is no cause for great alarm. However, PVCs can act as triggers for certain re-entry VT/VF. A high percentage of PVCs is cause for concern

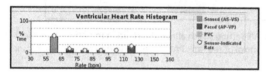

Fig. 24.2 Ventricular heart rate histogram. A vital part of event histogram diagnostics for CRT patients is the bar chart of color-coded ventricular events. The chart groups ventricular activity by rate, the circle shows the rate the activity sensor recommended.

tings might cause pacing rates that are higher than necessary.

If the patient has a rate-responsive CRT system, a Sensor Histogram reveals how much of the time (as a percentage) the sensor controlled the pacing rate. The sensor-driven rate refers to the time that the sensor (typically an accelerometer) showed that the patient required more rapid pacing support than would have normally been provided at the programmed base rate. For example, if the device was programmed to a base rate of 70 pulses/min and the Sensor Histogram revealed that the sensor drove the pacing rate 80% of the time, that means that 80% of the time the patient needed higher levels of rate support than 70 pulses/min (see Fig. 24.3).

There is no convenient formula that can tell a clinician how much rate support is appropriate, because patients have varying levels of activity. In fact, sensor parameters should be reviewed at every follow-up because changes in lifestyle, events in the patient's life and even seasons can make the patient more or less active and change rate response needs. In general, patients who are relatively fit and lead fairly active lives should have Sensor Histograms that reveal more sensor-driven pacing than very sedentary or frail patients.

If the patient's device offers the AF Suppression™ algorithm, diagnostics from that algorithm will reveal how frequently the algorithm went into effect. The Auto Mode Switch (AMS) log will also reveal important information on atrial tachyarrhythmias. The AMS function effectively disables the ventricular tracking of atrial activity when the patient's native atrial rate exceeds a programmable atrial rate cut-off. The AMS log will reveal the number of AMS episodes since the last follow-up and it presents data in the form of maximum and minimum rates and durations achieved from all of the episodes recorded (see Fig. 24.4).

When the AF Suppression™ algorithm is activated, the number of mode switch episodes should decrease sharply. AMS episodes are not ideal for the patient, in that they deprive him of one-to-one atrioventricular synchrony and some patients find the transitions in and out of mode switching noticeable or even unpleasant. However, they do protect the

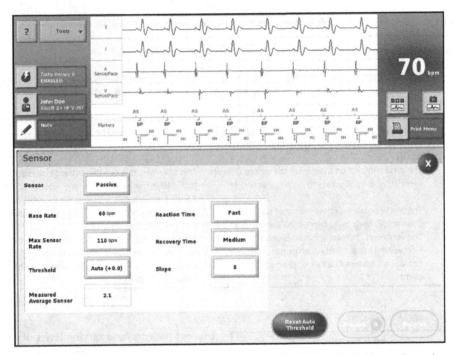

Fig. 24.3 Sensor parameters. The activity sensor allows a PASSIVE setting which allows the clinician to observe how the sensor would set the rate without actually giving the sensor control of the rate. PASSIVE helps to find appropriate sensor parameters.

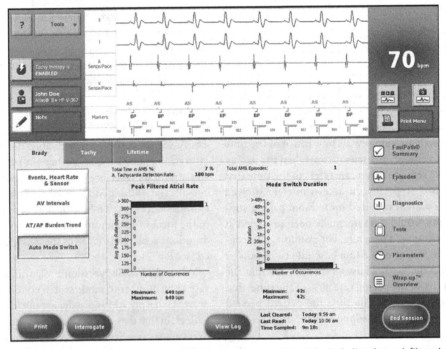

Fig. 24.4 Auto Mode Switch (AMS) diagnostics. The AMS screen captures AMS activity, including the peak filtered atrial rate, how many AMS episodes occurred, and how long they lasted.

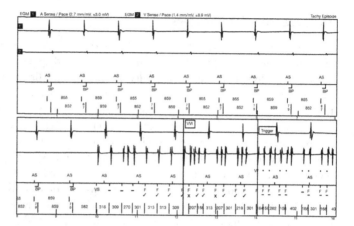

Fig. 24.5 Stored electrogram. In this example, an electrogram triggered by therapy delivery for a VF has been captured. This is a portion of the printout obtained from that diagnostic. It shows VF diagnosis on TRIGGER. Therapy delivery does not appear on this portion of the printout.

patient from rapid ventricular response to high-rate atrial activity.

Stored electrograms

Many CRT devices offer the ability to capture an intracardiac electrogram and store it in memory when a certain event occurs. These 'triggers' may be programmable and include such things as therapy delivery (CRT-D systems), entry into or out of AMS, when certain high atrial rates are reached, and so on (see Fig. 24.5). The stored electrogram can then be downloaded for review during follow-up. Unlike other forms of diagnostic data, the stored electrogram is not automatically erased when the device is programmed.

However, stored electrograms do eat up a large amount of device memory, so the device is unable to store unlimited amounts of lengthy tracings in its memory. Most devices store electrograms on the FIFO principle: first in, first out. This means that the newest data overwrite the oldest. In some devices, you may be able to program the electrogram memory to simply freeze when it reaches capacity. This preserves the stored electrograms, but it prevents new (and possibly very important) information from being recorded.

There are some good strategies to optimize device memory for getting the right types of stored electrograms:
- It may be possible to select one- or two-channel electrograms (atrial, ventricular, or atrial and ventricular). A two-channel electrogram uses

much more memory; however, it also provides much more data. Select that option only if you think that atrial data will be important in making patient care decisions.
- You may be able to program triggers on and off. The more triggers you select, the more likely you are to record electrograms. Use the triggers you need (for example, if the patient is known to have atrial tachyarrhythmias, you will want AMS information) but you do not necessarily have to select everything.
- There is probably an option to record 'pre-trigger' buffer information. This is the tracing right before the triggering event occurred. Very often, the pre-trigger buffer contains exactly the information you want! You can program how much pre-trigger information you want. While pre-trigger data consume memory, they are usually a good investment. Consider programming for several seconds of pre-trigger data.
- You may have options to limit the length of an electrogram. While this may vary with patients, generally you do not need extremely long tracings to see what happened right before, during and after a trigger.
- Consider what the patient is likely to experience when setting up triggers. Are you looking mostly to capture possible high-voltage rescue therapy? Or are you more interested in possible atrial tachyarrhythmias? Or PVCs?

Electrograms can be easily downloaded from the main or special programming screens. They are particularly useful for device troubleshooting.

Tachycardia diagnostics

Patients with CRT-D devices may very well experience therapy to address potentially life-threatening ventricular tachyarrhythmias. Tachycardia diagnostics provide insight into therapies. The best place to start is with a therapy summary (see Fig. 24.6), which reveals the number of episodes the patient has experienced in the follow-up period, along with how the device classified them and what, if any, therapy might have been delivered.

Things that should be considered when reviewing these tachycardia diagnostics:

- Is the device programmed to the right zone configuration? For example, a patient with a one-zone configuration who receives a lot of high-voltage therapy might be receiving high-voltage therapy for rhythm disorders that could be treated with antitachycardia pacing (ATP) or low-voltage shocks.
- Are the right supraventricular tachycardia (SVT) discriminators in place? A patient who receives frequent therapy delivery but has no SVT discriminators programmed may be getting inappropriate shocks. (The stored electrograms can help to confirm this.) If some arrhythmias were diagnosed but shocks inhibited appropriately, this confirms that the SVT discriminators are doing their job well.
- If the patient is receiving high-voltage therapy for ventricular tachycardia (VT) in the lower range, it might be worth considering activating ATP.
- If ATP is on, its success and failure rates are a good indication as to whether it ought to be fine-tuned or discontinued. In general, if ATP seems to fail frequently or accelerate VTs, it is wise to discontinue it. On the other hand, if ATP is frequently successful but sometimes failed, it may be possible to program some changes to make it even more effective.

Other tachycardia diagnostic reports include data on how many times the device charged and to what voltage level, the number of aborted therapies, and episode data. Episode data report on the diagnosis, type of arrhythmia, cycle length, what type of therapy was used (if any) with what results (see Fig. 24.7).

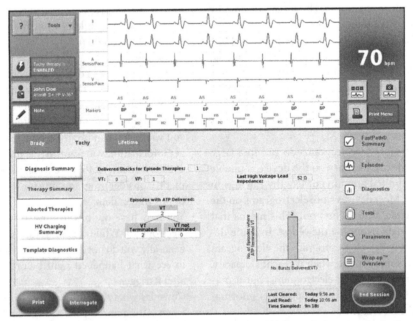

Fig. 24.6 Therapy summary. This overview screen shows the total number of high ventricular rate episodes the patient experienced in the follow-up period, how the device classified them, and what, if any, therapies were delivered. While high-voltage therapy tends to be a memorable event in the life of a cardiac resynchronization therapy (CRT)-D patient, do not rely on the patient's report as to what episodes he has received. In my own experience, there have been patients who received high-voltage therapy and did not know it! Antitachycardia pacing (ATP) is not often perceived by the patient. Some episodes may have been detected but resolved spontaneously before the patient realized there was a problem. In this example, only one shock was delivered for VF but the patient was twice successfully treated with ATP to convert VT.

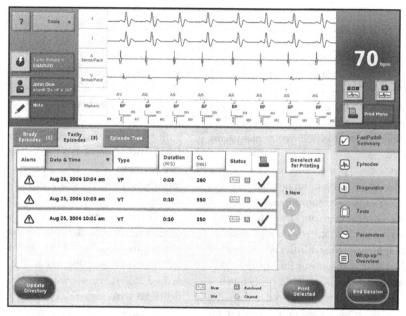

Fig. 24.7 Tachycardia episodes. This diagnostic report captures all of the high-ventricular rate episodes recorded in chronological order. The 'waveform' icon indicates there is a matching electrogram. Selecting a particular episode brings up the specifics on that episode. In this example, the patient experienced one episode of VF lasting 8 seconds and two earlier episodes of VT. From this screen, the clinician can access and print out stored electrograms and more detailed information on these events.

A companion stored electrogram may be available for certain episode reports.

Diagnostic data tips

There is good news and bad news about diagnostic data. The good news is that CRT device manufacturers around the world are building outstanding devices with a wealth of in-depth diagnostic information. The bad news is that manufacturers tend to name their diagnostic functions by slightly different names and programming techniques, although similar, may have subtle nuances that vary by company. Furthermore, a wealth of diagnostic information can create information overload, particularly in the fast-paced environment of most device clinics. Here are some tips to take advantage of diagnostic data without becoming overwhelmed or overburdened:

- Always access and print out all of the diagnostic data before you program anything.
- Check to see if the programmer is showing any alert or warning messages. Programmers are still

unique to manufacturers, but today's programmers are extremely intuitive. You should be able to rely on screen prompts to help you navigate even an unfamiliar programmer.

- Programmers may alert you that there are new electrograms stored. If they look to be of even possible interest, print them out.
- Look at overview diagnostic reports first and then drill down. Look at overall pacing activity and therapy summaries (CRT-D). Although devices store a lot of diagnostic information, you may not need to access all of it to do your job.
- Stored electrograms probably contain the most clinically significant information, but it is better for you to look at basic diagnostics first before advancing to the electrograms. That way you will know what you are looking for and not waste your time sorting through a lot of tracings of minimal interest.
- When in doubt, print it out!
- Remember that CRT is different from conventional pacing. With CRT, the goal is as close to 100% ventricular pacing as possible.

The nuts and bolts of diagnostics

- Fundamentally, device diagnostics are quite similar for implantable cardioverter-defibrillators (ICDs), pacemakers and cardiac resynchronization therapy (CRT) systems, but it is important to remember that the goal of CRT is to provide as close to 100% ventricular pacing as possible.
- Always review and print out all diagnostics before making any programming changes during follow-up. Programming new values will automatically clear (zero out) most diagnostics. This does not apply to stored electrograms.
- The best approach to diagnostics is to start at the highest level of diagnostic information and drill down as needed. There is probably much more diagnostic information stored in the device than the clinician will need for follow-up.
- To verify CRT stimulation, check the pacing diagnostics. The Event Histogram categorizes pacing by states while the Rate Histogram groups paced versus sensed activity by rate. CRT should pace the ventricle as much as possible.
- If the device has rate response, the Sensor Histogram indicates how much of the time the sensor controlled the pacing rate and what sort of sensor-driven rates occurred. This is needed to be sure that rate response parameter settings are programmed appropriately.
- The Auto Mode Switch (AMS) log shows how many times the AMS algorithm went into effect along with data on the number of AMS episodes and the highest and lowest rates and durations that occurred for AMS episodes.
- Stored electrograms offer some of the most clinically valuable information in follow-up. It may be possible to program what triggers an electrogram and the amount of pre-trigger buffer as well as the type of electrogram (one or two channels). When programming electrograms, balance the clinical need for information with the finite memory capacity of the device!
- The Therapy Summary reveals the total number of high-rate ventricular episodes diagnosed and how the device treated them. Drilling down, information is available on how the device arrived at its diagnosis, what therapies were delivered, what high-rate episodes occurred (this contains counter data and may have a companion stored electrogram) and even a summary of charging history for the device.
- Tachycardia diagnostics, in particular, can show if therapy is effective and appropriate. This is the best place to gain information to answer questions about the type and number of programmed supraventricular tachycardia discriminators, the appropriateness of the programmed device configuration (one, two or three zones) and the utility of antitachycardia pacing for that particular patient.
- Document, document, document. Print out everything you think might be useful.

Chapter 25

A Systematic Guide to CRT Follow-Up

For patients with implanted cardiac resynchronization therapy (CRT) devices, follow-up is part of routine life. Because follow-up becomes so ordinary to many CRT patients and their healthcare providers, it can be easy to overlook its tremendous importance to patient care and well-being. Follow-up verifies proper device operation, maximizes device longevity, ensures optimized CRT, addresses patient issues from anxiety to definite complaints, troubleshoots problems and documents information about how the patient and device have interacted over time. A systematic approach to follow-up can help time-stressed clinicians not only to meet these multiple objectives, but to do it in a reliable, relatively rapid format. The key to successfully following an implanted device – but especially a CRT system – is having a system.

What follows is a suggested system. Individual caregivers will be likely to modify it to meet their own objectives, clinical styles and needs of patients. What is more important than this particular system is having a system. A systematic approach assures that nothing is ever accidentally overlooked (easy to do in a busy clinic), that hidden or silent problems emerge, and that information needed to troubleshoot problems is available.

The patient interview

Every follow-up session should begin by addressing the most important part of any CRT system: the patient. While obtaining patient history is a good first step in any device follow-up session, there are special considerations for the CRT patient. Patients should be specifically asked about the medications they are taking. Most heart failure (HF) patients have multiple prescriptions and those under good medical management may have medications adjusted often as their conditions change. For patients

who find it burdensome to remember the names of their drugs, bringing pill bottles into the clinic can be a neat shortcut to be sure the files are updated. In particular, antiarrhythmic agents (amiodarone), β-blockers and digoxin are of interest to device therapy.

The patient should be asked about any complaints or changes. HF is a progressive disease and most CRT patients are elderly, so it is likely that patients will have numerous aches and pains. Remember, not all of these symptoms necessarily relate to the implanted device. Some of these side-effects may be related to drug therapy (for example, one fairly common side effect of β blockade is fatigue). Be aware that it is fairly common for device patients to attribute all of their symptoms to the device rather than drugs or other causes!

However, decreased cardiac output or suboptimal atrioventricular (AV) or VV timing may cause symptoms that device adjustment can address. Symptoms which might relate to the device include:

- Dizziness, light-headedness, feeling faint
- Palpitations, a 'racing heart,' pounding in the chest
- Shortness of breath
- Fatigue.

Associated signs include changes in skin color, respiratory rate and edema.

Examine the implant site for any signs of redness, infection or erosion. Check the neck veins (for distension), measure blood pressure, record the heart rate and listen to heart and lung sounds.

Many HF patients are under the care of more than one doctor. Be sure to ask the patient about other caregivers to be sure you have the whole picture of the procedures and pharmacological regimen the patient has. A multidisciplinary approach to HF patients is ideal.

Interrogation

Place electrodes on the patient for the surface ECG and then use the programmer to obtain a free-running ECG. Using basic ECG evaluation techniques, look at the ECG and see:

- Are there pacing spikes?
- Is there evidence of capture?
- Is there evidence of sensing? (There may not be.)
- Is there anything out of the ordinary?

Compare this ECG with any other ECGs on file for the patient to see if there are changes in QRS morphology. Changes in paced QRS morphology indicate that the device is pacing differently! This may indicate a problem, but at this point changes should only be noted.

Place the programmer wand over the implanted device and use the interrogation function to begin the programming session. Many devices today offer semi-automatic interrogation protocols. The device downloads basic information which will appear on the programmer screen. The programmer may also offer some prompts or pop-ups on screen that alert the clinician to new information, a new stored electrogram, or other remarkable conditions. It is possible to shortcut from this screen directly to go to the alert information. For a patient who appears at the clinic after a high-voltage shock, this may be all that is needed. For a more complete follow-up, the clinician should retrieve any alert information but then proceed through the rest of the steps.

While obtaining interrogation data, the programmer will alert clinicians if the device's internal battery is running low or if lead impedance values are out of range. These two conditions cannot be addressed by reprogramming the device.

If a low battery warning comes on-screen, the clinician should take immediate steps to schedule replacement surgery. If this is the first device replacement for the patient, they should be educated in terms of what to expect from the revision. Most devices allow considerable warning time before the battery is depleted, but it is wise to take immediate action for device replacement to be sure that therapy is not compromised.

Using telemetry, obtain and print out data on system parameters, with particular attention to lead impedance. For many devices, this is automatically part of the interrogation process, but it is crucial to check on lead impedance data with each follow-up. Lead impedance may be thought of as the resistance within the lead to the current flow; it is not a programmable value. Lead impedance values can and do vary by patient, by system configuration, and over time. Many programmers store previous lead impedance readings in memory and can compare current impedance values against previous values. If this is not an option, be sure to record lead impedance values each time in the patient's chart.

When evaluating lead impedance as part of routine follow-up, the clinician should look for significant (and relatively sudden) change rather than a specific value. Most leads have a very broad range of acceptable impedance values. While some fluctuation in these values is normal, any abrupt or large change (generally $>200\,\Omega$) strongly suggests that the lead has been compromised.

- A sudden increase of $\geq200\,\Omega$ in lead impedance suggests lead fracture (a break in the lead)
- A sudden decrease of $\geq200\,\Omega$ in lead impedance suggests damage to the insulation.

Lead impedance values must be contrasted with previous values. For example, if you know a patient has a lead with an impedance value of $400\,\Omega$ and the acceptable range for that lead is 200–$800\,\Omega$, the impedance value by itself does not tell you much. However, if you know that at the previous follow-up the patient's lead impedance value was $750\,\Omega$, then the 400-Ω reading this time strongly suggests a lead problem, most likely insulation breach. Yet both impedance values are technically within the normal range! Any lead impedance out-of-range is of concern, but even 'acceptable' values can indicate problems if there has been a big change.

If a sudden change in impedance values is noted, these steps should be followed:

- Obtain a second telemetry reading to confirm the first values.
- Lead problems are often best visualized on X-ray. A chest X-ray may be the next logical step.
- Check the paced ECG to see if there are pacing anomalies. Many lead problems can result in abnormal pacing and sensing. However, normal pacing and sensing do not rule out a potential lead problem.
- If the chest X-ray and pacing function are normal but there has still been a sudden significant change in lead impedance, the clinician should

still suspect that a possible lead problem. Such patients should be monitored closely.

In the event that a lead problem is detected, a device specialist should be consulted. In many cases, a new lead will have to be implanted.

Download diagnostics

Diagnostic data are available in a variety of different reports and formats; there is a tendency sometimes to dismiss this wealth of information as 'too much information', but it is crucial to download the diagnostic reports available. First and foremost, any programming changes made in follow-up will automatically clear most of the diagnostic counters, and data you might have wanted to consult will be lost. Second, information that may seem superfluous at first may turn out to be vital as you move through the steps of the follow-up. Third, good clinical practice involves keeping meticulous records, so it is very important to be sure the patient's file contains thorough records from each and every follow-up session.

Some clinicians prefer to deal with diagnostics as they work through the follow-up sequence rather than reviewing all diagnostics upfront. It is more important that clinicians develop a systematic approach than that they adhere to any one particular system. Thus, if it works better for a particular clinician to download diagnostics in a different sequence during follow-up, there is nothing wrong with that provided the clinician maintains that same sequence consistently with other patients. In my opinion, it is better to download diagnostics early in the sequence because it ensures diagnostic reports are properly downloaded and documented, it avoids unintentional loss of diagnostic data through programming, and it can help guide the further course of follow-up by giving the clinician some 'early warning signs' of things to look for. Naturally, downloading diagnostic data early does not mean that these reports should not be consulted—perhaps more exhaustively—during the course of the follow-up session.

There are numerous different types of diagnostic reports; manufacturers sometimes have slightly different names for them and even one manufacturer may have different names for different diagnostics in various device models. The main types of reports you should obtain are:

- Rate histograms (a record of how much pacing and sensing occurred and at what rates)
- Mode switch histogram, AT/AF Trend reports, AF Suppression log (records of how the device managed high atrial rates)
- Sensor histogram (for rate-responsive devices)
- Tachycardia episode tree (defibrillation activity in CRT-D systems)
- Stored electrograms.

Just as a systematic approach to follow-up requires you to move step-by-step through these procedures, you should also evaluate these diagnostics at this time with the same systematic process. Remembering the patient's condition and the programmed settings of the CRT system, review the diagnostic data with these questions in mind:

1 *Are the diagnostic data consistent with the goals of CRT?* There should be as close to 100% ventricular pacing as possible. For patients with CRT-D devices, potentially life-threatening ventricular tachyarrhythmias should be diagnosed and treated.

2 *Are the diagnostic data consistent with the programmed settings?* If supraventricular tachycardia (SVT) discrimination is programmed on, is it reducing inappropriate shocks? Is the pacing rate appropriately high? If mode switching or the AF Suppression™ algorithm is programmed on, there should not be a lot of rapid ventricular response to spells of high intrinsic atrial rates.

3 *Is there anything unusual showing up in the diagnostics?* Be sure to check any unusually high amounts of a specific type of activity (such as premature ventricular contractions, mode switch episodes, therapy deliveries, and so on). While some unusual activity may reflect suboptimal programming, unusual things that show up on diagnostics sometimes do not mean that anything is wrong.

4 *Are all of the programmed features functioning appropriately?* Check on mode switching, the AF Suppression™ algorithm, SVT discriminators, and rate response as well as other special algorithms or settings. For example, mode switching is intended to turn off atrial tracking in the presence of high-rate intrinsic atrial activity. This means that sensed atrial activity above the mode switch cut-off rate should not be tracked. SVT discriminators should reduce inappropriate shocks without decreasing specificity (treating appropriate shocks). Rate response should be sensitive enough to increase the rate in response to demand, but there should not be extended periods of sensor-driven high-rate pacing in a sedentary patient.

5 *Do the diagnostics provide any clues as to certain features or functions that might require fine-tuning or even troubleshooting?* Look for things such as rapid ventricular pacing in response to high sensed atrial rates, prolonged spells of very rapid intrinsic atrial activity, sensor-driven rates that seem too high or too prolonged for the patient's lifestyle, pacing rates that may be too slow, and less than near-100% ventricular pacing. It is also important to review the diagnostic data overall for anything that seems remarkable or unusual. Compare the diagnostic data from this follow-up with records from the last follow-up session or two. Have there been any significant changes? For example, several mode switch episodes may seem relatively insignificant, but if no mode switching had occurred previously, this could indicate the onset of atrial tachyarrhythmias.

Verify capture

In many ways, the sequence of systematic follow-up for a CRT system is not much different than for a pacemaker or implantable cardioverter-defibrillator, which means one of the key steps early in any follow-up session involves checking how the device is capturing the heart and how it senses.

Capture verification with a CRT device today is no more complicated than the capture testing in any other implanted device. Chapter 12 contains more extensive information on how to test for proper capture with a CRT system, but these are the important factors to remember:

- The goal of CRT pacing is biventricular (BV) pacing. This means capture verification is actually a two-phase process: the clinician must be sure the device is capturing both the right ventricle and the left ventricle.
- Capture thresholds for the right and left ventricle may be different—in fact, they usually are.
- The best approach to capture verification in a CRT system involves using the semi-automatic test. Capture testing in a tied-output device is more complicated (see Chapter 15), Tied-output systems are older devices that may still turn up at the clinic.

- QRS morphology is a very good indicator as to what is going on in the ventricle. A BV-paced complex will have a different morphology from an RV-only or an LV-only paced complex and all three will have a different shape from an unpaced QRS complex.

Another important aid in capture verification is the annotation function on rhythm strips from the programmer, which shows the clinician exactly how the device 'sees' the patient's cardiac activity. Annotations may not always be true to what is actually happening in the heart, but they are accurate representations of how the CRT system interprets the incoming signals.

Begin the capture test by confirming that capture is taking place. That can be done by watching an annotated rhythm strip to see if pacing spikes result in paced complexes. If capture is dubious, intermittent, or not occurring at all, increase the pacing rate prudently. The step-down test involves a series of very small decreases to the output pulse. If the device was properly pacing, at some point during step-down capture will be lost . The semi-automatic capture test will document results in both a tracing and a numeric value.

Record the capture thresholds for both ventricles in the patient's chart. If necessary, reprogram the RV and LV output pulses to assure consistent capture. As a general rule, it is more electrically efficient and effective to increase the voltage setting (pulse amplitude) than the duration (pulse width) of the output pulse. The dilemma in programming adequate output pulses for capture is the fact that capture thresholds are not stable. They are known to change with many factors, including drug interactions, time of day, postural changes and disease progression. As a result, the clinician must program a 'safety margin' to the output pulse to ensure that there is always sufficient energy to capture the heart reliably. After all, a CRT device that does not capture the heart does not provide the patient with needed therapy! The rule of thumb for safety margins is to program two or three times the capture threshold voltage. For example, if a patient has an RV threshold of 1 V, a 2 : 1 safety margin would require programming the output pulse to 2 V, while a 3 : 1 safety margin would demand 3 V. Clinicians may end up rounding a threshold such as 1.8 V to 5 V, for example.

If the CRT device is also pacing the atrium, an atrial capture threshold test should be attempted. Atrial capture testing is not always possible, because a capture test requires that the device be able to pace the atrium. For patients with persistent atrial tachyarrhythmias, it may be impossible or at least undesirable to try to pace the atrium. If atrial pacing occurs, a semi-automatic capture test can be performed. The test is an automatic step-down protocol. Results appear on-screen. A 2 : 1 or 3 : 1 safety margin is desirable. As a general rule, atrial thresholds are lower than ventricular thresholds.

Check sensing

Immediately after capture verification, it is important to check that the device is sensing cardiac activity appropriately. The sensing threshold is defined as the lowest sensitivity setting (which, rather counterintuitively, translates to the highest millivolt setting) at which the device can sense cardiac activity reliably. In order to determine what that value might be, it is crucial to observe and measure intrinsic activity.

Some devices offer a form of automatic P-wave and R-wave testing, which provides the amplitude values of intrinsic atrial and ventricular settings. Using these values, the clinician can then determine if the sensitivity settings are appropriate. For example, if a patient has an intrinsic R-wave of 2.5 mV, then the ventricular sensitivity should be set to around 1 mV, because that allows anything larger (like a 2.5-mV wave) to be seen. Since intrinsic signals are not necessarily of exactly the same amplitude at all times, a safety margin should be allowed. The general rule is that the programmed sensitivity setting should be about half (or less) than the intrinsic amplitude.

If there is no automatic method to obtain intrinsic signal amplitudes, the 'traditional approach' has been to decrease the pacing rate to the point that intrinsic activity starts to break through. If intrinsic activity can be viewed in this way, an annotated rhythm strip can help confirm whether such events are properly sensed (they will have annotations to that effect).

Note that the patient's lack of an underlying rhythm may make sensitivity testing difficult or even impossible. Patients with little or very slow intrinsic

cardiac activity may not be suitable candidates for this kind of testing. In such cases, it is best to use annotated rhythm strips and to check on programmed settings to verify what can be verified. Note in the patient's file if sensing threshold testing could not be done because of a lack of underlying rhythm.

ECG analysis

Paced ECGs were discussed in greater detail in Chapter 19. Some of the important things to remember during systematic follow-up are to run an annotated ECG and look 'past the annotations'. Annotations are very useful tools and they provide reliable information on what the device 'sees' and how it 'thinks'. However, never let an annotation be more important than the tracing. What you see on the rhythm strip is the 'real thing'. A good example of how annotations can miss a problem occurs when the CRT device oversenses (and under-paces) or undersenses (and over-paces). The annotations in these examples will see cardiac activity where the rhythm strip does not truly show it (oversensing) or will fail to identify genuine cardiac activity that the rhythm strip exhibits (undersensing).

Just as a systematic approach is invaluable in follow-up overall, so is a systematic approach to ECG evaluation. Here are the key points to analyze:

1 *Are the programmed settings consistent with what appears on the rhythm strip?* Look at rate, any special programmed features, pacing activity, and so on.

2 *Is there a depolarization associated with every pacing spike?* This suggests reliable capture. Spikes without depolarizations indicate that the device is trying to pace but the output is not capturing the heart.

3 *Is the device consistently pacing the ventricles?* The goal of CRT is as close to 100% ventricular pacing as possible.

4 *If it is a dual-chamber CRT system, is there atrial pacing? If there is not atrial pacing, what is the reason?* Atrial pacing may not occur if there is good native atrial activity or if there are atrial tachyarrhythmias.

5 *Is the QRS morphology indicative of BV pacing?* Since patients can vary considerably (and even the same patient can vary over time), it may be helpful to review previous rhythm strips for that patient. Any obvious change in QRS morphology indicates that something has changed with pacing—perhaps capture was lost in one chamber.

6 *Is sensing appropriate?* It may not be possible to observe this on all CRT strips, but note if there are intrinsic events and if they appropriately inhibit pacemaker output spikes.

7 *If the CRT device has an atrial lead, is pacing synchronous, in other words, is every atrial event associated with a ventricular event?* Note if there are isolated atrial or ventricular events.

8 *Is there evidence of any programmed algorithms or features and does it align with the programmed settings?* For example, if there is mode switching and the strip shows a run of atrial tachyarrhythmia, the mode switching should ensure that the atrial activity does not result in high-rate ventricular tracking.

9 *By the same token, are there things (like mode switching) that ought to be programmed on but are not on?*

Defibrillation features

The majority of CRT systems implanted in the USA are CRT-D or high-voltage systems. This requires a review of parameter settings and functions relating to defibrillation. Begin with the Therapy Summary screen, which should provide an overview of how many ventricular tachyarrhythmias occurred and how the device responded. If therapy was delivered, this should have caused an electrogram to be stored. These electrograms should be carefully reviewed to see if therapy was appropriate (i.e. if the patient truly had a ventricular tachyarrhythmia and not an SVT) or inappropriate (the therapy was administered to treat an SVT) and whether or not the therapy was successful.

In evaluating the therapy review, the clinician should go over these specific questions:

1 *Did the patient experience any ventricular tachyarrhythmias?* If so, the number and characteristics of these arrhythmias should be noted with a view to optimizing the device. If the patient seems to be having several episodes of 'fast' as well as 'slow' ventricular tachycardia (VT), it may be better to program a three-zone configuration (VT1 and VT2).

2 *If therapy was delivered, was it appropriate?* If inappropriate therapy was administered, the clinician should review SVT discrimination algorithms.

3 *Were any VTs treated with cardioversion or low voltage shock and what were the results?* If a lower-voltage shock successfully converts some VTs for a patient, it is a good option. However, if these lower-energy shocks do not seem to work or if they accelerate the VT, then the clinician should seriously consider programming higher-energy shocks.

4 *Were any VTs treated with antitachycardiac pacing (ATP) and what were the results?* ATP can be a very successful first line of defense, in particular for certain types of relatively slow and well-tolerated VT. However, ATP does not work on all types of VT; in some cases, it can even accelerate the VT. If results were less than successful, the clinician may wish to either revise the ATP protocol or program it off. On the other hand, if ATP works in a particular patient, it can be a very valuable part of the device arsenal, in particular because most patients do not even know they are receiving therapy with ATP and it does not cost a lot of battery energy.

5 *Should a defibrillation threshold (DFT) test be performed?* This is covered in more detail in Chapter 20, but there are many things to consider. From a purely academic standpoint, regular and frequent DFT testing is probably a good idea because defibrillation thresholds can and do change with time, drug interactions, disease progression and many other factors that are particularly true for HF patients. From a practical standpoint, DFT testing is time consuming, painful, and can be upsetting to the patient. For that reason, it is wise to stand a watchful middle ground. Review the therapy history. Did the patient require multiple shocks at maximum value in some cases? Is there evidence that the patient is not receiving adequate energy to defibrillate the heart? If so, renewed DFT testing may be warranted. For patients who receive no or very few shocks or who respond well to current defibrillation energy settings, DFT testing is not so urgent. This is a matter of clinical judgment.

In order to verify the proper function of the defibrillation lead in the right ventricle, it is useful to perform a high-voltage lead integrity check. In this test, the device is programmed to deliver a 12-V shock through the shocking electrodes of the defibrillation lead. During the test, the programmer will reveal the impedance value for the defibrillation lead. Note that these impedance values will probably not exactly match lead impedance values during actual therapy delivery, since actual therapy involves much greater amounts of energy. The clinician should observe the test carefully to be sure that the shock is delivered properly through the lead and to the patient; this verifies the lead's integrity.

At the very least, this test is uncomfortable for patients, who should be advised prior to the test that they will feel some twitching across the chest. Some patients experience the test as painful or even upsetting. For that reason, clinicians will have to use judgment as to how frequently defibrillation lead integrity should be checked with this method. In truth, 12 V is not a large amount of energy (in fact, many pacemakers can be programmed to deliver a 10-V output pulse). However, it is definitely a large enough amount of energy to be felt!

For patients with CRT-D systems offering Morphology Discrimination, the clinician should verify that the feature is programmed to provide automatic template updates. This automatic feature allows the templates to be revised frequently without programming intervention; the patient will not even be aware of what is going on. If the automatic feature was not programmed on, a manual update can also be performed. This is a quick, painless step. As a general rule, most patients should have the automatic update feature programmed on for their own safety as well as convenience.

Stored electrograms

Most CRT devices offer stored electrograms, which are identified on the programmer. If programmable triggers to initiate electrogram storage are offered, the clinician should review whether these triggers are appropriate. For example, entry into mode switching may be a programmable trigger that is not appropriate for all patients (e.g. patients without atrial tachyarrhythmias would not need this).

The clinician should review the available stored electrograms and download those that are of interest. These electrograms not only show how the patient and device are interacting, they can help guide programming considerations.

1 *In view of the stored electrograms, are the right features programmed?*

2 *If the patient received inappropriate therapy delivery, can SVT discrimination be adjusted?*

3 *If there are a many mode switch episodes, are there other programming changes that might be useful?* A patient in a prolonged Auto Mode Switch state might need the device reprogrammed permanently to a non-atrial-tracking mode, for example.

Programming

The bulk of any good follow-up session is really detective work: the clinician is trying to gather all of the clues to help understand what is going on between the patient and the device. In this next step, the clinician now needs to decide if there are any changes that can be made to the device that might provide even better therapy.

The first phase of programming any CRT system should involve timing optimization. The timing of the sensed and paced AV delay as well as the VV timing (LV and RV outputs) are crucial to CRT success. In fact, in many cases, the best way to convert a 'non-responder' to a responder is timing optimization. If the device offers the QuickOpt™ algorithm (covered more extensively in Chapter 15), timing parameters can be determined painlessly with a quick programming step. This algorithm will provide optimal settings which can be adjusted in this final step of the follow-up session.

If the CRT device does not offer the QuickOpt™ feature, timing optimization involves an echocardiogram. For that reason, the clinician would need to assess the need for timing optimization and take appropriate steps for the patient to receive an echocardiogram outside of the follow-up visit.

Other programming steps are based on what the clinician has discovered during follow-up fact-finding. The clinician should check mode, pacing rate, timing parameters, special features, SVT discrimination algorithms, pacing output parameters, shock output parameters and stored electrogram triggers. In all cases, the clinician should ask if current settings are appropriate or if the patient might require changes. New parameter settings can be entered and then programmed all at once in a step known as batch programming. Keep records of all programming changes.

One word of caution: most programmable parameters offer a wide range of very fine setting options. There is sometimes a tendency with clinicians to want to program large changes rather than very subtle shifts. In device therapy, small changes can have a big impact on the patient! Unless there is a compelling reason, avoid dramatic changes to parameter settings.

Note that sometimes programming one set of values may make other parameter settings unavailable. If this occurs, the programmer will notify the clinician about such incompatibilities.

Some clinicians print out two copies of the final device settings, one for the patient's chart and the other for the patient. Patients are asked to keep the printout in their wallets in the event that they ever need sudden medical treatment.

Final steps

Every follow-up session should begin and end with thorough documentation. Print out everything of interest for the patient's chart under the motto, 'When in doubt, print it out'. Follow-up can be made increasingly difficult (or much easier) depending on how much information from past sessions is available to the clinician.

Since most HF patients have multiple physicians and are likely to be involved in polypharmacy (taking multiple drugs), it may be useful to note that

information in the chart also. Many HF drugs are known to have potential impact on a CRT system. For example, β-blockers and digoxin can slow the heart rate, amiodarone can suppress ambient tachyarrhythmias, and Class I antiarrhythmics can have proarrhythmic effects. Device therapy can help mitigate some of the potential side effects of such drugs; in fact, some patients who require β blockade may end up with a permanent pacemaker to manage the drug-induced slowed heart rate.

At the conclusion of the session (if not before), be sure to talk to the patient and solicit questions. While device therapy is increasingly common around the world, CRT devices are relatively new and patients may be understandably confused about them. Device manufacturers offer excellent patient education materials which can also be distributed. In my opinion, it is important to spend a little time at the end of each follow-up to encourage patients to ask questions. Many patients who have genuine concerns and questions can hesitate to bring them up in a clinical situation. A little encouragement can help bring a patient's questions out. While I have no statistics to back this up, it has been my experience that an educated patient is usually more compliant and more positive about treatment.

The nuts and bolts of a systematic guide to CRT follow-up

- The purpose of follow-up is to verify proper function of the cardiac resynchronization therapy (CRT) device, to optimize parameter settings, to detect current or potential future problems with the system, and to address patient concerns.
- It is crucial for clinicians to develop a system for CRT follow-up and then to adhere consistently to that system. This chapter proposes some ideas for a system. The exact sequence of steps is not as important as the fact that the clinician has a systematic approach.
- A systematic approach ensures that no step is ever inadvertently omitted or overlooked and it forces a clinician to go through a sequence of steps rather than hurry through to deal with only obvious things. Many device problems show up in follow-up as 'little things' that can be

managed before they cause symptoms.
- Most CRT patients have multiple caregivers and are probably taking several different drugs. It is useful to obtain as complete information as possible about other physicians, other treatments, and especially the drugs the patient is taking. A few heart failure drugs (notably digoxin and β-blockers) can cause bradycardia; Class I antiarrhythmics have proarrhythmic effects.
- Interrogate the device and check lead impedance values. Lead impedance values are not programmable and should fall within a broad range of 'normal' values (see manufacturer's instructions to obtain the range for the lead). However, lead impedance values that change $>200\,\Omega$ in a short time (from one follow-up to the next) strongly suggest the possibility of lead damage … even if the impedance values are still

Continued.

Continued.

within the 'normal' or acceptable range.
- When the programmer warns about low battery status, an elective replacement procedure (to replace the generator, not the leads) should be scheduled.
- Download diagnostics before any programming is done. Diagnostic data can help guide programming choices; programming also zeroes out many diagnostic counters.
- Some of the most important diagnostic information includes rate histograms, mode switch histograms, sensor histograms (for rate-responsive devices), tachycardia episode tree or therapy summary, and stored electrograms.
- During follow-up, attempts should be made to verify capture and sensing and to perform a capture and sensing threshold test to be sure programmed settings are appropriate.
- An ECG should be obtained and analyzed with respect to annotations, pacing and sensing.
- For CRT-D devices, defibrillation activity should be reviewed (along with any relevant stored electrograms). From time to time, it may be useful to check the high-voltage lead integrity or to perform defibrillation threshold testing. Both of these things involve some degree of patient discomfort and should be performed only after careful clinical consideration; very frequent testing is probably not necessary for most patients.
- When reviewing defibrillation, it is important to check stored electrograms to confirm appropriate versus inappropriate therapy delivery and to verify supraventricular tachycardia discrimination algorithms.
- Programming should be done toward the end of the follow-up session, once the clinician has amassed the information needed to make wise programming choices. Programming changes can be entered and all new settings programmed at once.
- If the device has a QuickOpt™ feature, it can be used to optimize AV and VV timing without the need for any other testing (such as an echocardiogram). If this algorithm is available, it should be routinely used in follow-up. If timing optimization must be done with an echocardiogram, the clinician should use judgment in terms of how frequently this ought to be performed.
- Programming changes to the device is best done in very small steps. The idea that if a small amount is good, a larger amount is better does not apply to device therapy! Go slow with programming changes.
- Document, document, document!
- Encourage the patient to ask questions or express any concerns about therapy to you. Many patients wonder about their treatment but may hesitate to ask a seemingly 'busy doctor' or 'busy nurse' on a hectic day at the clinic. Take a few minutes to solicit questions.

Chapter 26

Troubleshooting

Troubleshooting a cardiac resynchronization therapy (CRT) system does not have to be as difficult as some clinicians have made it seem. I have a three-step approach to device troubleshooting:

- Identify the problem
- Identify the possible causes of such a problem
- Starting with the most likely cause, use a 'differential diagnosis' approach to explore each cause.

In truth, anyone who works with device patients long enough will occasionally encounter a very elusive or unusual problem. In such cases, you should not hesitate to call on the manufacturer's technical support: this may be the sales representative, a technical service person, or the technical support hotline most manufacturers maintain round-the-clock. However, the majority of issues that confront a device trouble-shooter have some typical causes. In fact, once you know the 'usual suspects', device troubleshooting can become almost routine.

What follows are, in the author's experience, some of the more likely scenarios a CRT device professional will encounter.

The patient does not seem to respond to CRT

Many patients are so-called non-responders, and there is good evidence that at least some non-responders can be converted to responders. There are several possible things that can reduce the effectiveness of CRT:

1 *The device is not pacing both ventricles.* Verify that there is capture in both ventricles.

2 *Atrioventricular (AV) timing or VV timing is not optimized.* Even very minor changes in these settings can increase the efficacy of CRT. If the device offers the QuickOpt™ algorithm, then timing optimization can be handled with a programming step. If the device does not have this feature, the patient should undergo echocardiography to help better time how the atrial output syncs up to the ventricular output and how the ventricular outputs are timed.

3 *The device is pacing the ventricles less than 100% of the time.* CRT is delivered only when the device paces the ventricle. Unlike a conventional pacemaker (which tries to inhibit itself in the presence of native cardiac activity), a CRT device should be programmed in such a way as to encourage pacing. Things to consider in this regard: an adequately high base rate, AV timing, appropriate capture.

4 *There is a problem with lead integrity.* Check lead impedance values to see if there has been a large magnitude change since the previous follow-up or if lead values are out of range. A chest X-ray is usually required to visualize better what is going on with the leads. A damaged, fractured, nicked or torn lead will require replacement (surgical intervention).

5 *There is a problem with lead placement.* This problem will typically show up early, if at all. It may be that because of where the lead is placed in the left ventricle, it is difficult for the lead to capture the heart reliably. Pacing performance is notoriously location dependent; thresholds can vary dramatically with even slight changes in lead placement. Unfortunately, this problem requires surgical revision to correct. If the lead is truly placed in an inopportune location, it should be revised.

The patient is responding (at least somewhat) to CRT but there is less than 100% ventricular pacing

If the CRT system is not pacing the ventricles consistently, it is probably because spontaneous ventricular activity is breaking through.

1 *The base rate should be programmed at a rate above the patient's native ventricular rate, if at all possible.*

Evaluate the patient's intrinsic ventricular rate and adjust the base rate accordingly.

2 *AV timing should be optimized.* By moving up the ventricular output with respect to the atrial output pulse, the ventricles have less opportunity to beat on their own.

3 *Verify capture.* It is possible that the device is trying to pace at an appropriate rate but not all of the output spikes are capturing the heart. Verify capture with the semi-automatic capture test function and double check output pulse parameters, that is, the pulse amplitude (V) and pulse width (ms).

4 *The device is sensing far-field P-waves.* This occurs when the LV lead picks up paced or sensed atrial signals and inappropriately interprets them as native ventricular events, which inhibit ventricular pacing. This should show up as RV pacing [no LV and thus no biventricular (BV)], with atrial output spikes occurring at the appropriate times to inhibit the LV output. This can often be corrected by making the LV lead less sensitive (and thus more immune to stray atrial signals). In some cases, far-field P-wave sensing occurs because of the location of the LV lead. In such cases, the lead may have to be moved.

5 *The patient may be experiencing runs of ventricular tachycardia (VT).* High-rate ventricular activity can be caused when the device tries to pace the ventricle to keep up with an atrial tachyarrhythmia (atrial tracking). Verify what is going on in the atrium. If the patient is experiencing a lot of high-rate atrial activity, program the mode switch algorithm, the AF Suppression™ algorithm, or change the mode to a non-atrial-tracking mode (DDDI, DDIR, VVI or VVIR). The patient might also have VT at rates too slow for antitachycardia pacing (ATP) or defibrillation therapy. Using clinical judgment, determine the right cut-off rate for the patient. For example, if the patient is experiencing runs of VT at 100 beats/min, the device could either be programmed to pace at 105 pulses/min or the clinician could program pacing to 90 pulses/min and then set up a three-zone configuration in a CRT-D system with a VT1 cut-off rate of 100 beats/min. In such cases, ATP might be a good choice for therapy for VT1.

6 *There is a problem with the leads.* The leads may be damaged (check the lead impedance values and then verify on X-ray) or placed in a suboptimal location. This requires surgical revision to correct.

BV capture is unreliable, intermittent, or not happening!

BV capture refers to the CRT device's ability to pace both right and left ventricles successfully. Since these chambers are paced by different leads and typically have different thresholds, there is more margin for error here than with a conventional device.

1 *There is a problem with capture.* Conduct a capture threshold test and determine the thresholds for both ventricles. Verify that the device outputs (pulse amplitude in voltage and pulse width in milliseconds) are appropriate to capture the heart. A 2 : 1 or 3 : 1 safety margin should be programmed.

2 *There is a problem with the leads.* If you cannot capture one or both ventricles despite high output pulses, there may be a problem in getting that energy to the heart. Verify lead impedance values and check the leads on a chest X-ray if lead impedance values (or sudden changes) make you suspicious. Lead placement can also hamper capture; in such cases, the lead may require surgical revision.

3 *There is a problem with sensing.* Oversensing can lead to under-pacing. Oversensing occurs when the device is so sensitive, it actually starts to 'sense' native cardiac activity that is not there! The result is that the device thinks the ventricles have beat on their own and thus it inhibits the output pulse. Verify the sensing threshold and review the sensitivity setting. Remember, sensitivity programming can seem counter-intuitive: a high millivolt setting is less sensitive than a low millivolt setting. Another sensing problem can occur when the device starts to 'see' atrial pacing outputs and inappropriately categorizes them as native ventricular activity. Far-field P-wave sensing involves an overly sensitive LV lead; reduce LV lead sensitivity.

The CRT-D system is delivering inappropriate therapy

This painful and alarming condition occurs when the device delivers high-voltage therapy to supraventricular tachycardias (SVTs) rather than true VTs. In such cases, retrieve the stored electrogram for therapy delivery and study the annotations. This will tell you what the device 'saw', while the tracing itself will tell you what was going on in the heart.

1 *The device saw a rapid ventricular rate but did not realize it was an SVT.* The device may not always be able to differentiate an SVT from a true VT without proper programming. In such cases, a therapy episode summary will show that a VT or ventricular fibrillation was detected when, in truth, the arrhythmia was an SVT. In such cases, it is useful to review the programmed SVT discrimination algorithms and adjust them as appropriate. Be sure that AV rate branch and Morphology Discrimination are on (with automatic template updates); some patients may need the added protection of Sudden Onset or Interval Stability. Sudden Onset is useful for patients who experience sinus tachycardia, while Interval Stability benefits those who are prone to episodes of atrial fibrillation.

2 *The device saw a VT that was not there at all.* This can be caused by a phenomenon known as 'double-counting', which occurs when some events (not ventricular events) end up being perceived by the device as ventricular events. This may occur when far-field P-wave sensing is going on (P-waves get counted inappropriately as ventricular events) or when some other form of oversensing is occurring (such as counting T-waves as ventricular events). Another scenario involves potential interference, such as entering an environment with a lot of electromagnetic interference (ask the patient about where they are when inappropriate therapy occurs). Retrieve the stored electrograms and check the annotations. Electromagnetic interference is best handled by avoidance. Double-counting or oversensing require an adjustment to the sensitivity settings and may require sensing threshold testing.

The device does not defibrillate when appropriate

This is one of the most dangerous scenarios for a CRT-D patient, although fortunately not the most common. When a potentially life-threatening ventricular tachyarrhythmia occurs but is not treated, the patient runs the risk of serious injury or death. This usually happens because the device fails to detect and diagnose the arrhythmia.

1 *The device is undersensing.* This occurs when the device simply does not recognize or count all of the ventricular activity that is going on. Retrieve the annotated stored electrogram to verify whether the ventricular complexes were 'seen' by the device and counted. If not, try to get a reading on the patient's intrinsic atrial and ventricular depolarizations. Compare the programmed sensitivity values with these native signal amplitudes to confirm that sensing parameters are adequate. Most defibrillators rely on a self-adjusting sensitivity algorithm. If you confirm that sensing values are appropriate for the size of the patient's signal but that sensing in the device is inadequate, contact the device manufacturer's technical services department. Sensitivity in a device can be reprogrammed, but this requires care and technical expertise. It is not recommended that clinicians attempt to do this without consulting with technical support and certainly clinicians relatively new to device therapy should avoid undertaking this kind of step without technical consultation.

2 *The detection parameter settings or SVT discriminators are not appropriate for the patient.* Look at how the device is programmed. Is the VT detection rate appropriate? If it is too high (for example, 200 beats/min) then VT at lower rates would not be treated (for example, 190 beats/min). Programming very restrictive SVT discrimination algorithms or too many algorithms may cause a device to classify a true VT as an SVT. This can be verified by reviewing therapy information on the programmer. If this is the case, review and reprogram the SVT discrimination algorithms.

3 *There is a problem with the leads.* If it appears that the device properly diagnosed the VT and delivered therapy but the therapy was ineffective, there may be a problem. Perform a high-voltage lead integrity check and note lead impedance values. An out-of-range impedance value or a big change in impedance value suggests lead damage; verify this on a chest X-ray. Damaged leads require replacement.

4 *The shock output parameters are too low.* If the device properly diagnoses a VT and properly delivers adequate therapy, it may be that the energy is insufficient to defibrillate the heart. Review the output parameters of high-voltage therapy and consider doing defibrillation threshold (DFT) testing. DFTs can change over time, with drug use, and with disease progression. It may be that the 10-J shock that once successfully defibrillated the patient is no longer adequate. If possible, increase the energy output.

If the shocks appear ineffective even though they are at maximum value, there are adjustments that can be made to maximize defibrillation efficacy (see Chapter 20) or consult with a manufacturer's representative. In particular, changing tilt values can be helpful.

Conclusion

Troubleshooting CRT device problems is an important process and one that is best approached systematically. Clinicians who deal even occasionally with devices need to be aware of basic troubleshooting techniques. As a rule of thumb, the most likely problems are the ones that occur most often. While unusual cases do occur (and provide lots of material for the medical journals and professional conversations), in actual clinical practice, common problems occur most commonly. Thus, troubleshooting should start with the most likely causes and expand from there.

Clinicians who are relatively new to device therapy should not hesitate to seek the advice and guidance of more experienced colleagues (if available) or to call on the manufacturer's representative for assistance. Manufacturers produce a lot of material about the proper use of their products and may also offer training opportunities to use the devices better. Some of the best device experts have learned about troubleshooting and device therapy by being mentored by colleagues and taking advantage of what manufacturers have had to offer in terms of training.

The nuts and bolts of troubleshooting

- Define the problem, identify potential causes, and then sort through them. Remember the most likely causes of a problem are those that occur most often.
- While lead problems are relatively rare, they are potentially devastating and they can cause any number of possible device problems. A damaged or badly positioned lead can cause problems with pacing, sensing and therapy delivery.
- Lead problems should be confirmed on X-ray and then referred to a device specialist. As a general rule, a problem with a lead requires a new lead to be implanted.
- Sensing and pacing problems can often be seen on annotated tracings. Retrieve any relevant stored electrograms and contrast what the device thinks it saw (annotations) and what the heart was actually doing (tracing).
- Discuss the problem with the patient. Some problems can be caused by electromagnetic interference (EMI). If a patient experiences inappropriate shocks only in certain environments, it is possible that there is EMI in that location. EMI may not always occur where you think it should. Electronic surveillance equipment in department stores, dental equipment used in manicure salons and the proliferation of electronic equipment in society cause EMI to occur in seemingly benign locations.
- The best way to manage EMI is to avoid it, if at all possible. Site surveys of potential EMI locations may be required; sometimes a manufacturer's technical staff will be able to assist with this.
- Check how the device is programmed. In some cases, it is doing exactly what it was programmed to do … it was just not programmed appropriately.
- Atrioventricular and VV timing optimization may be required to optimize CRT systems. This requires echocardiography and is a fairly time-consuming, elaborate and expensive step. An alternative is the QuickOpt™ algorithm, which is available in certain devices. This algorithm allows timing optimization with a routine programming step.

Glossary

AAA   See **antiarrhythmic agent**.

ablate and pace   A nickname for **AV nodal ablation** and subsequent implantation of a permanent cardiac rhythm management device.

ACE   See **angiotensin-converting enzyme**.

ACE inhibitor   A drug that inhibits the angiotensin-converting enzyme from changing angiotensin-I (A-I) into angiotensin-II (A-II). Since A-I is an inactive substance and A-II is a powerful vasoconstrictor, this drug helps keep low the otherwise overly high level of A-II in a heart failure patient. ACE inhibitors reduce mortality in heart failure patients and have a class effect.

active can   See **hot can**.

acute heart failure (AHF)   (1) A sudden worsening of heart failure symptoms, typically characterized by pulmonary or peripheral congestion (or both). (2) Sometimes used to describe new-onset cases of heart failure.

adrenergic system   Part of the body's sympathetic nervous system (SNS) which governs the body's 'fight-or-flight' response to danger. The adrenergic system is further subdivided into the α-**adrenergic system** and the β-**adrenergic system**. Adrenergic activity can include increased heart rate and elevated blood pressure.

AF   See **atrial fibrillation**.

AFl   See **atrial flutter**.

afterload   The amount of resistance against which the heart must work to pump blood. Blood pressure and the state of the vasculature influence afterload.

AHF   See **acute heart failure**.

aldosterone   A chemical substance in the body (technically a steroid hormone) which acts to regulate fluid retention (sodium and water) in the body.

all-cause mortality   Death for any reason, including being hit by a bus. Many large randomized clinical trials for heart failure use all-cause mortality as an end-point.

α-adrenergic system   A portion of the body's sympathetic nervous system (SNS) which regulates vasoconstriction, digestion and certain other functions. See also β-**adrenergic system**.

amiodarone   The main antiarrhythmic agent not contraindicated for heart failure patients. Amiodarone is a Class III AA prescribed to suppress tachyarrhythmias. While many heart failure patients may benefit from amiodarone, it has not been shown to confer mortality benefits.

angina pectoris   Chest pains typically caused by coronary artery disease blocking blood supply to the heart.

angiotensinogen   A protein in the blood which can be converted into angiotensin-I in the presence of the enzyme renin. See also **renin–angiotensin–aldosterone system**.

angiotensin   A chemical substance (technically a kinin) produced by the body. There are two types of angiotensin: angiotensin-I (A-I) and angiotensin-II (A-II). A-I is largely inactive and is converted by another enzyme (the angiotensin-converting enzyme) into A-II, which has significant physiological effect on the body. See also **angiotensin-I** and **angiotensin-II**.

angiotensin-I   A chemical substance (kinin) produced when renin (an enzyme) acts upon (hydrolyzes) a blood protein called angiotensinogen. Angiotensin-I or A-I is an inactive substance and can be converted by another enzyme into angiotensin-II (A-II), which is a powerful vasoconstrictor. A-I may be thought of as the inactive but necessary precursor of A-II. See also **angiotensin-II**.

angiotensin-II   A chemical substance (kinin) produced when a special enzyme known as the angiotensin-converting enzyme acts upon angiotensin-I, an inactive kinin produced when renin

191

acts upon angiotensinogen (a plasma protein). Angiotensin-II is a powerful vasoconstrictor. See also **angiotensin-I**.

angiotensin-converting enzyme   A chemical substance (enzyme) in the body which acts upon angiotensin-I and changes it to angiotensin-II. Abbreviated **ACE**.

angiotensin-receptor blocker   Abbreviated ARB. A drug that blocks the ability of angiotensin-II (A-II) from being effective by jamming or blocking the receptor cells. Unlike an ACE inhibitor, which lowers the level of A-II in the blood, an ARB does nothing to decrease the amount of A-II but renders it ineffective. ARBs should be prescribed to heart failure patients who do not tolerate ACE inhibitors.

anode   The positive pole.

antiarrhythmic agent   Abbreviated **AAA**. Any of many classes and types of drugs given to patients in an effort to control rhythm disorders. Many AAAs have the paradoxical side effect of proarrhythmia, i.e. they may induce or make the patient more susceptible to other rhythm disorders. As such, most AAAs are contraindicated for heart failure patients with the exception of **amiodarone**.

antitachycardia pacing   Abbreviated **ATP**. A type of therapeutic response to ventricular tachycardia which uses programmed stimulation at low voltages (typical pacing outputs) to terminate a rhythm disorder. ATP is recommended only for the treatment of re-entrant monomorphic VT in patients who tolerate that VT well and do not suffer hemodynamic compromise during the VT. ATP is only used to treat VT; it is never appropriate to use ATP to treat VF.

aorta   The body's main 'conduit' for blood. Blood from the left side of the heart is pumped into the aorta for distribution to the entire body.

aortic outflow   A parameter measured on echocardiography and used for CRT device optimization, particularly AV delay timing and VV timing. It measures how rapidly blood is ejected out of the left ventricle and into the aorta (and thus, out to the body).

aortic stenosis   A narrowing of the aortic valve, a valvular disease commonly associated with heart failure. When aortic stenosis is present, the left ventricle has an increased load against which it

must work to pump oxygenated blood out into the body.

aortic valve   The valve between the left ventricle and the aorta.

AP–VP   One of the four states of dual-chamber pacing in which a paced atrial event is followed by a paced ventricular event. This means the device paces the atrium and then paces the ventricle. Such states are desirable in CRT systems. See also **pacing state**.

AP–VS   One of the four states of dual-chamber pacing in which a paced atrial event is followed by a sensed ventricular event. This means the device paces the atrium and the impulse conducts to the ventricle naturally and causes a ventricular depolarization resulting in a sensed ventricular event. Such states should be minimized in CRT systems. See also **pacing state**.

appropriate therapy   For CRT-D (and ICD) devices, high-voltage therapy delivered in response to a true ventricular tachycardia. See also **inappropriate therapy**.

ARB   See **angiotensin-receptor blocker**.

arrhythmia   An abnormal heart rhythm, also called a **rhythm disorder** or dysrhythmia.

arrhythmogenesis   Provoking, causing or contributing to the start of an arrhythmia. Factors associated with arrhythmogenesis in heart failure patients include mineral and chemical imbalances, high rates of circulating catecholamines, myocardial lesions from prior heart attacks, and increased refractoriness due to stretched heart muscles.

AS–VP   One of the four states of dual-chamber pacing in which a sensed atrial event is followed by a paced ventricular event. This means the SA node generated a natural electrical impulse, which failed to conduct and cause ventricular depolarization; as a result, the device paces the ventricle. Such states are desirable in CRT systems. See also **pacing state**.

AS–VS   One of the four states of dual-chamber pacing, in which a sensed atrial event is followed by a sensed ventricular event. This means the device did not pace the heart at all but was inhibited or in standby mode. Such states should be minimized in CRT systems. See also **pacing state**.

AT   See **atrial tachycardia**.

ATP   See **antitachycardia pacing**.

artificial left bundle branch block A condition induced by conventional pacing from the right ventricle which alters electrical conduction through the heart in such a way that the paced heart appears to have a form of left bundle branch block and exhibits a characteristically wider QRS complex on the surface ECG.

atrial contribution to ventricular filling The atrial contraction following the passive filling of the ventricles, which forces an additional quantity of blood into the already-filled ventricles. Nicknamed **atrial kick**.

atrial diastole The repolarization and relaxation of the heart's upper chambers (atria). Atrial diastole can be observed on a surface ECG as the PR segment.

atrial fibrillation Abbreviated **AF**. A cardiac rhythm disorder characterized by very rapid and seemingly disorganized atrial activity, some of which conducts to the ventricle and provokes a rapid ventricular response. AF is a comorbidity to heart failure.

atrial flutter Sometimes abbreviated **AFl**. A form of atrial tachycardia that is rapid but very regular and is characterized by a sawtooth pattern on the ECG.

atrial kick See **atrial contribution to ventricular filling**.

atrial systole The depolarization and contraction of the heart's upper chambers (atria). Atrial systole can be observed on a surface ECG as the P-wave.

atrial tachyarrhythmia A broad general term for any abnormally high atrial rhythm. This rhythm disorder originates in the atria but frequently involves a rapid ventricular response, which may, in fact, be the source of symptoms.

atrial tachycardia Abbreviated **AT**. A broad term for an abnormally high atrial rhythm that is not atrial fibrillation.

atrioventricular node A specialized collection of cells located in the approximate center of the heart which slows the electrical conduction of an impulse through the heart. Abbreviated **AV node**.

atrium One of two of the heart's upper chambers, plural atria.

automaticity The property of cardiac cells to generate an electrical impulse spontaneously. The sinoatrial node is best known for its automaticity, but actually all cardiac cells possess some degree of automaticity.

AV block A mechanism associated with bradyarrhythmias in which an impulse from the sinoatrial (SA) node occurs at the right time but is unable to pass through the atrioventricular (AV) node at the right speed to conduct to the ventricles. Although the condition is called AV block, impulses may be delayed (first-degree AV block), intermittently blocked (second-degree AV block), or totally blocked (third-degree AV block). Advanced AV block is a pacemaker indication. Also called **heart block**.

AV conduction delay In many heart failure patients, a form of electrical dyssynchrony that occurs when the normal electrical conduction from the atria to the ventricles is delayed.

AV delay A timing parameter in CRT devices which defines the length of time after an atrial output pulse is delivered (RA) to the time that a ventricular output (RV or LV or both, depending on whether there are independently programmable values) is delivered. The AV delay may require **optimization** to find the ideal value for a particular patient. The sensed AV delay involves the time from a sensed atrial event to the ventricular output, while a paced AV delay involves a paced atrial event.

AV node See **atrioventricular node**.

AV nodal ablation A procedure, typically performed using a radiofrequency ablation catheter, in which portions of tissue in the AV node are destroyed in such a way that it severs the electrical conduction pathway linking atria to ventricles. An AV nodal ablation is performed to help manage chronic AF. It works by dissociating atria from ventricles; the atria keep fibrillating but there is no longer a rapid ventricular response. Such patients usually get a permanent cardiac rhythm management device to pace the ventricle. The procedure has been nicknamed **ablate-and-pace**.

azotemia A condition in which there is too much nitrogen in the blood. This condition can be caused by kidney dysfunction. Some heart failure patients develop pre-renal azotemia as a result of too much diuretic.

baroreceptors Special nerve cells in the body which respond to changes in blood pressure. Baroreceptors are located in the walls of large arteries (e.g. in the carotid sinus and the aortic arch) and monitor the stretch of the vessel wall. When baroreceptors sense high or low blood pressure, they can cause the body to respond with compensatory mechanisms, such as vasoconstriction or dilation.

β-adrenergic system   A portion of the body's sympathetic nervous system (SNS) which regulates vasodilation, heart rate, bronchial activity and other functions. See also **α-adrenergic system.**

β-blocker   A general term given to drugs that block the β-adrenergic system (and sometimes the α-adrenergic system as well). These drugs have a positive chronotropic, positive dromotropic and positive inotropic effect (they increase heart rate, increase electrical conduction speed and increase the vigor of the cardiac contraction). They are considered a mainstay of drug therapy for all heart failure patients, even those without symptoms. β-Blocker generic names end in 'olol' and some of the best known are carvedilol, bisoprolol and metoprolol. β-Blockers do not have a class effect and some have been proven to have both a morbidity and a mortality benefit for heart failure patients.

biphasic   Having two phases. Modern CRT-D devices deliver defibrillating energy in a biphasic waveform. The biphasic waveform has an initial positive phase followed by a negative phase; in many cases, the second phase is shorter in pulse duration than the first. Clinical evidence suggests that biphasic waveforms are more effective at defibrillating the heart than monophasic waveforms of the same energy.

bipolar   A type of electrical configuration which describes leads (and pulse generator configuration) in which the electrical circuit is formed by the tip and ring electrodes on the lead. See also **unipolar.**

biventricular pacing   Another term for cardiac resynchronization therapy. Biventricular or BV (sometimes BiV) pacing is an older term; CRT is the preferred term.

blood pressure   A measurement of the pressure or force of the blood against the artery walls expressed in millimeters of mercury. A typical blood pressure reading consists of two numbers, a systolic (or maximum) blood pressure value followed by a diastolic (or minimum) blood pressure value. A typical way of writing a blood pressure reading would be 120/80 mmHg.

blood count   A routine blood test for heart failure patients which measures the amount of hematocrit and plasma protein in the blood, thus conveying information about the blood's viscosity.

bradyarrhythmia   A broad general term for any abnormally slow heart rhythm   There are two main causes of bradyarrhythmias: sinus node dysfunction and AV block. Also called **bradycardia.**

bradycardia   See **bradyarrhythmia.**

CAD   See **coronary artery disease.**

can   A slang term for **pulse generator.**

cannulation   A general term for the insertion of a tube (cannula). In CRT implantation, cannulation is the process of placing a sheath or catheter into the coronary sinus to facilitate passage of the LV lead from the right atrium, through the coronary sinus, and then out into the coronary venous system on the exterior of the left ventricle.

capacitor   An electronic component within a pulse generator (defibrillator) which stores an electrical charge until it reaches the desired proportions and then discharges it all at once. Capacitors allow devices with low-voltage batteries to deliver large, high-voltage outputs.

cardiac cycle   The four phases of a single 'heart beat' that must occur in proper sequence for normal cardiac function. It begins with the contraction of the heart's upper chambers (atrial systole) followed by a very brief period of relaxation (atrial diastole). The third phase is ventricular contraction (ventricular systole) followed by ventricular relaxation (ventricular diastole).

cardiac index   The cardiac output of an individual divided by their body surface area. Cardiac index relates cardiac output (an absolute value) to the patient's size. For example, a very small person might be well served with a cardiac output value that would be inadequate for a large person.

cardiac output   The volume of blood the heart can pump through the body's system in 1 min, measured in milliliters. An average cardiac output might be 5000 ml/min. Abbreviated **CO.**

cardiac resynchronization therapy (CRT)   A type of device-based treatment that involves pacing right and left ventricles in an effort to resynchronize or better time the left-ventricular contraction. A popular misconception of CRT is that it only synchronizes right and left ventricles. It synchronizes the left-ventricular contraction, so that it contracts as a unified whole.

cardiomyopathy A disease of the heart muscle (myocardium). The most common forms of cardiomyopathy are **dilated cardiomyopathy** and **hypertrophic obstructive cardiomyopathy**.

cardioversion In CRT-D devices or ICDs, shock therapy at less than maximum energy settings, for example, shocks of 20 J.

cathode The negative pole.

charge time The amount of time it takes for a CRT-D device from diagnosis to charge to full capacity and deliver therapy. Charge times can vary with device age, battery status and the state of the capacitor.

CHF See **congestive heart failure**.

chronic AF See **permanent AF**.

chronic heart failure A term mainly used to distinguish permanent heart failure from acute heart failure. Chronic heart failure refers to the permanent or long-term state.

chronotropic incompetence The inability of the heart to increase (or slow) its rate to meet the patient's metabolic demands. Heart failure patients frequently suffer from chronotropic incompetence, because their hearts cannot beat fast enough to sustain many ordinary activities (such as going up stairs, etc.), although their hearts may beat rapidly enough to support them at rest. Chronotropic incompetence often requires pacing support with a rate-responsive device.

class effect A condition when different drugs of the same class all have the same effect. When there is a class effect, one drug in that class can be substituted from another easily. ACE inhibitors have a class effect; β-blockers do not.

CO See **cardiac output**.

committed The characteristic of a CRT-D system which means it will deliver therapy once an arrhythmia is diagnosed, i.e. once diagnosed, therapy cannot be aborted. See also **non-committed**.

comorbidity A condition or disease which is frequently associated with another seemingly unrelated condition or disease. Comorbidities do not 'cause' each other and may develop independently. It is typical for comorbid conditions to form a vicious cycle, one exacerbating the other. Heart failure and atrial fibrillation are comorbid conditions.

compensatory mechanism In heart failure, any change in the heart adapted specifically to make up for deficits encountered because of an injury or impairment to the heart's ability to pump effectively. For example, if cardiac output is reduced because of less-than-optimal contractility, the heart may try to compensate for this defect by increasing its rate. In that case, the faster heart rate is a compensatory mechanism.

complete heart block A nickname for third-degree AV block, the most severe form of AV block.

concentric hypertrophy A type of ventricular remodeling experienced in some heart failure patients in which the heart becomes more rounded in shape as the interior ventricular walls get thicker. The thicker ventricular walls limit the capacity of the pumping chambers and make the heart more rigid. The heart loses its ability to relax effectively during diastole, which results in diastolic dysfunction. See also **eccentric hypertrophy**.

congestive heart failure (CHF) Heart failure with significant fluid accumulation. At one time, all heart failure was thought to be congestive heart failure, in that fluid accumulation was the main way to diagnose the syndrome. Today, we realize that heart failure can be present in patients who are not yet congested.

connector (1) On a pulse generator, the clear epoxy portion on the top with ports into which leads are inserted. This is nicknamed **header**. (2) On the lead, the metal pin portion of the lead that inserts into the port.

contractility The property of muscle cells, in particular cardiac cells, to contract and to contract more vigorously when they are stretched vigorously. Note that the stretching can only be done to a point. Overstretching a contractile cell can cause it to stretch out of shape. However, within reasonable limits, a vigorous stretch leads to a vigorous contraction, similar to the way a rubber band snaps back more vigorously the more it is stretched.

conventional pacemaker A term often used to describe a pacemaker with one or two leads (in the right ventricle and/or right atrium).

conventional pacing A term increasingly used to describe pacing from a lead placed in the apex of the right ventricle or in the right ventricular outflow tract. This is the main form of pacing in standard pacemakers today, but there is growing evidence that it induces a form of artificial left bundle branch block that may worsen systolic dysfunction in patients with a compromised left ventricle. There is at this time no evidence that patients with a standard pacing indication and normal ventricular function experience such negative effects. Also called **RV pacing**.

coronary arteries A network of vessels that send blood out from the heart muscle itself. They wrap around the exterior of the heart much like a 'crown,' from which they take their name.

coronary artery disease Abbreviated **CAD**. A disease in which the coronary arteries become occluded or blocked because of a build-up of fatty deposits and plaque. CAD is one of the most common causes of heart failure.

coronary sinus Abbreviated **CS**. A small structure within the heart, located between atria and ventricles, and through which deoxygenated blood flows into the right atrium to enter the cardiac cycle. The CS is about 3 or 4 cm in length and continues to the exterior of the heart, where it becomes the great cardiac vein (GCV), with many small tributaries. The LV lead is placed by cannulating the coronary sinus and passing the lead from the right atrium, through the coronary sinus, and into the coronary venous system on the exterior of the left ventricle.

CRT See **cardiac resynchronization therapy**.

CRT-D A cardiac rhythm management device that offers CRT therapy and defibrillation.

CRT-P A cardiac rhythm management device that offers CRT therapy in a pacemaker form (no defibrillation capability).

Decay Delay A programmable parameter in defibrillation that allows the dynamic sensitivity algorithm to plateau at the Threshold Start for a specified (and programmable) period of time. See also **Threshold Start**.

decompensated heart failure A type of advanced heart failure in which the heart is no longer able to pump effectively. A patient with decompensated heart failure often requires emergency hospitalization.

decompensation The inability of the heart to compensate for conditions that make it difficult to pump blood. In the early stages of heart failure,

the heart is often able to compensate for problems and can pump blood relatively efficiently. As heart failure progresses, these compensatory mechanisms actually change the shape of the heart and introduce other problems, so that the heart eventually cannot pump efficiently.

defibrillation threshold Abbreviated **DFT**. The lowest amount of energy (in joules or volts) required to defibrillate the heart reliably.

delta A value that quantifies change, often as a degree or percentage, but sometimes as an absolute value (in milliseconds, for example). Many SVT discrimination algorithms require the clinician to program a delta value to help assess the suddenness of arrhythmia onset or the stability of R–R intervals.

depolarization A change in charge caused by the inflow or outflow of charged ions through a semipermeable cell membrane in a cardiac cell. Depolarization occurs at the cellular level and causes the muscle cells to contract, resulting in a cardiac contraction.

device configuration The number of zones or diagnostic categories programmed in a CRT-D or ICD system. Counting the category of normal sinus rhythm (NSR) as zero, typical configurations are 1 zone (NSR and VF), 2 zones (NSR, VT and VF) and 3 zones (NSR, VT1, VT2 and VF). In the three-zone configuration, VT1 is 'slow' VT and VT2 is 'fast' VT.

DFT See **defibrillation threshold**.

DFT management The ability to make an implanted defibrillator (CRT-D or conventional ICD) compensate for high or rising energy requirements to defibrillate the heart. The patient's DFT cannot be managed in and of itself; however, the device may be optimized or reprogrammed to help compensate for high DFTs.

DFT testing Testing done during CRT-D or ICD implantation to establish the patient's minimum defibrillation energy requirements. In some cases, DFT testing is not performed and the maximum outputs are programmed automatically.

diastole The resting phase of the cardiac cycle when the heart passively fills with blood.

diastolic blood pressure The lowest amount of pressure exerted against the artery walls by the force of blood through the vessels, typically expressed as the second figure in blood pressure readings. For example, if a person has a blood pressure reading of 160/90 mmHg, 90 mmHg is the diastolic value. See also **systolic blood pressure**.

diastolic heart failure   Heart failure associated with the filling of the ventricles with blood, i.e. the diastolic portion of the cardiac cycle. Diastolic heart failure is more common in females.

diastolic mitral regurgitation   The backward flow of blood in the left side of the heart, up from the left ventricle over the mitral valve and into the left atrium that occurs when the left ventricle is at rest. Many heart failure patients experience diastolic MR, particularly when they have an abnormally prolonged AV conduction delay.

digoxin   A cardiac glycoside which can make the heart contract more vigorously and may slow the heart rate. While many heart failure patients take digoxin, it is not considered one of the 'mainstays' of heart failure drug therapy.

dilated cardiomyopathy   A disease which causes the heart muscle (myocardium) to become flabby, oversized and floppy. This flabby heart cannot pump blood effectively. A patient with dilated cardiomyopathy will eventually experience a heart that changes shape (remodels) into an enlarged, rounded shape. Although it is not known why, dilated cardiomyopathy is more common in men than in women.

dispersion of refractoriness   Technically, the location, at any given moment in time, of the refractory tissue in the beating heart. The term is more commonly used to refer to a disadvantageous arrangement of refractory and responsive tissue in the beating heart. During the cardiac cycle, the heart depolarizes and repolarizes; there is a period of refractoriness (when the tissue can no longer be stimulated to depolarization) immediately after depolarization. When a heart is fibrillating, particularly when many foci of stimulation fire in the atria in rapid succession, the dispersion of refractoriness may be such that the atria are not uniformly refractory and then uniformly responsive. Instead, segments of the atria are refractory at any given moment. It is believed that atrial pacing can help reduce atrial arrhythmias by reducing the dispersion of refractoriness.

diuretic   A type of drug that provides symptomatic relief of congestion by increasing urinary output and ridding the body of excess fluid. The main types of diuretics are the milder thiazide and metolazone and the more potent **loop diuretics**.

discrimination   For CRT-D and ICDs, the ability of the device to differentiate ventricular tachycardias (VTs or rhythm disorders that originate in the ventricle) and supraventricular tachycardias (SVTS or rhythm disorders that originate above the ventricles). Sometimes called **SVT discrimination**. Discrimination is accomplished through algorithms in the device. Examples of these specific discriminators include **Sudden Onset, Interval Stability, Rate Branch** and **Morphology Discrimination**. Note that discriminators may vary by manufacturer and even by models from a single manufacturer.

double-counting   Any device behavior in which diagnostic counters count inappropriate signals as well as what they ought to be counting (and thus count 'double'). Double-counting may occur when a CRT system experiences far-field P-wave sensing and counts both true ventricular events and inappropriately sensed atrial events as true ventricular events. Double-counting in a CRT-D system can lead to inappropriate therapy delivery.

dropsy   An old name for heart failure.

dyspnea   Shortness of breath, one of the most frequent symptoms of heart failure.

dysrhythmia   See **arrhythmia**.

dyssynchrony   A process in some heart failure patients in which the ventricles get out-of-sync. Dyssynchrony can be interventricular (the right ventricle contracts before the left ventricle instead of simultaneously), intraventricular (the left ventricle contracts in waves or segments instead of as a unified whole) as well as mechanical (the ventricles contract out of sequence) and electrical (the electrical conduction system is abnormal). CRT devices address the problem of ventricular dyssynchrony.

eccentric hypertrophy   A type of ventricular remodeling experienced in some heart failure patients in which the ventricles progressively dilate, so that the heart muscle becomes enlarged and flabby. This reduces myocardial contractility and leads to a lowered ejection fraction (systolic dysfunction). See also **concentric hypertrophy**.

ECG   Electrocardiogram or electrocardiography. Sometimes **EKG** (to avoid confusion between similar-sounding terms ECG and EEG).

EDI   See **end diastolic index.**

EF   See **ejection fraction.**

ejection fraction   The amount of blood (stated as a percentage of total volume) that the ventricles eject or pump out in one cardiac cycle. Abbreviated **EF** Note that the EF score most frequently cited is the **left-ventricular ejection fraction** or **LVEF.** A normal EF score is considered to be around 50%.

EKG   See **ECG.**

electrical dyssynchrony   See **ventricular dyssynchrony.**

electrical remodeling   Changes in the conduction pathways of the heart and impulse generation as a result of heart failure. Electrical remodeling is believed to occur at the cellular level and can affect impulse generation (sinus node dysfunction), slower conduction, re-entry mechanisms, and changes in the ventricular repolarization and relaxation phase.

embolism   A blood clot which breaks free of the vessel and lodges somewhere in the body other than the heart. When an embolism lodges in the brain, it can cause a stroke.

end diastolic index   A measurement of how much blood is contained in the ventricle by square millimeter of ventricle. Abbreviated **EDI.**

end-point   A specific and measurable objective that defines the point at which data are collected in a clinical trial. The PAVE study used as its end-point the distance patients could walk in the 6-min walk test at 6 months. Clinical trials often have primary and secondary end-points.

delivered energy   The amount of electrical energy that a CRT-D device can actually deliver to the heart. Delivered energy is always lower than stored energy. Delivered energy is a more clinically relevant value than stored energy. See also **stored energy.**

far-field   In CRT devices, the term for the other channel. For example, if the atrial lead senses ventricular activity (from either the LV or RV), that is called 'far-field R-wave sensing'. Likewise, if the LV lead picks up atrial signals, that is called 'far-field P-wave sensing'. Far-field sensing occurs when a lead in one chamber (either atrium or one or the other ventricle) picks up signals from the other chamber (atria to ventricles or ventricles to atria).

far R   See **far-field R-wave sensing.**

Far-field P-wave sensing   Behavior unique in CRT systems in which the LV lead picks up atrial signals (pacing output pulses or intrinsic signals) and inappropriately counts them as sensed ventricular events. Far-field P-wave sensing occurs when the LV lead is located close enough to the atria to pick up those signals and may often be remedied by adjusting LV sensitivity.

far-field R-wave sensing   Behavior by the CRT system in which a ventricular output pulse is inappropriately sensed by the atrial channel of the device and mistakenly counted as an intrinsic atrial event. This type of behavior (sometimes called far R or crosstalk) can cause the device to miscount atrial activity and inappropriately pace the ventricle in response. There are programming steps that can reduce the risk of far-field R-wave sensing, including the **PVAB** and **PVARP** settings.

fluoroscope   A live moving X-ray image or the equipment used to produce it. Fluoroscopic equipment usually involves a C-arm that allows the 'camera' to shoot at different angles. The main angles in use are AP (anterior-posterior), LAO (left-anterior-oblique), RAO (right-anterior-oblique), cranial (from skull down), and caudal (from feet up). For CRT device implantation, the most common fluoroscopic images are AP, LAO 30 (at a 30° angle) and RAO 40 or 45.

fusion   A phenomenon of paced rhythm that occurs when an output pulse 'collides' with an intrinsic contraction. The result is that the output pulse contributes but does not entirely cause the contraction. A fusion (or fused) beat has a unique morphology, unlike a true paced or a true sensed event. Fusion confirms capture but it is an inefficient type of pacing. Fusion is typically a timing problem (the paced rate is about the same as the intrinsic rate); however, occasional fused beats may not be a source of concern. See also **pseudofusion.**

guidewire   A wire used in lead placement (for both right and left sides of the heart) to serve as a placeholder and to facilitate lead passage, but which is not intended to remain in the body. Typically, a guidewire is inserted first into the vein and it 'guides' the pacing lead into the venous system.

header A slang term for **connector** (the clear epoxy connector on top of the pulse generator).

heart block See **AV block**.

heart failure A complex syndrome, i.e. a constellation of symptoms, which occurs when the heart loses its ability to pump blood effectively. Its most common symptoms are shortness of breath, fatigue and fluid accumulation.

heart rate The frequency of cardiac activity, typically assessed by number of cardiac contractions in one minute (usually abbreviated beats/min). In healthy individuals, heart rate varies over the course of a day, with activity, stress and other factors.

heart rate variability The natural changes in heart rate that occur in patients in response to changes in activity, metabolic demand and other factors. For example, healthy individuals may have a resting heart rate of 60 beats/min, a heart rate that drops to 52 beats/min when they are asleep, a heart of 80 beats/min walking around the yard, 100 beats/min going upstairs, and 120 beats/min playing tennis. Heart failure patients have significantly depressed heart rate variability.

hematocrit A red blood cell.

hemodynamic monitoring An invasive electrophysiological procedure involving measurements of pulmonary capillary wedge pressure.

hemodynamics The properties and characteristics governing the flow and circulation of blood through the body.

hemostasis valve A small plastic valve, often included in a left-heart delivery system, which prevents blood from flowing out backward through the system.

high-output device A CRT-D system capable of delivering a relatively high amount of energy, expressed in joules. A high-output device might offer 36 J delivered energy.

high-voltage therapy In CRT-D systems and ICDs, defibrillation therapy at maximum energy output settings, often 32–36 J.

HOCM See **hypertrophic obstructive cardiomyopathy**.

hot can Slang term for a programmable defibrillation configuration which allows defibrillating energy to travel from a coil on the defibrillating (RV) lead to the CRT-D can itself. Sometimes called **active can**. See also **shocking vector**.

hyperkalemia Having high levels of potassium in the body.

hypernatremia Having high levels of sodium in the body.

hypertension High blood pressure.

hyperthyroidism A condition related to an overactive thyroid.

hypertrophic obstructive cardiomyopathy Abbreviated HOCM. A disease of the heart muscle (myocardium) which causes the walls of the heart, in particular the walls of the left ventricle, to become very thick and the myocardium itself to become stiff and rigid. When HOCM is present, the pumping capacity of the heart is drastically reduced, in that the heart holds much less blood in its chambers. HOCM can be genetic.

hypertrophy The excessive development (especially an increase in bulk) of an organ or part of the body. Heart failure patients can develop cardiac hypertrophy, an enlarged heart. See also **concentric hypertrophy** and **eccentric hypertrophy**.

hypokalemia Having low levels of potassium in the body.

hyponatremia Having low levels of sodium in the body.

hypotension Low blood pressure.

hypothyroidism Underactive thyroid.

hypovolemic A state in which the patient is in fluid overload, i.e. congested.

hysteresis A programmable function in conventional pacemakers which encourages intrinsic conduction (unpaced activity) to prevail as much as possible. Hysteresis works by imposing a hysteresis rate which is slightly lower than the programmed base rate. For example, if the base rate was programmed to 70 pulses/min and the hysteresis rate was programmed to 60 pulses/min, the pacemaker would be inhibited if the patient's rate was 60 beats/min or above. However, when the pacemaker paced, it would pace at 70 pulses/min. Hysteresis is not of value in CRT patients, since they need as close to 100% ventricular pacing as possible. See also **negative AV hysteresis**.

iatrogenic Caused or induced by a physician. For example, AV nodal ablation results in iatrogenic heart block.

idiopathic A disease or condition of unknown origin.

inappropriate therapy   For CRT-D (and ICD) devices, high-voltage therapy delivered to treat something other than a true ventricular tachycardia, typically the rapid ventricular response to a supraventricular tachycardia. Inappropriate therapy exposes the patient to the stress of shock therapy, which can put a drain of the device battery. See also **appropriate therapy**.

incidence   The number of new cases of a disease or syndrome each year.

index   An attempt to relate one variable (such as cardiac output) to the patient's size. For example, a cardiac output that is adequate for a small person would be inadequate for a large one. Indexing is a way to create a value that can be used without taking the patient's size into account.

insufficiency   Any condition in which a vessel or organ cannot work as efficiently as required.

Interval Stability   A discrimination algorithm in CRT-D (and ICD) devices which compares a number of R–R intervals (intrinsic ventricular events) during a tachycardia in an X out of Y pattern, for example, 8 out of 12 consecutive intervals, and compares the interval with a programmable delta value. If the R–R intervals in the sequence change by more than the delta value, the intervals are not stable; if the R–R intervals change by less than the delta value, the intervals are stable. Interval stability strongly suggests a true ventricular tachycardia, while unstable intervals are more likely to be the result of rapid ventricular response to atrial fibrillation.

interventricular   Involving the right and left ventricles. For example, interventricular dyssynchrony occurs in some heart failure patients when the right ventricle contracts before the left ventricle, instead of at the same time.

interventricular mechanical delay   Abbreviated **IVMD**. A measurement that can be taken on an echocardiographic study which defines the time from electrical activation of the ventricles (either by an output pulse from a CRT device or a natural electrical impulse) until the point at which blood flows out of the heart (from LV into the aorta or from RV into the pulmonary artery). As a general rule, the IVMD value should be < 40 ms.

intraventricular   Involving the totality of one ventricle only. For example, some heart failure patients have intraventricular dyssynchrony, which means their left ventricles contract in sections or segments, rather than as a unified whole.

ischemia   The condition that results when a condition or disease blocks the supply of oxygen and causes damage to certain tissue in the body. A heart attack is an ischemic disease, in that it creates damage to the myocardium by depriving it of oxygen.

IVMD   See **interventricular mechanical delay**.

J   See **joule**.

joule   Abbreviated **J**. A unit of energy used to describe defibrillation energy in CRT-D devices. Specifically, 1 J is the amount of energy it takes to do the work by a force of one Newton acting through a distance of one meter. Typical CRT-D devices may offer maximum delivered energy of 25–36 J.

lead   A thin, insulated wire designed to be implanted in the human body for use with a permanent CRT system. A lead has a connector at the proximal end (to plug into a port in the connector portion of the CRT pulse generator) and is placed within the heart. Leads deliver electricity to the heart and transmit signals from the heart back to the pulse generator.

lead revision   A surgical procedure to fix a problem with a lead. Lead revision may involve removing a lead and replacing it with a new one; it may involve adding a new lead and disconnecting the old lead by unplugging it from the pulse generator and capping it; or it may involve repositioning the indwelling lead or reconnecting it more securely to the pulse generator.

LBBB   See **left bundle branch block**.

left bundle branch block   Abbreviated **LBBB**. A conduction disorder which affects the electrical pathways in the left fascicles of the heart. LBBB commonly occurs in heart failure patients (although it also occurs in people without heart failure) and appears on the surface ECG as a widened QRS with a characteristic notch.

left heart   The left atrium and left ventricle.

left-heart delivery system   A general name for a package of tools useful in cannulating the coronary sinus and implanting an LV lead. Most CRT manufacturers offer one or more of these 'systems', which may include steerable or non-steerable catheters, sheaths, introducers, an occlusive balloon, a hemostasis valve and other equipment.

The main purpose of a left-heart delivery system is to provide a convenient kit of useful equipment.

left-sided heart failure An infrequent term to describe heart failure with significant damage to the left side of the heart. Left-sided heart failure involves left-ventricular dysfunction and manifests as congestion in the pulmonary veins. See also **right-sided heart failure.** Note that it is possible for one person to have both left-sided and right-sided heart failure; they are not mutually exclusive.

left-ventricular ejection fraction The amount of blood (stated as a percentage of total contents) pumped out of the left ventricle during one contraction. A normal score might be around 50%. Abbreviated **LVEF.**

left-ventricular lead Abbreviated **LV lead.** The stimulation lead that distinguishes a CRT device from a conventional device and which is placed in such a way that it can stimulate the lateral (outside) free wall of the left ventricle. Despite its name, the LV lead is not actually placed within the left ventricle; it is inserted into the right atrium, through the coronary sinus, and then out to the coronary venous system in such a way that it lodges in a vein and can pace the left ventricle from the outside. LV leads pace but usually do not sense; they cannot defibrillate. Unlike leads for the right side of the heart, an LV lead does not have an active-fixation or passive-fixation mechanism, but instead lodges in place owing to its shape at the distal end. Typical LV leads are curved, S-shaped, or angulated.

loop diuretic The most powerful form of diuretic drug, an agent that works at the loop of Henle to relieve congestion in heart failure patients.

loop of Henle A 'sodium pump' within the tubule of each individual nephron or kidney cell that encourages the body to retain sodium. Loop diuretics work at the loop of Henle, encouraging the body to release sodium and, with it, fluid.

LV Left ventricle or left-ventricular.

LV lead Left-ventricular lead.

LVEF See **left-ventricular ejection fraction.**

macrodislodgement A noticeable physical change in the position of a permanently implanted lead in the heart, including a lead becoming 'un-fixated' in the myocardium. In most instances, macrodislodgement involves a change in lead position

significant enough to show up clearly on an X-ray. Macrodislodgement of a lead will also be evident on rhythm strips. Macrodislodgement of a lead (sometimes just called lead dislodgement) almost always requires surgical revision.

maximum sensor rate Abbreviated **MSR.** A programmable parameter which defines the highest rate the device will pace in response to activity sensor input.

maximum tracking rate Abbreviated **MTR.** A programmable parameter which defines the highest rate the device will pace the ventricle in response to sensed atrial activity.

mechanical dyssynchrony See **ventricular dyssynchrony.**

metolazone A mild diuretic drug.

MI See **myocardial infarction.**

microdislodgement A very small shift or change in the position of a permanently implanted lead in the heart. A microdislodgement of the LV lead may not be noticeable on an X-ray but could cause changes on the ECG.

mitral inflow Doppler velocity A parameter measured on echocardiography that is used for CRT optimization, particularly finding the ideal AV delay value for a particular patient. This parameter measures how fast blood flows into the LV over the mitral valve.

mitral regurgitation A backward flow of blood from the left ventricle upward into the left atrium. Abbreviated **MR.**

mitral valve The valve between the left atrium and the left ventricle.

mitral valve insufficiency A general term for any condition which impairs the ability of the mitral valve to open and close well and to prevent the backward flow of blood.

monophasic Having one phase. A defibrillating waveform may be monophasic if it has only one (positive) phase. Early ICDs had monophasic waveforms, but today most implantable defibrillators and CRT-D systems use biphasic waveforms. See also **biphasic.**

morphology In general, the shape of something. On an ECG, morphology refers to the shape of particular waveforms, such as QRS morphology. Morphologies on the ECG can vary widely in CRT patients and may even vary over time in an individual patient.

Morphology Discrimination   A discrimination algorithm in some CRT-D (and ICD) devices which compares a template of the individual patient's QRS complex in normal sinus rhythm with QRS complexes which occur during tachycardia. The match is indicated as a programmable percentage value, for example, a 60% match is counted as a match. If the programmed number of matches in a programmed number of consecutive intervals (an X out of Y pattern) are matches, then the morphology is determined to be a match and an SVT (normal sinus rhythm). If the programmed number of intervals do not match, then the morphology is determined to be non-sinus and, thus, a ventricular tachycardia.

MR   See **mitral regurgitation**.

MSR   See **maximum sensor rate**.

MTR   See **maximum tracking rate**.

myocardial infarction   Abbreviated **MI**. The medical term for a 'heart attack', in which blood flow to the heart via the coronary arteries is blocked and starves certain regions of the myocardium for oxygen. The result is that a portion of the myocardial tissue dies (infarct site) and lesions (scar tissue) form in that area. An MI can be mild, severe, or even fatal depending on how much tissue is damaged.

myocardium   The heart muscle.

myocyte   A heart muscle cell.

negative   In ECG evaluation, a deflection or curve downward from the baseline. See also **positive**.

Negative AV hysteresis   A programmable function in CRT systems which works to encourage maximal ventricular pacing. (In this way, it is the antithesis of hysteresis in conventional pacemakers, which encourages maximal intrinsic activity.) Negative AV hysteresis automatically shortens the A–R or P–R interval whenever it detects an intrinsic ventricular event during the AV delay. The device maintains that shortened AV delay for the next 32 cycles. If no other intrinsic ventricular events are detected, then the previous AV delay setting is restored.

nephron   A kidney cell. The body has about a million nephrons.

neurohormonal model   A relatively new way of understanding the complex mechanisms and progression of heart failure in that the sympathetic nervous system (SNS) becomes overactive in heart failure patients, flooding the body with neurohormones. These neurohormones exert a profound effect on the heart and can lead over the long term to ventricular remodeling and other serious consequences. Drug therapy for heart failure is based on the neurohormonal model.

neurohormones   Chemical substances produced by the body's nervous system which transmit messages and cause specific physical responses. Although a neurohormone, technically, is a hormone produced by or acting upon a nervous tissue, in heart failure discussions, the term neurohormone is sometimes used to describe other similar substances that may not technically be hormones (these are sometimes called neuromodulators). An example of a true neurohormone is norepinephrine. Angiotensin is not technically a neurohormone, but is often included in discussions of the neurohormonal model of heart failure.

neurotransmitter   A chemical substance used to help relay (transmit) messages from nerve cell (neuro) to nerve cell.

non-committed   The characteristic of a CRT-D system which means that it will abort therapy after an arrhythmia is diagnosed if sinus rhythm is restored before the shock can be delivered. See also **committed**.

non-responder   A CRT patient who fails to derive benefit from the implanted CRT system. There is no official consensus on a single measure for non-response to CRT, but in general, a non-responder is a person who meets at least one of the following three criteria: (i) worsening heart failure post-CRT device implant, (ii) no improvement in NYHA class 6 months post-implant with increased ventricular remodeling, or (iii) initial favorable response to CRT but currently worsening symptoms. About a third of CRT patients can be considered non-responders, but many can be converted to responders with proper troubleshooting. See also **responder**.

normal sinus rhythm   Abbreviated **NSR**. (1) A healthy intrinsic rhythm in which the atria drive the heart rate and there is one-to-one AV synchrony. (2) In CRT-D devices and ICDs, a term which refers to native cardiac activity within a specified rate range, regardless of the actual rhythm. For example, a clinician can program that a CRT-D device consider any intrinsic activity at rates between 60 and 100 beats/min to be normal sinus rhythm.

NSR See **normal sinus rhythm**.

NYHA New York Heart Association.

NYHA Class I A category of heart failure in which a patient has symptoms of heart failure (shortness of breath and fatigue) with exertion that would limit normal individuals. Class I is the mildest stage of heart failure in the NYHA Classification System.

NYHA Class II A category of heart failure in which a patient has symptoms of heart failure (shortness of breath and fatigue) with ordinary exertion.

NYHA Class III A category of heart failure in which a patient has symptoms of heart failure (shortness of breath and fatigue) with less than ordinary exertion.

NYHA Class IV A category of heart failure in which a patient has symptoms of heart failure (shortness of breath and fatigue) even at rest. Class IV is the most severe category of heart failure.

NYHA Classification System The most commonly used method to categorize or classify patients with heart failure based on symptoms produced during exertion. There are four classes (I, II, III and IV), with I the mildest and IV the most severe. Note that NYHA classes are not necessarily permanent; patients may change classification (improving or worsening) with various treatments.

occlude To form a blockage. Plaque can occlude the coronary arteries, which, in turn, blocks blood flow.

OPT See **optimal pharmacological therapy**.

optimal pharmacological therapy Abbreviated **OPT**. The ideal and state-of-the-art drug regimen for an individual heart failure patient. OPT is highly specific and changes over time with disease progression, but generally involves a diuretic, β-blocker, ACE inhibitor (or, if not tolerated, an angiotensin-receptor blocker) and possibly such other drugs as digoxin, spironolactone or amiodarone. Most randomized clinical trials of heart failure patients require all patients, even those in the device groups, to be on OPT at baseline and throughout the study. OPT is considered the foundation of any heart failure treatment.

optimization The adjustment of an implanted CRT system to establish or increase the heart failure patient's response. CRT optimization typically involves timing cycle adjustments, such as finding the ideal AV delay value.

os A slang term for the **ostium**, in particular, the ostium of the coronary sinus.

ostium In general, an inlet to a larger structure. In CRT terminology, the ostium is the entry to the coronary sinus. Sometimes nicknamed **os**.

OTW See **over-the-wire**.

output The stimulus delivered by the pulse generator, defined in pulse amplitude (voltage) and pulse width or pulse duration (milliseconds).

over-the-wire Abbreviated **OTW**. The quality of a lead or catheter which is placed in the heart by first inserting a guidewire or stylet and then advancing the lead 'over-the-wire'. When the lead is in place, the stylet is then withdrawn. Over-the-wire leads are popular for left-ventricular use. See also **stylet-driven**.

overdrive pacing Atrial pacing intended to 'control' the atrial rate in such a way that high-rate intrinsic atrial events do not occur. When there is forced atrial pacing (i.e. the atrial pacing rate is programmed in such a way that it is more rapid than native atrial activity), it is very difficult for atrial tachyarrhythmias to occur. Many pacemakers, ICDs and CRT devices have overdrive algorithms.

P-wave. The portion on a surface ECG that represents the intrinsic atrial depolarization and contraction.

pacemaker-mediated tachycardia Abbreviated **PMT**. A rapid ventricular rate facilitated by the presence of a pulse generator system. A PMT is not caused by the system but once a re-entry tachycardia gets started, the device acts like a re-entry pathway. There are programming options to help manage PMTs, including programming a long PVARP setting. This should be done with caution in CRT patients, since a long PVARP may discourage some ventricular pacing.

pacing state A term borrowed from bradycardia pacing which defines dual-chamber events by initials: AS is an atrial sensed event while AP is an atrial paced event. Likewise, VS is a sensed ventricular event while VP is a paced ventricular event. Programmer annotations may describe pacing states as AS–VP, AP–VP, and so on.

pacing system analyzer Abbreviated **PSA**. A small portable device often used in CRT or other cardiac rhythm management device implantation which allows the implant team to test the implanted leads prior to connecting them with the pulse generator.

parasympathetic nervous system Part of the body's nervous system which might be considered the 'peaceful twin' of the sympathetic nervous system (SNS). In healthy individuals, the parasympathetic nervous system (PSNS) is dominant and serves as the check-and-balance system for the SNS. In heart failure patients, the role of the PSNS becomes subordinate to the SNS.

paroxysmal AF Atrial fibrillation that starts suddenly and resolves without medical intervention. Episodes of AF are typically very short and may not even cause symptoms. Paroxysmal AF is the first and mildest stage of this progressive rhythm disorder.

passive filling of the ventricles The period during diastole or rest when blood flows into the heart.

PCWP See **Pulmonary capillary wedge pressure.**

peelable The quality of an introducer, catheter or sheath which allows it to be torn or pulled apart (peeled away) to facilitate removal after lead placement. See also **slittable**.

perfusion (1) Pumping a fluid through an organ or tissue. (2) The degree of saturation of tissues with oxygen-rich blood. Poor renal perfusion is a consequence of heart failure which occurs when the kidneys are deprived of an adequate supply of oxygenated blood.

permanent AF Atrial fibrillation that does not resolve spontaneously and no longer responds to medical intervention. This is the final and most severe stage of this progressive rhythm disorder. Also called **chronic AF**.

persistent AF Atrial fibrillation that requires medical intervention to resolve, typically chemical or electrical cardioversion. This is the second stage of progressive AF and frequently involves symptoms. At this stage of AF, the rhythm disorder can still be medically managed.

plaque A mixture of cholesterol, fatty deposits and other waste materials that form in the blood and build up in the blood vessels. Patients with coronary artery disease have plaque in the coronary arteries, which occludes those vessels.

PNS See **parasympathetic nervous system.**

polypharmacy Taking multiple medications, a common situation for most heart failure patients.

port The cavity or area in the epoxy connector of the pulse generator into which leads are to be plugged.

positive In ECG evaluation, a deflection or curve upward from the baseline. See also **negative.**

post-shock pacing Abbreviated **PSP**. Special temporary pacing parameters that can be used for a short period of time right after therapy delivery by a CRT-D device (or ICD) to pace tissue that may be 'traumatized' by a recent shock. In general, PSP parameters involve higher outputs, a lower base rate and no rate response. PSP parameters should go into effect a few seconds after therapy delivery and be used only for a few minutes. PSP values are programmable.

post-ventricular atrial refractory period Abbreviated **PVARP**. A programmable parameter in a CRT system which blanks the atrial channel for a programmable amount of time immediately after a ventricular event (paced or sensed) occurs. The purpose of the PVARP is to prevent far-field R-wave sensing (the atrial channel 'seeing' the ventricular output as an intrinsic atrial event). For CRT patients, the PVARP should be programmed to a relatively short value (to encourage ventricular pacing). However, a very short PVARP can open the door to pacemaker-mediated tachycardias.

PR interval The time between an intrinsic atrial event (natural contraction of the atrial) and the subsequent intrinsic ventricular event. Some heart failure patients have a prolonged PR interval.

PR segment The portion on a surface ECG between the P-wave and the QRS complex, typically represented by a short straight line, that represents the period of atrial diastole or repolarization and relaxation.

preload The amount of blood that flows into the heart for each cardiac cycle, defined in terms of the end diastolic index, which affects how much the heart muscle must stretch to accommodate it. High or low preloads can affect the heart's ability to pump effectively.

premature ventricular contraction Abbreviated **PVC**. Sometimes called a premature ventricular event or **PVE**. An intrinsic ventricular event which occurs without an associated atrial event.

prevalence The number of cases of a disease or syndrome at any given time.

preventricular atrial blanking period Abbreviated **PVAB**, sometimes called Pre-VAB. A programmable parameter which blanks the atrial channel for a short (programmable) period of time immediately before a ventricular output pulse is delivered. The purpose of PVAB is to reduce the risk of far-field R-wave sensing (i.e. having the atrial channel mistakenly 'think' a ventricular output pulse is an intrinsic atrial event). A typical PVAB setting is very short, for example, around 16 ms.

primary prevention Describes a patient or therapy given to treat a condition for which the patient is at risk but for which there is no documented evidence in that patient. Prophylactic ICD therapy in heart failure patients at risk for sudden cardiac death but who have never experienced an arrhythmia is considered primary-prevention therapy. Many recent large clinical trials have supported device therapy as primary prevention in certain types of heart failure patients (e.g. SCD-HeFT). See also **secondary prevention**.

PSA See **pacing system analyzer**.

pseudofusion A phenomenon of paced rhythm that occurs when an output pulse falls directly 'on top of' an intrinsic contraction. The result is that the output pulse is wasted and the heart beats on its own. Pseudofusion beats look like intrinsic beats but with a pacemaker spike on top. Pseudofusion neither proves nor disproves capture. Pseudofusion wastes energy (the pacemaker output pulse contributes nothing to the heart's contraction); however, occasional appearances of pseudofusion on an ECG may not be a source of concern. Pseudofusion is a timing problem; it occurs because the paced rate is about the same as the intrinsic rate. See also **fusion**.

PSP See **post-shock pacing**.

pulmonary capillary wedge pressure A measurement taken in hemodynamic monitoring (an electrophysiological procedure) in which a balloon capillary is wedged into the pulmonary artery in order to measure blood pressure in the left atrium. Abbreviated **PCWP**.

pulmonary valve The valve between the right ventricle and the pulmonary artery. Blood from the right side of the heart is pumped out through the pulmonary valve and over the lungs.

pulmonary veins A network of vessels that collects blood from the lungs and sends it back to the left side of the heart.

pulse generator The can-shaped device implanted in the pectoral region which contains the electronic circuitry and battery of the CRT system. Nicknamed **can**.

pulse pressure The difference between systolic and diastolic blood pressure values. For example, a person with a blood pressure reading of 120/80 mmHg has a pulse pressure of 40 (120−80). Pulse pressure is sometimes used to indicate the degree of severity of heart failure.

PVAB See **preventricular atrial blanking period**.

PVARP See **post-ventricular atrial refractory period**.

PVC See **premature ventricular contraction**.

PVE Premature ventricular event, see **premature ventricular contraction**.

quality of life Abbreviated **QOL**. In clinical studies and other areas of evidence-based medicine, a quantifiable measurement of how patients subjectively assess their own status, in particular with regard to psychological well-being, physical well-being and the ability to go about their normal lives.

quality of life questionnaire A standardized test vehicle which captures the patient's subjective assessment of their life in terms of psychological and social well-being, physical well-being and lifestyle. QOL questionnaires quantify these assessments for analysis.

QOL See **quality of life**.

QRS complex The portion of the surface ECG that represents ventricular systole (depolarization and contraction of the ventricles). It is the largest portion of a normal ECG because the ventricular contraction creates the most electrical energy.

QRS duration The amount of time, typically expressed in milliseconds, that the surface ECG shows for the ventricular depolarization and contraction, i.e. the QRS complex. In the healthy heart, the QRS complex is typically < 120 ms in duration. Many clinical trials use QRS durations of > 120 ms to be lower boundary for 'wide QRS'. Wide QRS is a marker of some disputed accuracy for the severity of HF and the presence (and possibly degree of) ventricular dyssynchrony.

R-wave   This term may either be the first deflection of the QRS complex or be an abbreviated way to refer to the entire QRS complex.

RA   Right atrium or right atrial.

RAA system   Renin–angiotensin–aldosterone system.

rate adaptation   See **rate response**.

Rate Branch   A discrimination algorithm in dual-chamber CRT-D (and ICD) devices, which compares the intrinsic atrial rate with the intrinsic ventricular rate and uses that information to help the device decide whether to deliver or inhibit therapy. The three main branches are (i) atrial rate greater than the ventricular rate (A > V), which indicates atrial fibrillation or atrial flutter (an SVT); (ii) atrial rate the same as the ventricular rate (A = V), which indicates a sinus tachycardia (an SVT); and (iii) atrial rate less than ventricular rate (A < V), which indicates a ventricular tachycardia. Only the third branch would allow the device to proceed to therapy. While Rate Branch is a very useful and fundamental discrimination algorithm, some rhythm disorders can be somewhat deceptive. For that reason, Rate Branch is often used in conjunction with other discriminators in patients with known multiple rhythm disorders.

rate control   A type of approach to the management of atrial fibrillation which seeks to control the rapid ventricular response and does not try to convert the atrial fibrillation to normal sinus rhythm. Ablation for AF is a form of rate control approach. See also **rhythm control**.

rate cut-off   Any value in beats or pulses per minute that defines or helps to define a rate range; it may be a maximum, minimum or boundary setting. If a clinician programs the device to mode switch at atrial rates > 120 beats/min, then 120 beats/min may be called the rate cut-off.

rate modulation   See **rate response**.

rate response   A type of pacemaker feature included in the pacing function of many advanced ICDs and CRT systems which incorporates a sensor and allows for pacing rates to increase in response to the patient's needs, typically measured in terms of activity level. Most rate-responsive ICDs use an activity sensor (typically an accelerometer) and increase the rate based on patient movement. Rate response is indicated by an 'R' in the fourth position of the pacemaker code (for example, DDDR is a DDD device with rate response). Also called **rate modulation** and **rate adaptation**.

rate-responsive PVARP   A pacemaker parameter which automatically reduces the PVARP setting when the patient's native atrial rate exceeds 90 beats/min. Rate-responsive PVARP thus shortens the atrial refractory period as the patient's atrial rate increases. A typical rate-responsive PVARP setting might be 'low', which reduces the PVARP by 1 ms per atrial beat/min over 90. Thus, if the patient's intrinsic atrial rate was 150 beats/min, the rate-responsive PVARP would decrease the PVARP temporarily by 60 ms (150 − 90 = 60). For this particular parameter, the term 'rate-responsive' has nothing to do with the device's activity sensor.

re-entry   A mechanism for tachyarrhythmias in which an impulse gets 'trapped' in an endless loop, in which it circulates at a high rate of speed. Re-entry tachycardia requires a re-entry pathway (a 'loop' where one side conducts faster than the other side), a trigger (typically a premature cardiac event) and exact timing. Not all people have the pathways suitable for sustaining a re-entry tachycardia (substrates). Re-entry is the most common mechanism behind atrial and ventricular tachyarrhythmias.

reforming   The process of improving capacitor performance by charging the capacitor completely and allowing the charge to painlessly dissipate (bleed off). Reforming the capacitor improves the state of the dielectric component within the capacitor. Capacitors can be reformed manually or automatically.

remodeling   See **ventricular remodeling**.

remote patient monitoring   Any number of systems that allow a patient with an implanted device to have information stored in the device downloaded and transmitted, either using telephone lines or the internet, to a station that can interpret the downloaded information. Remote patient monitoring only downloads data; parameter settings cannot be changed remotely. Remote patient monitoring allows a patient to 'check in' with the clinic from the privacy of their own home. Data are transmitted either to a clinic (or doctor's office, hospital, etc.) or to a special service that may receive, forward or even interpret the data.

renin–angiotensin–aldosterone system A portion of the body's sympathetic nervous system (SNS) which is activated primarily when renal perfusion decreases. This triggers a cascade of events in the renin–angiotensin–aldosterone (RAA) system, such that angiotensin-II is created (a powerful vasoconstrictor) and aldosterone is released (which prompts the body to store sodium and water).

renin A blood enzyme that is produced by the body's RAA system (secreted by kidney cells), which acts on a plasma protein known as angiotensinogen to produce angiotensin-I. An angiotensin-converting enzyme (ACE) then acts on angiotensin-I to produce angiotensin-II, a powerful vasoconstrictor.

repolarization Restoration of the original charge in a cell following a depolarization (charge reversal) caused by the inflow or outflow of charged ions through semipermeable cell membrane in a cardiac cell. Repolarization occurs at the cellular level and causes the muscle cells to relax, resulting in a cardiac relaxation (diastole).

responder In CRT therapy, a patient who derives a significant degree of symptomatic relief from a CRT device. Not all heart failure patients indicated for CRT are responders.

resynchronization To restore the proper timing of cardiac functions or synchrony, in particular to restore an efficient unified ventricular contraction and relaxation. Although resynchronization may involve resynchronizing right and left ventricles, it more often involves the restoration of a unified, coherent left ventricular contraction. A dyssynchronous heart often has a left ventricle that contracts in sections rather than as a whole. As a result, portions of the left ventricle are contracting as other portions are relaxing. This sectionwise contraction means that blood sloshes back and forth in the heart instead of being pumped outward. Most resynchronization devices compel the left ventricle to contract all at once, causing more efficient pumping of blood.

responder A CRT patient who derives benefit from the CRT system. There are varying ways to assess CRT response, including 'soft measures,' such as symptoms or functional status (improvement in distance covered in 6-min walk) or those who meet objective criteria (such as oxygen uptake at the anaerobic threshold during exercise or reduction of LV diameter). An improvement in NYHA classification is often used as a way of determining CRT response, but heart failure patients can sometimes be deemed 'responders' if their NYHA class stabilizes and does not worsen. See also **non-responder**.

response For CRT patients, a significant degree of symptomatic relief obtained from a CRT system. Not all heart failure patients respond to CRT therapy.

revascularization A general term for cardiac surgeries that repair vessel damage. The best-known type of revascularization is the coronary artery bypass graft or CABG procedure.

reverse remodeling A restoration of the size, shape and functionality of the myocardium in a patient who had experienced ventricular remodeling as a result of heart failure or other disorder. There is growing evidence that ventricular remodeling is reversible with proper treatment.

rhythm control A type of approach to the management of atrial fibrillation which seeks to convert the rhythm disorder back to normal sinus rhythm which, in turn, would help slow the rapid ventricular response. Pharmacological therapy for AF is often a form of rhythm control approach. See also **rate control**.

rhythm disorder See **arrhythmia**.

right-sided heart failure An infrequent term to describe heart failure with significant damage to the right side of the heart. Right-sided heart failure impairs the body's ability to pump blood out over the lungs. It is associated with congestion in systemic circulation. Cases of true right-sided heart failure are rare; most people with right-sided heart failure also have left-sided heart failure. See also **left-sided heart failure**.

RV Right ventricle or right-ventricular.

RV pacing See **conventional pacing**.

SA node See **sinoatrial node**.

SCA See **sudden cardiac arrest**.

SCD See **sudden cardiac death**.

secondary prevention   Describes a patient or therapy given to treat a condition for which there is documented evidence in that particular patient. For example, a patient who survived an episode of potentially life-threatening ventricular fibrillation might receive an ICD as secondary prevention. The first ICD indications were all secondary prevention, but expanding indications are defining indications for certain primary-prevention patients as well. See also **primary prevention**.

septal to posterior wall motion delay   Abbreviated **SPWMD**. An echocardiographic measure (in milliseconds) which defines the time lag between the contraction of the interventricular septum (the wall inside the heart between right and left ventricles) and the contraction of the back wall of the left ventricle. As a general rule, a SPWMD value of < 130 ms is a good predictor of a favorable response to CRT.

sheath   A simple tube, sometimes used in LV lead placement to cannulate the coronary sinus.

shocking vector   The path that defibrillating energy takes through the heart. For CRT-D patients, the shocking vector may form a current pathway from the two coils of the defibrillating (RV) lead or from one coil of the lead to the CRT-D generator itself ('hot can' or 'active can').

sick sinus syndrome   See **sinus node dysfunction**.

sinoatrial node   A small, specialized group of cells located in the high right atrium of the healthy heart which spontaneously generates electrical impulses that cause the heart to depolarize and contract. In a healthy heart, the sinoatrial node is sometimes known as the heart's natural pacemaker. Abbreviated **SA node**.

sinus bradycardia   An abnormally slow heart rate caused by slow impulse formation in the sinoatrial (SA) node. Symptomatic sinus bradycardia is often an indication for a pacemaker.

sinus node dysfunction   A disorder in the heart's sinoatrial (SA) node, the heart's natural pacemaker, which causes impulses to be formed too slowly to support metabolic need. Sinus node dysfunction leads to sinus bradycardia, an abnormally slow heart rate originating from the SA node. Also called **sick sinus syndrome**.

sinus tachycardia   A rapid ventricular rate which is triggered by a rapid atrial rate and may be a response to exercise, exertion or stress. During athletic activity, sinus tachycardia with 1 : 1 atrial–ventricular activity is often appropriate.

slittable   The quality of an introducer, catheter or sheath which requires it to be cut with a device (a slitter, like a scalpel or razor) to allow for removal after lead placement. See also **peelable**.

SND   See **sinus node dysfunction**.

SNS   See **sympathetic nervous system**.

spironolactone   An aldosterone blocker, which also acts as a relatively mild potassium-sparing diuretic.

SPWMD   See **septal to posterior wall motion delay**.

SSS   Sick sinus syndrome. See **sinus node dysfunction**.

ST segment   The portion on the normal surface ECG after the QRS complex and before the T wave, typically shown as a short flat line, which represents a moment following ventricular contraction and before relaxation commences. It is very brief.

steerable   The quality of a catheter that allows the implanting physician to move the distal tip by controlling the handle. A steerable catheter may move in one direction only (in which the implanter controls the 'curl' of the tip) or in two directions (in which the implanter can cause the tip to go to the right or left).

stenosis   A pathological thickening of a vessel or valve so that it is unable to work as efficiently as intended.

step-down test   A type of test in which a relatively high value is tested first and then is decreased in small increments. Capture testing of CRT systems is typically done as a step-down test until capture is lost.

stored energy   The amount of electrical energy that a CRT-D device can store in its capacitors. Stored energy is always higher than delivered energy. See also **delivered energy**.

stratification   A way of sorting data, particularly clinical study data, by category. For example, after PAVE data were collected, they were stratified by NYHA HF classification and it was found that the greater the NYHA Class, the more benefit a patient derived from CRT versus conventional pacing.

stroke volume   The amount of blood that the heart can pump out in a single cardiac cycle.

stylet A thin metal wire that can be inserted into the lumen (center) of a pacing lead, giving it the stiffness required to allow the implanting physician to maneuver it through the veins and into the heart. The stylet is withdrawn when the lead is in place.

stylet-driven The quality of a lead or catheter which is being manipulated into the heart by having a stylet inserted into it. See also **over-the-wire**.

substrate An abnormal pathway in the cardiac conduction system which can form adjacent to a lesion caused by a myocardial infarction. A substrate can facilitate and maintain re-entry circuits, which makes certain types of tachyarrhythmias possible.

sudden cardiac arrest See **sudden cardiac death**.

sudden cardiac death Abbreviated **SCD**. A form of death which occurs within 24 h from onset of symptoms and is caused by cardiac events, typically (but not exclusively) from ventricular fibrillation. SCD is a major cause of death in heart failure patients and the rate of SCD increases with NYHA heart failure class. Also called **sudden cardiac arrest**.

Sudden Onset A discrimination algorithm in CRT-D systems (and ICDs) which uses a programmable delta value and then compares a series of tachycardia intervals (in an X out of Y pattern, for example, in 8 out of 12 consecutive intervals) with the delta to determine if the tachycardia started suddenly (the intervals showed less than the delta value of change) or gradually (the intervals showed more than the delta value of change). A sudden-onset tachycardia is more likely to be a ventricular tachycardia.

supraventricular tachycardia Abbreviated **SVT**. A tachycardia which originates above the ventricles, typically in the atria or AV node. Although the arrhythmia is often atrial in origin, it frequently involves rapid ventricular response to the high atrial rate. An example of a typical SVT is atrial fibrillation.

SVT See **supraventricular tachycardia**.

SVT discrimination See **discrimination**.

SVT Discrimination Timeout A programmable feature in some CRT-D (and ICD) devices which sets a timer, after which the device automatically proceeds to deliver high-voltage therapy. The timer commences when the device determines a rhythm disorder is an SVT and inhibits therapy delivery. **SVT Timeout** (as it is sometimes called) is used when the device is programmed to a two-zone or three-zone configuration (VT and VF or VT1, VT2 and VF) and SVT discrimination algorithms are used in one or both of the VT zones. When an SVT discriminator inhibits therapy for a VT, the timer commences; when it expires, the device automatically goes to high-voltage therapy. The purpose of SVT Discrimination Timeout is to protect the patient from prolonged exposure to a rapid ventricular rate.

sympathetic nervous system Part of the body's nervous system which regulates many of the bodily functions not under conscious control, such as respiration, digestion and heart rate. In a healthy individual, the sympathetic nervous system (SNS) controls the body's 'fight-or-flight' response, which floods the body with specific chemicals to enable it to withstand great exertion or stress. In a heart failure patient, the SNS becomes overly active, even dominant, exposing the patient to a long-term flood of stress hormones. See also **parasympathetic nervous system**.

syndrome A group of symptoms associated with a specific condition. A syndrome is not the same as a disease. Heart failure is a syndrome rather than a disease.

systole The period of cardiac contraction.

systolic blood pressure The maximum amount of pressure exerted against the artery walls by the force of blood through the vessels, typically expressed as the first figure in blood pressure readings. For example, if a person has a blood pressure reading of 140/80 mmHg, 140 mmHg is the systolic value. See also **diastolic blood pressure**.

systolic heart failure A type of heart failure associated with systolic action, i.e. with pumping blood out. Left-ventricular (LV) impairment is associated with systolic heart failure.

T-wave The portion on the surface ECG that represents ventricular repolarization and relaxation.

telemedicine A broad general term that describes a variety of technologies and approaches to treating patients not present in the clinic. Telemedicine can involve remote patient monitoring (checking on patient status using telephone lines or the internet) or it may involve treating or even surgical interventions on patients who are at a distant location.

thiazide   A mild diuretic.

Threshold Start   A programmable parameter used in defibrillation that defines the initial value of the sensitivity setting for a cardiac cycle. CRT-D devices employ automatic and dynamic sensitivity algorithms; Threshold Start is the initial value for sensitivity at the start of each cardiac cycle. It is established by a percentage (programmable) of the peak value taken during the previous sensed refractory period. For example, if the largest signal in the last sensed refractory period was 6 mV and the Threshold Start was programmed to 50%, then the Threshold Start would begin at 3 mV (50% of 6 mV).

thrombus   A blood clot which breaks free of the vessel and lodges in the heart. Note that if that same clot were to lodge elsewhere in the body, it would be called an **embolus**.

tied-output device   An older type of CRT system tin which right and left ventricular outputs were one output, that is, occurred at the same time and defined by the same parameters. Today, CRT systems offer independent outputs for right and left ventricles.

tilt   The amount that a defibrillation waveform decreases in energy (stated as a percentage decrease from initial value) over time. Tilt may be programmable in CRT-D systems and is a way to program indirectly the pulse width of the defibrillating waveform. Typical tilt settings are around 50% or 65%, with 50% correlating to the shorter pulse width. For example, a 50% tilt sets a pulse width that allows the initial energy to decrease 50%.

tricuspid valve   The valve in the heart that separates the right atrium from right ventricle. A transvenous right-ventricular pacemaker lead has to pass through the tricuspid valve at implant.

unipolar   A type of electrical configuration which describes leads (and pulse generator configuration) in which the electrical circuit is formed by the tip electrode of the lead and the pulse generator. See also **bipolar**.

variability   See **heart rate variability**.

vasoconstriction   The ability of the body to narrow the diameter of blood vessels. Vasoconstriction can be a compensatory mechanism of the body to help elevate blood pressure when the body senses that blood pressure is too low. See also **vasodilation**.

vasodilation   The ability of the body to widen or expand the diameter of blood vessels. Vasodilation can be a compensatory mechanism of the body to help decrease blood pressure when the body senses that blood pressure is too high. See also **vasoconstriction**.

vector   See **shocking vector**.

ventricle   One of two of the heart's lower chambers.

ventricular diastole   The repolarization and relaxation of the heart's lower chambers (ventricles). Ventricular diastole can be observed on a surface ECG as the T-wave.

ventricular dyssynchrony   The condition that CRT devices address, the inefficient and out-of-sync contraction and relaxation of the ventricles. Although ventricular dyssynchrony can involve out-of-sync right and left ventricles, it more commonly involves a left ventricle that contracts in sections rather than as a unified whole. Not all patients with heart failure have ventricular dyssynchrony, but many do. The most commonly accepted marker for the presence and, to some degree, the severity of ventricular dyssynchrony is a wide QRS (> 120 ms). Also called **mechanical dyssynchrony**.

ventricular fibrillation   Abbreviated **VF**. A dangerous form of ventricular tachyarrhythmia characterized by very rapid and wildly disorganized ventricular beats at rates of ≥ 200–300 beats/min. During VF, no individually distinct QRS complexes appear on the screen. The heart tries to beat so rapidly that it can no longer fully contract and relax; instead, it just quivers. VF can be fatal in a few moments, if left untreated. It is believed that VF is the mechanism responsible for many cases of sudden cardiac death.

ventricular remodeling   Changes to the shape and muscle quality of the myocardium caused by heart failure. There are two main types of ventricular remodeling: **concentric hypertrophy** (diastolic dysfunction) and **eccentric hypertrophy** (systolic dysfunction). There is growing evidence that ventricular remodeling can be reversed with proper treatment. See also **reverse remodeling**.

ventricular systole   The depolarization and contraction of the heart's lower chambers (ventricles). Ventricular systole is represented on a surface ECG as the QRS complex.

ventricular tachyarrhythmia An arrhythmia originating in the ventricles and characterized by a rapid ventricular rate. Ventricular tachyarrhythmia is a broad general term that covers two main types of arrhythmias: **ventricular tachycardia** and **ventricular fibrillation**.

ventricular tachycardia Abbreviated **VT**. An arrhythmia originating in the ventricles and characterized by a rapid ventricular rate, typically in the range of around 100 beats/min up to 300 beats/min. A VT many be monomorphic (originating from one focus in the ventricles and having QRS complexes of one same shape) or polymorphic (originating from more than one foci and having different-looking QRS complexes). Clinicians sometimes find it useful to differentiate between 'fast VT' and 'slow VT' with somewhat arbitrary cut-off rates. VT is a dangerous and potentially even life-threatening arrhythmia.

VF See **ventricular fibrillation**.

viscosity The thickness of a liquid. For heart failure patients, this refers to the thickness of blood in the body.

volume For heart failure patients, volume refers to the quantity of blood in the body. Blood volume is affected by congestion or fluid accumulation.

VT See **ventricular tachycardia**.

VT Therapy Timeout A programmable feature in some CRT-D (and ICD) devices which sets a timer, after which the device automatically proceeds to deliver high-voltage therapy. The timer commences with tachycardia detection and is used when the device is programmed to respond first with less-than-high-voltage therapy (either antitachycardia pacing or cardioversion). When the timer expires, the device automatically goes to high-voltage therapy. The purpose of VT Therapy Timeout (sometimes called **VT Timeout**) is to protect the patient with VT from prolonged exposure to ineffective therapy.

VT Timeout See **VT Therapy Timeout**.

warfarin An anticoagulation drug often used in patients with permanent AF.

wide QRS The term applied to QRS durations on a surface ECG that are considered excessively long and indicative of some degree of ventricular dyssynchrony. In randomized clinical trials, 'wide QRS' is often defined as any QRS duration > 120 ms or > 150 ms.

zone A diagnostic category of defibrillation defined by rate. Zones in CRT-D devices may include NSR (normal sinus rhythm), VT1 (slow VT), VT2 (fast VT) and VF. The number of zones programmed (from 1 to 3) is called the device configuration.

Index